AF787329

Liver Disease and Surgery

Edited by Georgios Tsoulfas and Luis Rodrigo

Published in London, United Kingdom

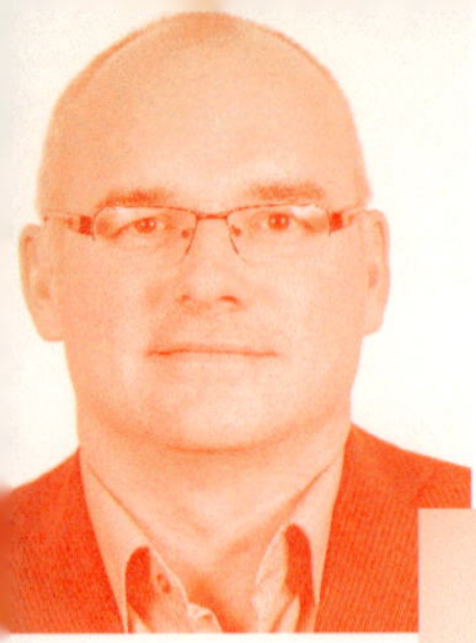
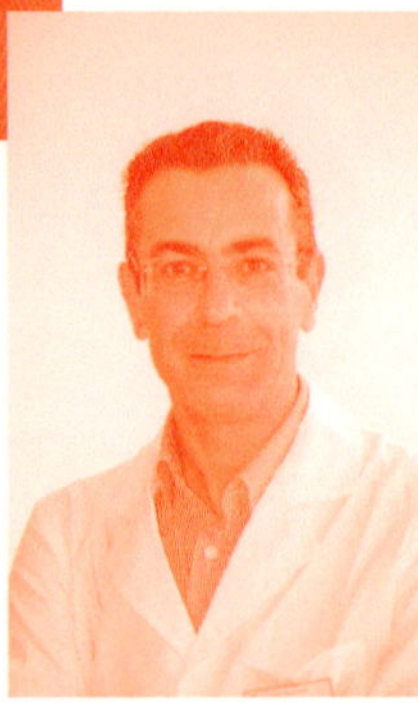
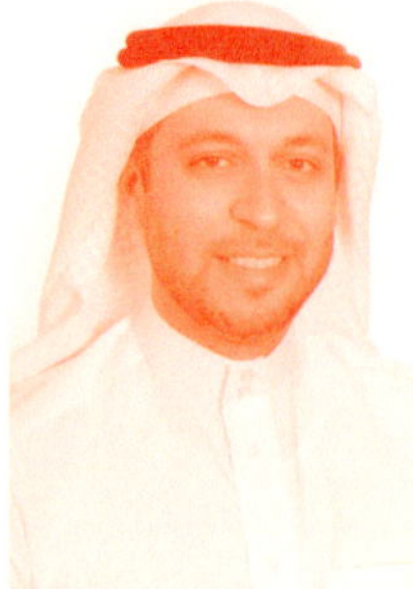
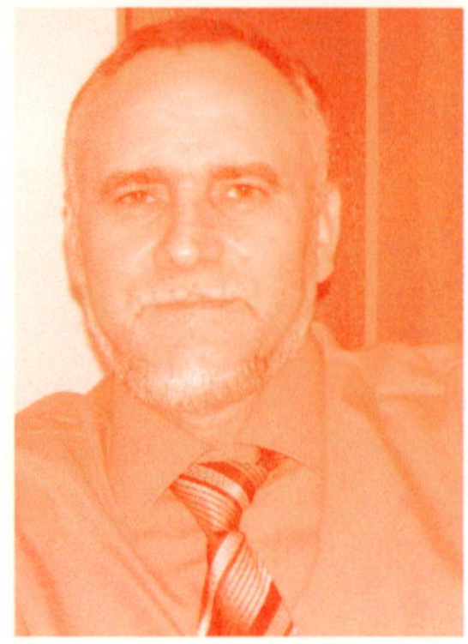
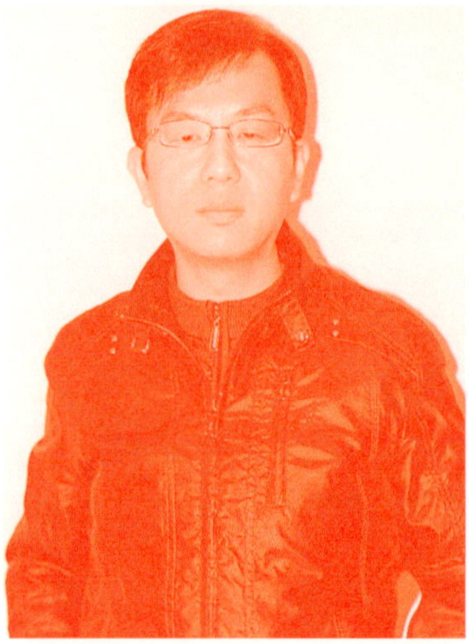
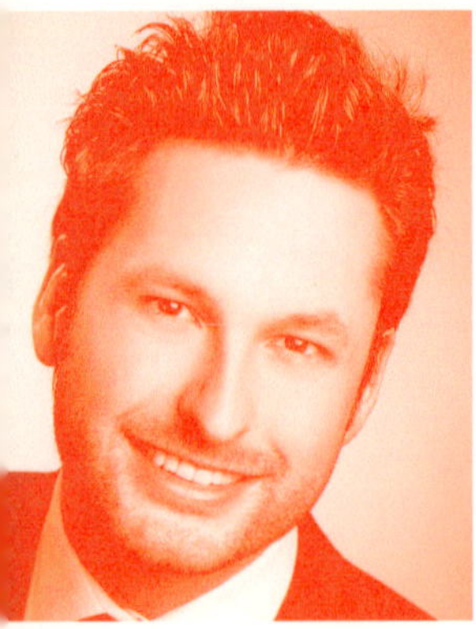
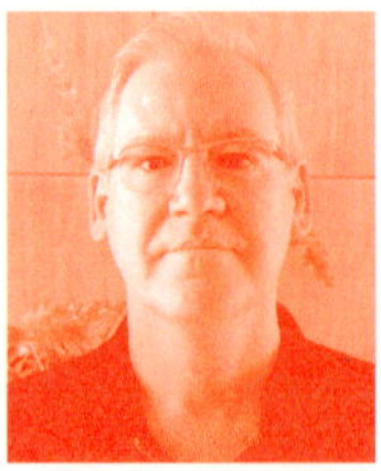

IntechOpen

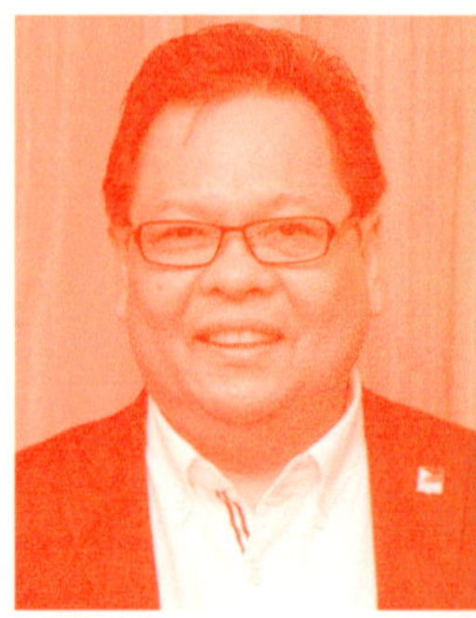
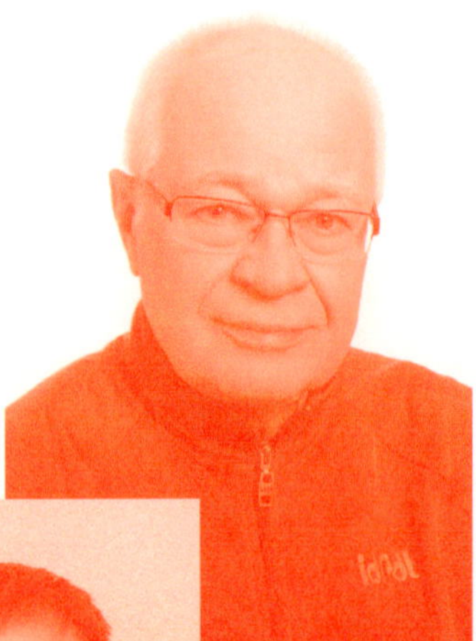
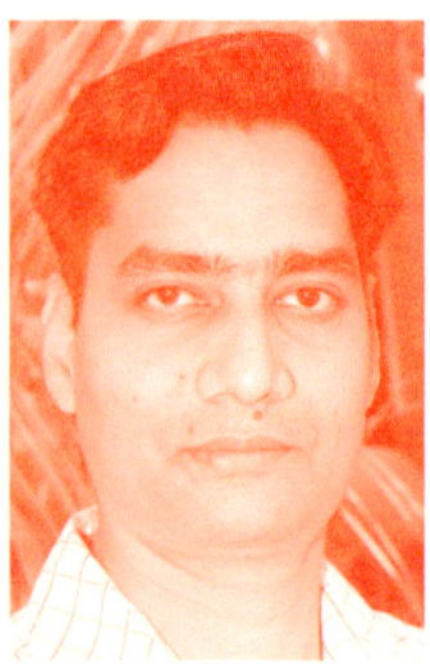
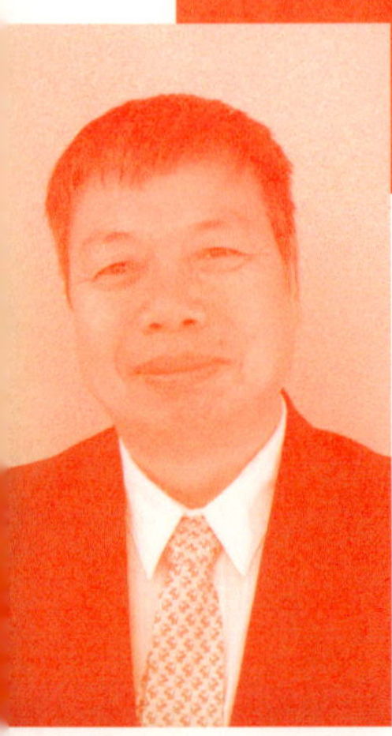
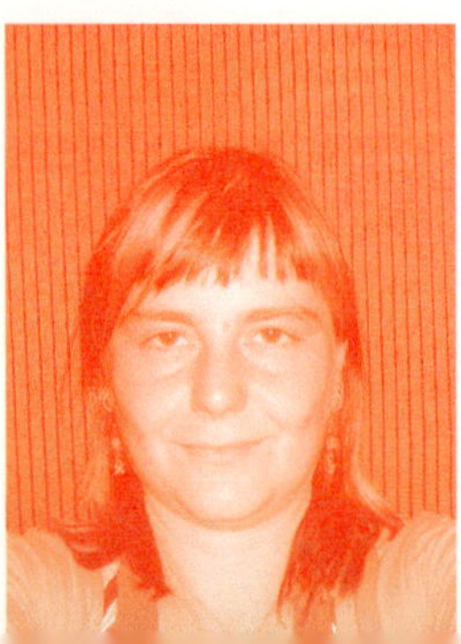
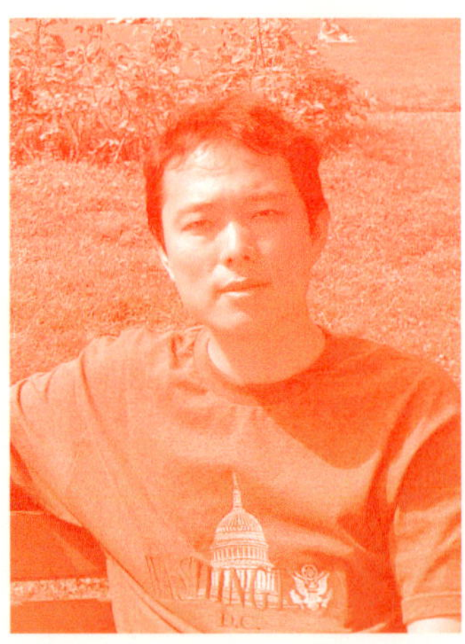

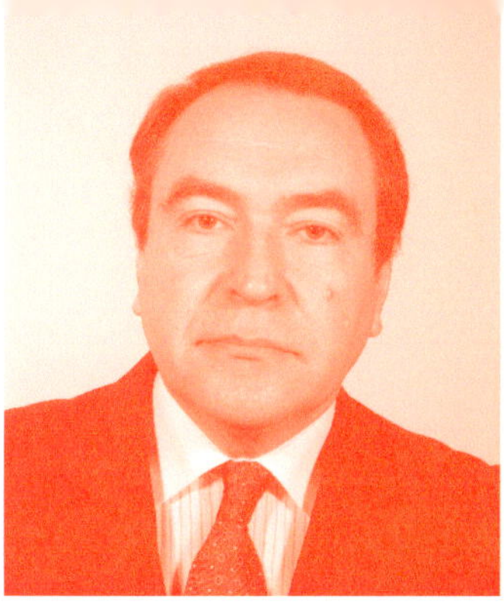
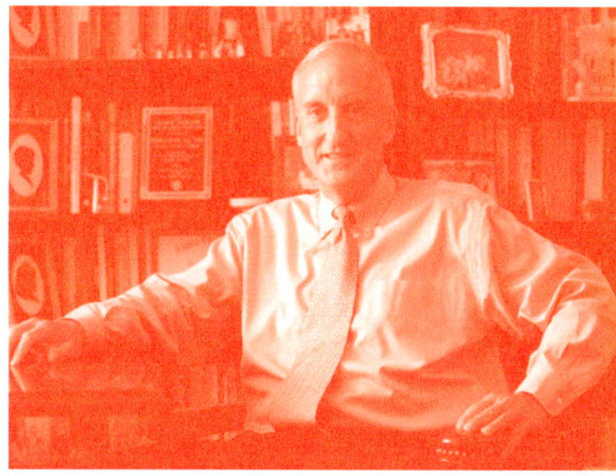
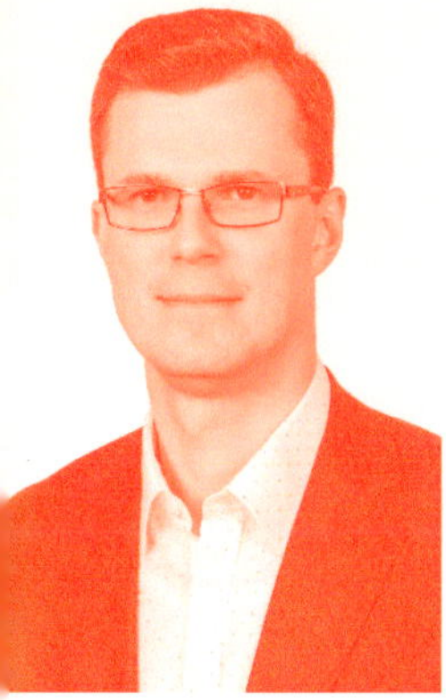
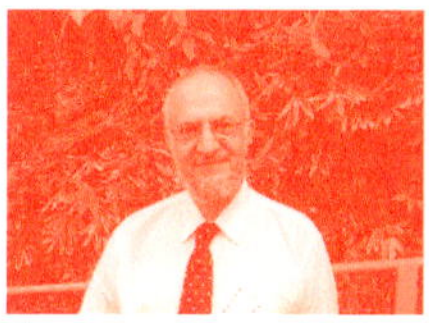
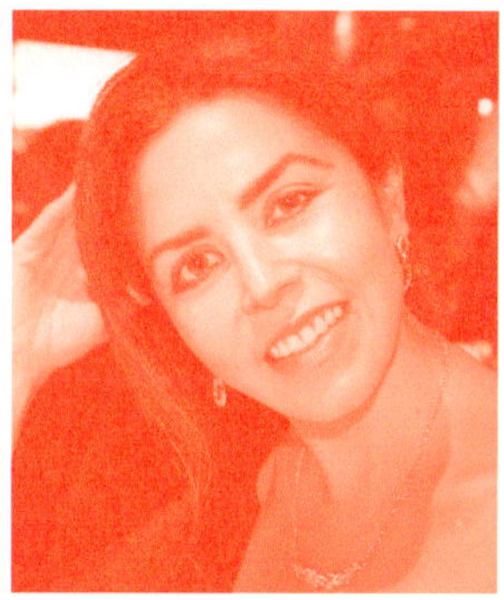

Supporting open minds since 2005

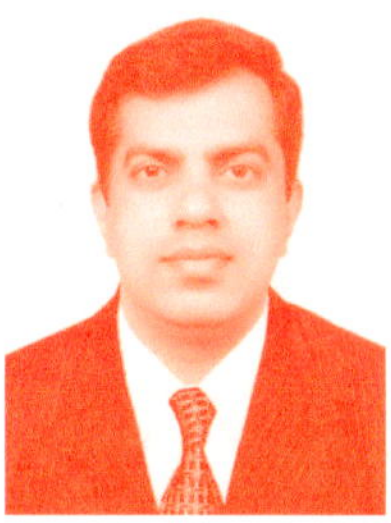
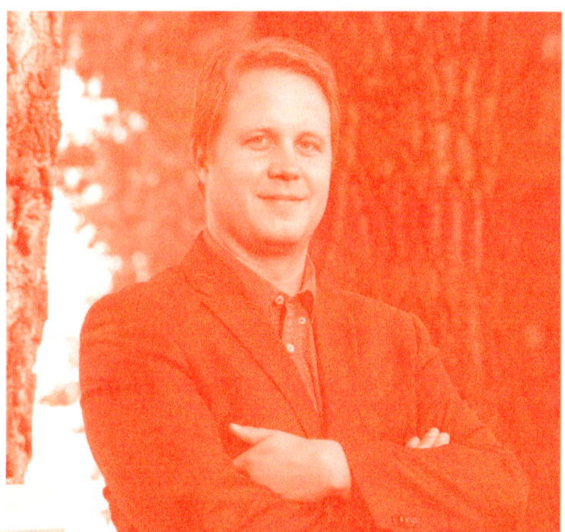
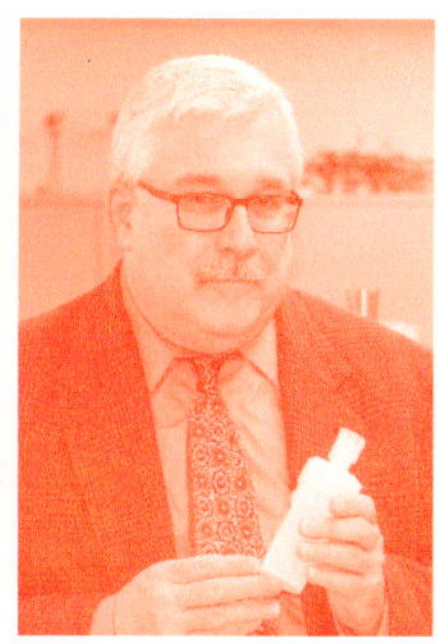
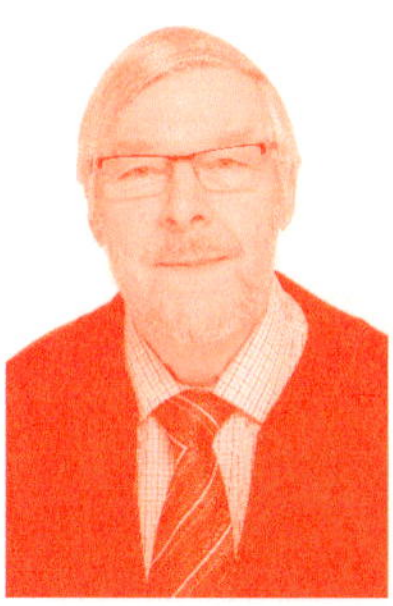
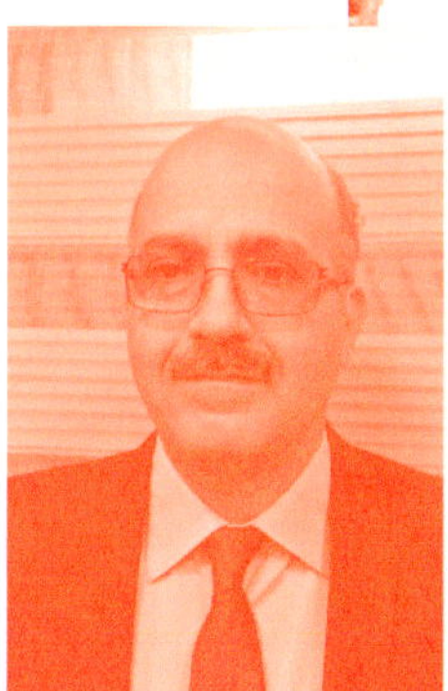
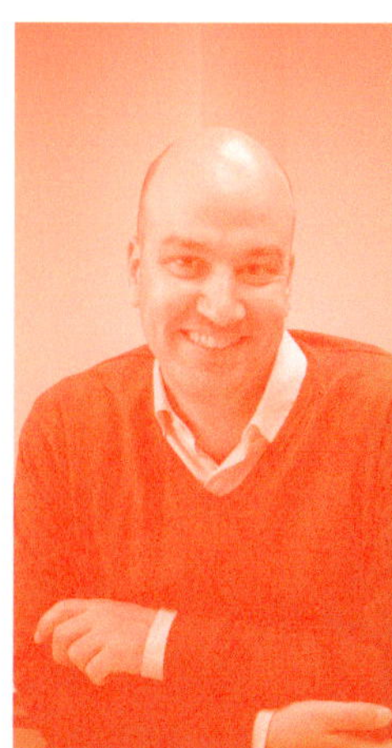
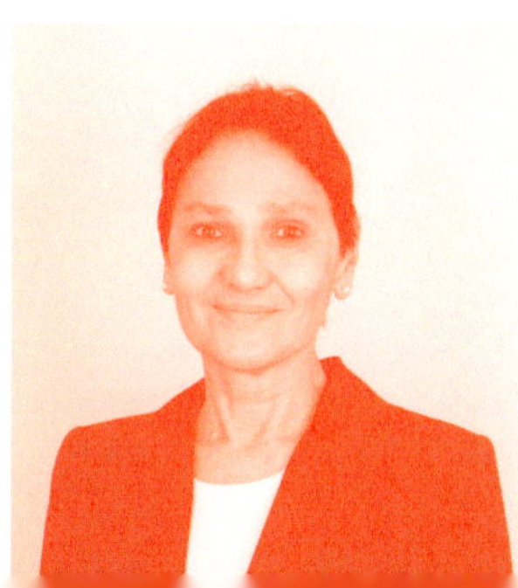

Liver Disease and Surgery
http://dx.doi.org/10.5772/intechopen.77694
Edited by Georgios Tsoulfas and Luis Rodrigo

Contributors
Fabio Uggeri, Mauro Scotti, Enrico Pinotti, Mattia Garancini, Marco Braga, Fabrizio Romano, Simone Bini, Chiara D\'Alterio, Stefania Brozzetti, Leonardo Luca Chiarella, Chiara De Lucia, Katia Fazzi, Michele Di Martino, Monjur Ahmed, Carmen Peralta, Maria Eugenia Cornide Petronio, Mónica B. Jiménez-Castro, Jordi Gracia-Sancho, Luis Burgos San Juan, Hector Losada, Cesar Muñoz, Marcelo Klein, Pablo Guzman, Jorge Silva, Ricky Harminder Bhogal, Stephanos Pericleous, Aamir Khan, Areti Karapanagiotou, Achillefs Pitsoulis, Maria Vasileiou, Nikolaos Voloudakis, Nasser Mousa, Gamal Shiha, Mirela Patricia Sirbu Boeti, Beatrice Tivadar, Lupescu Ioana, Mirela Boros, Vlad Herlea, Dana Tomescu, Brasoveanu Vladislav, Daniel Simplicio Torres, Jefferson Abrantes, Carlos Eduardo Brandão-Mello, Jonathan Huang, Edwin Lee

© The Editor(s) and the Author(s) 2019
The rights of the editor(s) and the author(s) have been asserted in accordance with the Copyright, Designs and Patents Act 1988. All rights to the book as a whole are reserved by INTECHOPEN LIMITED. The book as a whole (compilation) cannot be reproduced, distributed or used for commercial or non-commercial purposes without INTECHOPEN LIMITED's written permission. Enquiries concerning the use of the book should be directed to INTECHOPEN LIMITED rights and permissions department (permissions@intechopen.com).
Violations are liable to prosecution under the governing Copyright Law.

(cc) BY

Individual chapters of this publication are distributed under the terms of the Creative Commons Attribution 3.0 Unported License which permits commercial use, distribution and reproduction of the individual chapters, provided the original author(s) and source publication are appropriately acknowledged. If so indicated, certain images may not be included under the Creative Commons license. In such cases users will need to obtain permission from the license holder to reproduce the material. More details and guidelines concerning content reuse and adaptation can be found at http://www.intechopen.com/copyright-policy.html.

Notice
Statements and opinions expressed in the chapters are these of the individual contributors and not necessarily those of the editors or publisher. No responsibility is accepted for the accuracy of information contained in the published chapters. The publisher assumes no responsibility for any damage or injury to persons or property arising out of the use of any materials, instructions, methods or ideas contained in the book.

First published in London, United Kingdom, 2019 by IntechOpen
IntechOpen is the global imprint of INTECHOPEN LIMITED, registered in England and Wales, registration number: 11086078, 7th floor, 10 Lower Thames Street, London, EC3R 6AF, United Kingdom
Printed in Croatia

British Library Cataloguing-in-Publication Data
A catalogue record for this book is available from the British Library

Additional hard and PDF copies can be obtained from orders@intechopen.com

Liver Disease and Surgery
Edited by Georgios Tsoulfas and Luis Rodrigo
p. cm.
Print ISBN 978-1-78985-065-9
Online ISBN 978-1-78985-066-6
eBook (PDF) ISBN 978-1-83880-273-8

For EU product safety concerns:
IN TECH d.o.o., Prolaz Marije Krucifikse Kozulić 3, 51000 Rijeka, Croatia, info@intechopen.com or visit our website at intechopen.com.

We are IntechOpen, the world's leading publisher of Open Access books

Built by scientists, for scientists

4,400+
Open access books available

117,000+
International authors and editors

130M+
Downloads

151
Countries delivered to

Our authors are among the
Top 1%
most cited scientists

12.2%
Contributors from top 500 universities

WEB OF SCIENCE™

Selection of our books indexed in the Book Citation Index in Web of Science™ Core Collection (BKCI)

Interested in publishing with us?
Contact book.department@intechopen.com

Numbers displayed above are based on latest data collected.
For more information visit www.intechopen.com

Meet the editors

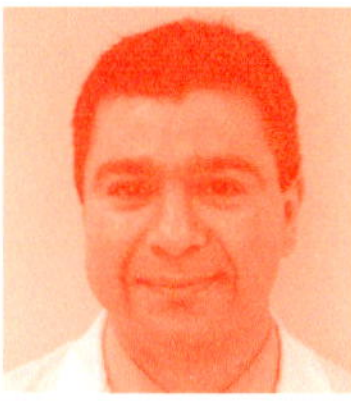

Dr Georgios Tsoulfas received his medical degree from Brown University School of Medicine and completed his general surgery residency at the University of Iowa Hospitals and Clinics, as well as a transplant research fellowship at the Starzl Transplant Institute at the University of Pittsburgh. He then completed a two-year transplantation surgery fellowship at the Massachusetts General Hospital, Harvard Medical School and then joined the Division of Solid Organ Transplantation and Hepatobiliary Surgery at the University of Rochester Medical Center as an Assistant Professor of Surgery. He has currently moved back to Greece, where he is an Associate Professor of Surgery at the Aristoteleion University of Thessaloniki. He has published over 90 papers in peer-reviewed journals and in PubMed, as well as 29 book chapters. He is a reviewer for over 60 international journals and is on the editorial board of several others. His clinical and research interests include hepatobiliary surgery, primary and secondary hepatic malignancies, ischemia/reperfusion injury, as well as medical/surgical education and the use of technology.
He is currently the Vice Chair of the International Relations Committee of the American College of Surgeons and the World President of the International College of Surgeons.

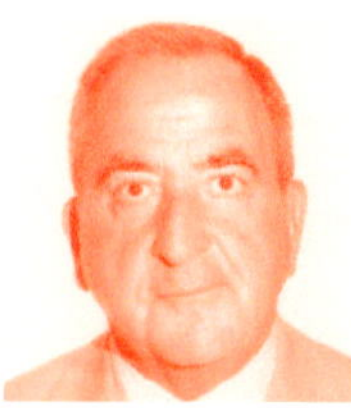

Dr. Luis Rodrigo MD was Emeritus Professor of Medicine at the University of Oviedo (Spain). He has been the Chief of Gastroenterology Service at the HUCA Hospital in Oviedo for more than 40 years. He obtained his PhD in 1975 and has a long teaching and research career. He has published a total of 585 scientific papers, 310 written in English with the rest in Spanish. He has participated as main investigator in a total of 45 clinical trials and has directed 40 doctoral theses. He has contributed actively to the formation of approximately one hundred specialists in gastroenterology working in his hospital and other hospitals in Spain and abroad. He has written approximately 35 chapters in books of several subjects and has been the editor of 22 books in his specialty and related diseases.

Contents

Preface

The complicated nature of hepatic anatomy and physiology, as well as the variety of challenging diseases affecting the liver, have all contributed to the field of hepatic surgery being a highly demanding surgical specialty. The training of a liver surgeon consists of achieving technical expertise, a deep understanding of the intricacies of hepatic anatomy and physiology, experience with acute and chronic liver disease ranging from trauma, infections, benign lesions to primary and metastatic malignancies, as well as knowledge of the continuously evolving technologies. This foundation is necessary to be able to correctly choose from a variety of different treatment methods and different hepatectomy techniques that would be best suited to a specific patient and a specific health problem. The multitude of hepatic surgery techniques involve strategies such as ablation, electroporation, resection with several different instruments and, last but not least, liver transplantation. At the same time, the physician dealing with these complex issues needs to be aware of the right mix of treatments, as well as the proper sequence of administration. Additionally, it is imperative to have an understanding of the molecular biology of hepatic function and the evolution of the various diseases to be able to provide patient-targeted therapies.

This book provides an overview of all the above with chapters presenting the intricacies of liver physiology, the challenges and current update on complex hepatic diseases such as hepatocellular carcinoma and cholangiocarcinoma, discussion about the role of robotic surgery and descriptions of the indications and techniques for some of the more demanding hepatic surgeries involved in the treatment of both benign and malignant liver diseases. The book's value lies in the fact that the authors present us with their distilled wisdom, which is the result of substantial experience and daily involvement in this most difficult field of medicine and surgery.

This book should be a useful resource for any physician, whether they are in training or in practice, treating patients with hepatic diseases.

Dr. Georgios Tsoulfas, MD, PhD, FICS, FACS
Associate Professor of Surgery,
Aristotle University of Thessaloniki,
Thessaloniki, Greece

Dr. Luis Rodrigo, MD
University of Oviedo,
Spain

Section 1

Hepatic Physiology Affecting Hepatic Surgery

Chapter 1

Minimal Hepatic Encephalopathy: Silent Tragedy

Gamal Shiha and Nasser Mousa

Abstract

Hepatic encephalopathy (HE) is brain dysfunction caused by both acute and chronic liver diseases that produces a spectrum of neuropsychiatric symptoms in the absence of other known brain diseases. Minimal hepatic encephalopathy (MHE) is the mildest form of this spectrum. MHE is defined as HE without symptoms on clinical or neurological examination, but with deficits in the performance of psychometric tests, working memory, psychomotor speed, and visuospatial ability. Minimal hepatic encephalopathy is associated with impaired driving skills and increased risk of motor vehicle accidents and has been associated with increased hospitalizations and death. Despite its clinical importance, a large number of clinicians had never investigated whether their cirrhotic patients might have MHE. Although, there is no single gold standard test for diagnosis of MHE, a combination of two neuropsychological tests or psychometric hepatic encephalopathy score battery test and/or neurophysiological test is standard for diagnosis of MHE. It was found that, treatment for MHE improves neuropsychiatric performance and quality of life and decreases the risk of developing overt HE (OHE). The agents used to treat OHE have been tested in patients with MHE. In particular, lactulose, rifaximin, probiotics and L-ornithine and L-aspartate (LOLA) have all been shown to be beneficial, with documented improvement in psychometric performance after treatment.

Keywords: liver cirrhosis, hepatic encephalopathy, minimal hepatic encephalopathy, ammonia, neuropsychological testing, motor vehicle accident, lactulose and rifaximin

1. Introduction

Hepatic encephalopathy (HE) is a serious clinical problem of portal hypertension and cirrhosis that is characterized by neurologic and neuropsychiatric abnormalities. It is manifested by personality changes, cognitive dysfunction, and altered level of consciousness [1, 2]. Based on the severity, HE is classified into two groups: overt HE (OHE) presents episodically or continuously with obvious and clinically detectable symptoms; in contrast, covert HE (CHE) combines the two lowest grades of HE (minimal HE (MHE) and HE grade 1) [3]. Therefore, under the new classification (**Table 1**), OHE starts with grade 2 or with evidence of asterixis and disorientation. MHE is characterized by subtle cognitive and psychomotor deficits in the absence of recognizable clinical symptoms and signs of HE and is documented by neuropsychometric (NP) tests and neurophysiological tests, but HE grade 1 is defined by the presence of mild clinical alterations like euphoria, anxiety, or a shortened attention span. Although the consequences are serious, mostly CHE

IntechOpen

Classification	Covert HE		Overt HE		
	MHE	Grade I	Grade II	Grade III	Grade IV
Description	* Absence of recognizable clinical symptoms and signs * Impairments only measurable with psychometric tests (psychomotor speed/ executive functions or neurophysiological alterations)	* Minor lack of awareness * Euphoria or anxiety * Shortened attention span * Altered sleep rhythm	* Fatigue, apathy, or lethargy * Slight disorientation for time and place * Obvious personality change * Inappropriate behavior * Asterixis	* Somnolence to semi-stupor * Confused * Marked disorientation to time and place *Aggression	* Coma * Signs of increased intracranial pressure

Table 1.
New classification combining covert and overt HE.

is often unnoticed or even neglected in routine clinical practice due to only very mild symptoms associated with grade 1, or no diagnostics in case of MHE [4, 5].

Minimal hepatic encephalopathy may have a bad impact on quality of life, risk of road traffic accidents, and can progress to overt HE [6, 7]. Still, there are no current guidelines for the ascertained diagnosis of MHE. The Working Group on HE endorsed that, at least two of the following neuropsychologic tests should be used for diagnosing MHE: number connection test-A (NCT-A), NCT-B, block-design test (BDT), and the digit-symbol test (DST) [4]. The existing definition of MHE is built on psychometric test results that are two SDs more than normal on at least two psychometric tests [8]. Therapy for MHE is targeted toward the gut, due to the ammoniagenic role of the gut contents, which have been hypothesized to play a part in MHE pathogenesis. Guidelines for HE in chronic liver disease do not recommend routine treatment of MHE. However, they state that when a patient has clear cognitive impairment, or deterioration of quality of life (QoL), skills for driving, or ability to perform jobs that require manual labor or have high public risk, the patient should be treated [3, 9].

2. Prevalence of MHE

MHE is considered as a part of wide spectrum of typical neurocognitive alterations in liver cirrhosis, mostly involving the areas of attention, alertness, response inhibition, and executive functions [10, 11]. Depending on the population studied, patient level of education, age of the patients, and the diagnostic tool used, MHE incidence varies from 20 to 80% of cirrhotic patients [12–15].

3. Physiopathology

The pathogenesis of MHE is nearly similar to that of OHE [16]. The ammonia toxicity remains the key factor, but recently there is increased evidence that, hyperammonemia acts synergistically with systemic inflammation, oxidative stress, and gut microbiota [17, 18]. Numerous investigators suggested that, hepatic encephalopathy is a disorder of astrocyte function that plays a role in the detoxification of ammonia [19].

3.1 The role of ammonia

Ammonia is a key intermediate product in the metabolism of proteins. It is manufactured by the bacterial metabolism of amino acids and purines that are consumed in the human diet [20]. Under physiological environment, about 90% of the ammonium is primarily cleared by the synthesis of urea in the liver (by the Krebs cycle) and subsequently cleared by the kidneys and to a lesser extent by the muscles (**Figure 1**). Ammonia is also consumed in the conversion of glutamate to glutamine, a reaction that depends upon the activity of glutamine synthetase [21]. In liver cirrhosis, there are two factors that contribute to hyperammonemia: the first is a decrease in the healthy hepatocytes, resulting in deficiency of NH_3 detoxification; the second is the existence of porto-systemic shunting that results in shifting of NH_3-rich portal blood to the systemic circulation without hepatic detoxification—subsequently, the extrahepatic metabolization of ammonia by the brain and skeletal muscle cells becomes more important [17, 22, 23]. The skeletal muscle plays a significant role in ammonia metabolism as it contains glutamine synthetase. However, the muscle wasting that is clear in advanced cirrhosis may increase hyperammonemia. The kidneys express glutaminase and, somewhat, play a role in ammonia production. Similarly, the kidneys express glutamine synthetase and play a key role in ammonia metabolism and excretion [20]. Ammonia crosses the blood-brain barrier and is metabolized in the astrocytes by glutamine synthetase, which converts NH_3 and glutamate to glutamine [17]. Increasing glutamine in astrocytes produces an osmotic gradient (**Figure 2**), promotes water shift into astrocyte producing edema [23], and generation of reactive oxygen species,

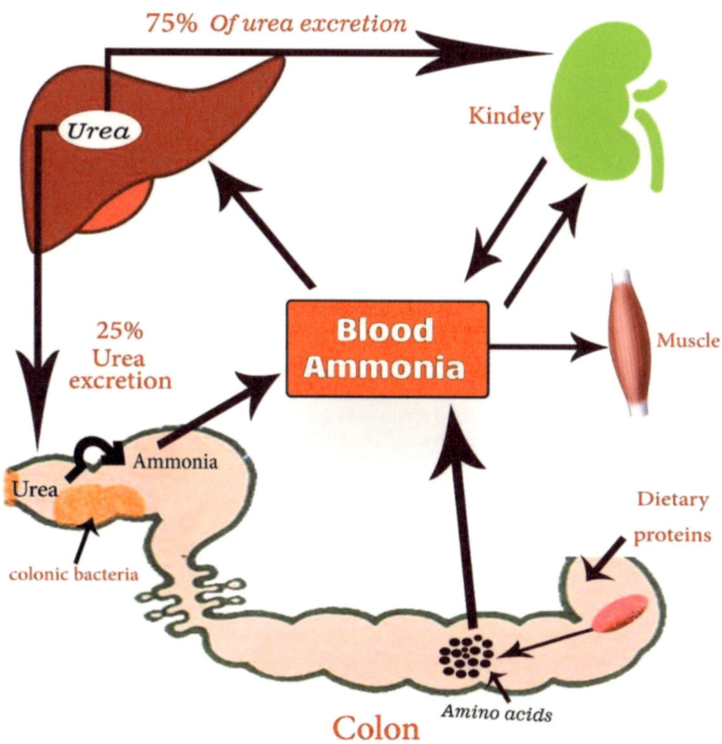

Figure 1.
Ammonia is produced primarily in colon from breakdown of amino acids and urea by bacteria. The ammonia is taken up by hepatocytes and converted, in the urea cycle, to urea, which is passed into blood. Urea is primarily excreted in the kidneys (75%) and the intestine (around 25%).

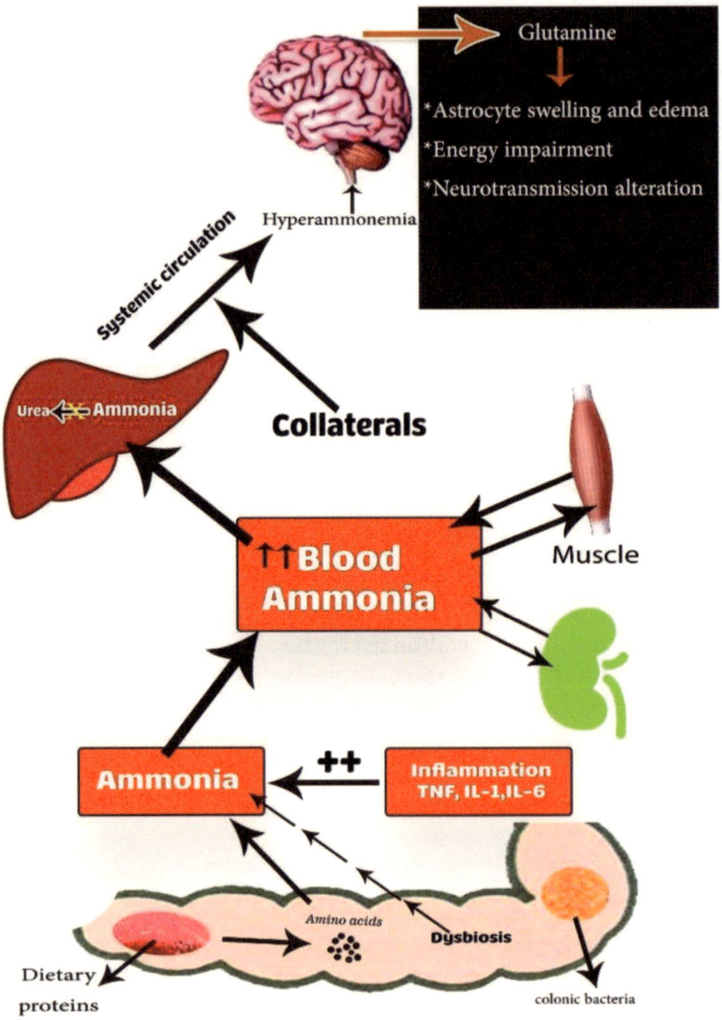

Figure 2.
Pathogenesis of hepatic encephalopathy. In normal conditions, gut release of ammonia results in high portal vein ammonia levels. Microbiota is also responsible for the formation of ammonia, endotoxins. In liver cirrhosis, the liver extracts portal venous ammonia poorly. The subsequent increase of arterial ammonia levels leads to increased disposition of ammonia in other tissues. Both the brain and muscle lack a complete urea cycle and rely on the formation of glutamine. Thus, the brain and muscle become ammonia-uptake and glutamine-releasing organs. In the brain, astrocytes metabolize ammonia through glutamine synthetase, converting glutamate and ammonia to glutamine which is osmotically active and promotes water shift into the astrocyte, thus producing intracellular swelling and edema.

thereby contributing to the cerebral dysfunction seen in HE [17]. The high-energy consumption by this process leads to oxidative stress which is accompanied by cellular dysfunction and disruption of neurotransmission predominantly of glutamate and γ-aminobutyric acid [24]. In the brain, NH_3 produces inactivation of neuronal chloride extrusion pumps; these processes result in inhibition of both axonal conduction and excitatory postsynaptic potentials, subsequently suppressing inhibitory postsynaptic potential formation and depolarizing neurons [25, 26].

3.2 Inflammation

Studies demonstrated that, severity of MHE might not correlate with severity of liver disease or the level of ammonia, proposing the existence of other pathogenic stimuli. Inflammation is one such stimulus that may add to the advancement of MHE and its progression to overt HE [27]. The studies suggested that, inflammation plays a synergistic role with ammonia in producing and modulating MHE [27–29]. Studies in patients with cirrhosis have documented higher levels of proinflammatory cytokines like tumor necrosis factor (TNF)-α, interleukin (IL)-1β and IL-6. This reflects the possibility of developing a systemic inflammatory response that alters the blood-brain barrier (BBB) permeability and allows diffusion of ammonia moreover [30, 31].

3.3 Microbiota

Studies suggested that, many interactions with gut microbiota can play an active role in MHE (**Figure 2**). Microbiota changes have been linked with impaired cognition, endotoxemia, and inflammation. With the progression of cirrhosis, there is dysbiosis (unfavorable change in the composition of the microbiome) with decreased levels of autochthonous taxa (native Firmicutes) bacteria and increased levels of other taxa (Bacteroidetes, Actinobacteria). The native bacteria are important for the harmony of the gastrointestinal flora and for the well-being of the entire body. The autochthonous bacteria produce short-chain fatty acids that feed the colonic mucosal cells and reduce local colonic inflammation, and produce anti-bacterial peptides [32]. In patients with minimal HE, stool microbiota studies demonstrated an increase in *Streptococcus salivarius* [33]. Zhang et al. found worse dysbiosis in all cirrhotic patients versus healthy controls and also found over-representation of two bacterial families, Streptococcaceae and Veillonellaceae, in cirrhotic patients with and without MHE as compared with controls. Moreover, patients with MHE had an overabundance of *Streptococcus salivarius*. This dysbiosis could increase ammonia production due to its urease activity, and its count positively correlated with ammonia levels and cognitive testing in patients with MHE [34]. The cirrhosis dysbiosis ratio (CDR) is the ratio of autochthonous to non-autochthonous taxa in cirrhosis. The lower the CDR the more the endotoxemia and more decompensated the cirrhosis [35].

4. Natural history of MHE

The incidence of MHE increases with progression of liver disease. With time, MHE may improve or progress to OHE [36, 37]. The rate of progression to overt HE was much higher in patients with MHE and Child-Pugh score > 6 than in those with MHE and Child-Pugh score ≤ 6 [38]. Moreover, MHE in patients with large portal-systemic shunts had a better outcome due to preserved hepatocytes [39]. Real probability of OHE at 3 years was 56% in patients of liver cirrhosis in the presence of MHE and 8% for those without MHE [37]. In addition, existence of MHE in cirrhosis associated with shorter survival time and increased mortality rate compared to those without MHE [40–43].

5. Clinical significance

MHE has a significant impact on daily activities. It decreases patients' quality of life (QoL) [43, 44] and driving impairment due to the attention and visuomotor coordination deficits [45–47]. The Sickness Impact Profile was studied in a group of patients with cirrhosis to evaluate QoL indicators such as sleep, rest, eating, work, home management, recreation, ambulation, daily care, movement, and emotional behavior. All scales were significantly decreased in patients with MHE compared with individuals without MHE [48]. Moreover, those patients suffer from falls [49] and have a high risk of development of episodic HE [2].

5.1 Health-related quality of life (HRQoL)

Quality of life is a multidimensional index that reports all aspects of human well-being, including physical and cognitive capabilities, functional behavior, emotional status, and psychosocial adjustment [50]. The American Association for the Study of Liver Diseases survey conducted in 2007 demonstrated that, most clinicians believe MHE to be a significant problem. However, only 50% of clinicians had examined whether their patients might have MHE, and 38% had never studied their patients with liver cirrhosis [51]. Several evidences show that, HRQoL may seem to be influenced by the coexistence of MHE [48, 52–56]. MHE increases the incidence of disability, and has a negative effect on daily activities. The impact of the perception of the disease, in the form of a "Sickness Impact Profile," has been studied in cirrhotic patients to assess the indicators of QoL. Each profile was significantly reduced in patients with MHE compared to individuals without MHE [48]. In addition, in the presence of MHE, QoL indicators, such as the capacity to drive a car, and the incidence of sleep disorders were also negatively affected [57, 58].

5.2 MHE and falls

Minimal hepatic encephalopathy is significantly associated with high risk of falls explaining the increased healthcare and hospitalization rate in patients with MHE compared to cirrhotic patients without MHE [49, 59, 60]. The presence of cognitive impairment was the only independent factor predictive of a fall. The chance of a fall in 1 year was found to be significantly higher in patients with MHE compared to those without MHE. Urios et al. demonstrated that, MHE patients show impaired balance, mainly on an unstable surface with eyes open, with longer reaction and confinement times and lower success in stability test limits compared to patients without MHE [61].

5.3 Effect of MHE on driving

Traffic accidents are more common in patients with MHE compared to normal individuals, as the driving process in patients with MHE is affected by defects in many factors such as, defects in attention and information processing, slow reactions, improper estimation of traffic conditions, and lack of coordination [48, 62]. As many as 33% of MHE patients reported a traffic accident or violation within the past year [63]. Interestingly, treatment with lactulose could substantially reduce societal costs by preventing motor vehicle accidents [64].

5.4 Risk of overt HE

MHE has been found to predict the development of overt HE in cirrhotic patients [2]. A recent study demonstrated that, CHE and elevated blood NH_3 levels contributed to OHE development in cirrhotic patients [65]. The results of Wang et al. showed that, solely serum albumin level < 30 g/L is the predictor for developing OHE in CHE patients [66]. In a study of Thomsen et al., that enrolled 106 clinically stable cirrhotic patients with no previous history of OHE and followed them for 230 ± 95 d, it was found that, 13.3% of CHE patients developed OHE [67]. In a multicenter study by Patidar et al., a total of 170 cirrhotic patients were followed for a mean of 13 months. They found that 30% of cirrhotic patients developed at least one OHE episode, and that CHE increased their risk of developing OHE, hospitalization, and death/transplant [36].

6. Diagnosis of MHE and CHE

There is no single optimal measure for diagnosis of MHE because none of the diagnostic strategies covers all aspects of deficits that are present in MHE [68, 69]. Testing approaches can be divided into two major types: psychometric and neurophysiological [70, 71]. As MHE affects many elements of cognitive functioning, which may not be impaired to identical degrees, the International Society for Hepatic Encephalopathy and Nitrogen Metabolism (ISHEN) recommends the use of at least two tests, based on the local population norms and availability, and if possible, with one of the tests being more widely accepted to serve as a comparator [72].

6.1 Diseases associated with minimal hepatic encephalopathy

The diagnosis requires the indication of tests in subjects who appear normal, but may suffer from cirrhosis, as the physician usually does not observe MHE [73]. Further group of patients who are not cirrhotic and may develop MHE are those with porto-systemic shunts of inborn origin or secondary to portal thrombosis. The available data of the neuropsychological characteristics of these patients indicate that cognitive abnormalities are indistinguishable from MHE [74].

6.2 Indications for testing

There is no consensus on patients to test for MHE. Some physicians recommend screening of all cirrhotic patients. However, testing should be completed in patients at risk (**Table 2**) for MHE such as, cirrhosis or porto-systemic shunts [5]. Special attention should be given to active drivers, patients handling heavy machines or reporting decline in work performance [75, 76].

6.3 Neuropsychological (paper-and-pencil) tests

The American Association for the Study of Liver Diseases (AASLD) and the European Association for the Study of the Liver recommended neurophysiological

Patients at risk of accidents • Risks at work, e.g., machine worker • Driving accident within the past year • Unprovoked falls
Patients who complain of cognitive symptoms • Psychomotor performance: "I have difficulty in carrying out fine motor tasks." • Decreased attention: "I am frequent feelig of confused." • Poor memory: "I forget a lot".
Patients with decline in work performance observed by relatives or colleagues
Patients with previous history of episodic HE

Table 2.
Patients with cirrhosis, portal vein thrombosis, or porto-systemic shunts who should undergo tests for MHE.

Test	Tested domain	Time required (minuets)	Advantages	Disadvantages	Impact factor
NCT-A	Psychomotor speed	1–2	Gold standard for MHE diagnosis validated internationally	Learning effects	Age and culture
NCT-B	Psychomotor speed, set shifting, divided attention	1–3	Validated internationally	Learning effects	Age and culture
DST	Psychomotor speed, attention	4	Very sensitive and is an early indicator	Learning effects	Age and culture
BDT	Visuospatial reasoning, praxis, psychomotor speed	10–20	It can be used for dementia testing as well	Learning effects	Age and culture
SDT	Psychomotor speed	1–2	Only tests psychomotor speed, a higher sensitivity	Learning effects; only tests psychomotor speed	Age and culture
LTT	Psychomotor speed, visuomotor ability	2–4	Tests a balance between speed and accuracy	Learning effects, outcomes are errors and time	Age and culture
Animal-naming test	Semantic fluency test, verbal retrieval and recall	1	Easy test that has the required characteristics of simplicity, speed, for illiterate patients	Less validated test	
CFF	Visual discrimination and general arousal	10	Easy administration, application by a non-specialist, and results are independent of literacy and age, test can be administered at bedside	Not suitable for red-green blindness and visual impairment	Age
ICT	Response inhibition, working memory, vigilance, attention	15–20	Simple administration, higher sensitivity/specificity	Need highly functional patients, not suitable for non-English-speaking patients	Age and education
Stroop test	Psychomotor speed and cognitive alertness	10	Quick to explain to patients, and simple to score and evaluate	Should be familiar with iPhone/iPad	Age and education
The SCAN Test	Working memory, vigilance, attention	15–20	Simple administration	Learning effects	Age and education
CDR assessment battery	Reaction time, memory, and recognition	15	Appreciable test-retest reliability	Learning effects	Age, education, and culture
EEG	Generalized brain activity	10–15	Can be done in comatose patients, no need of patient cooperation or risk of a learning effect	Nonspecific and may be influenced by accompanying metabolic disturbances	Requires neurological expertise in evaluation

Table 3.
Psychometric tests recommended for diagnosing minimal hepatic encephalopathy.

and psychometric tests to diagnose MHE [3, 51]. Many tests are used for diagnosis of MHE (**Table 3**); however, the gold standard and the most frequently used psychometric test for MHE diagnosis is psychometric hepatic encephalopathy score (PHES) [3, 4, 42].

6.3.1 Standard neuropsychological assessment

Neuropsychological testing is a useful methodology for quantifying cognitive impairment. These tests directly measure cognitive functions that are directly related to activities of daily living. These include the number connection test A (NCT-A), number connection test B (NCT-B), figure connection test (FCT A), figure connection test B (FCT B), digit symbol test (DST), and serial-dotting test (SDOT) [77].

6.3.1.1 Number connection tests

The NCT-A accesses the visual-spatial orientation and psychomotor speed. Twenty-five circles numbered from 1 to 25 are scattered randomly on a sheet of paper. The patients must connect the numbers in order in the shortest time possible without mistakes. If a mistake is made, the subject must stop, correct the error, and then continue without stopping the clock. The test score is the time needed to perform the test, including the time needed to correct all errors. Poorer performance is shown by a longer time for completion (**Figure 3**). In the NCT-B (**Figure 4**), the numbers from 1 to 13 and the letters from A to L were included in circles. The patient is asked to connect numbers and letters in alternating manner, that means go from 1-A-2-B-3-C and so on. Test outcome is the time needed by the patient to perform the test, including error correction time. Besides visuospatial orientation and psychomotor speed, this test is suitable to study the ability to shift attention [78].

According to the guidelines of the International Society for Hepatic Encephalopathy and Nitrogen Metabolism [79], the results of NCT-A will be considered abnormal when the test scores are more than the mean + 2 standard deviations (SDs) from the age-matched normal values. A newly developed electronic number connection test (eNCT) was developed. This test flashes the numbers 1–25 on a screen and needs the participant to click them in order while being timed [80]. These tests are time-consuming, and their results are influenced by age and educational status. However, these tests are recommended for diagnosis of MHE [42, 81].

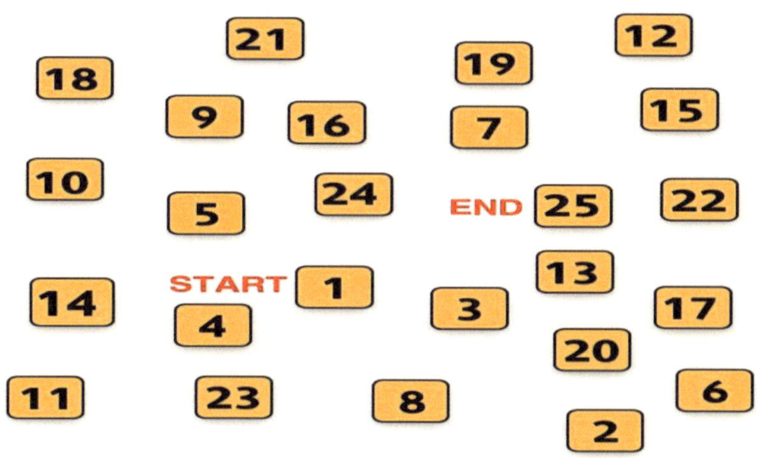

Figure 3.
Number connection tests-A.

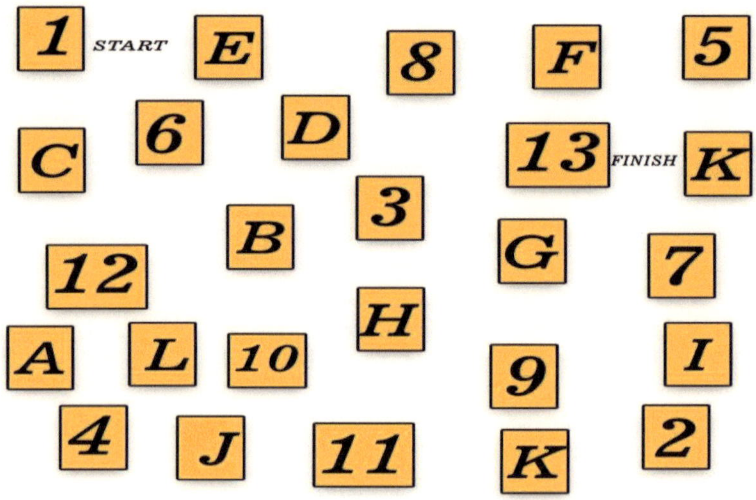

Figure 4.
Number connection tests-B.

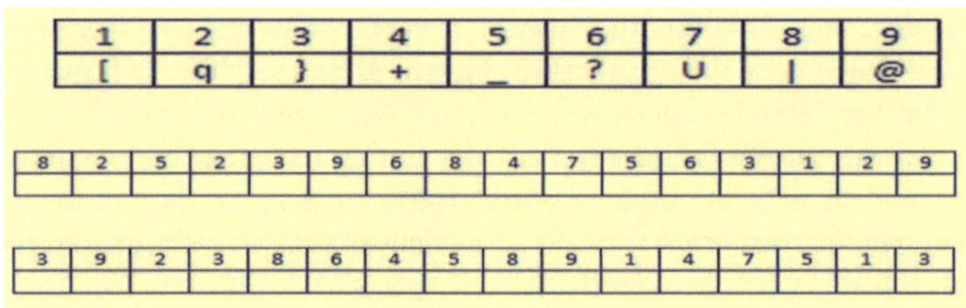

Figure 5.
Digit symbol test.

6.3.1.2 Digit symbol test DST

Nine fixed pairs of numbers and symbols are present at the top of the test sheet. The patient is given a series of double boxes with a number given in the upper part. The target is to draw a symbol related to this number into the lower part of the boxes. The test result is the number of boxes correctly filled in 90 s (**Figure 5**). Pathological test results indicate a deficit in visuoconstructive abilities. [82]. DST will be considered abnormal when the test scores are less than the mean − 2 SDs from the age-matched normal values [79].

6.3.1.3 Block design test

This test recorded speed and accuracy. The task is to take 6–9 blocks that have all white sides, all red sides, and red-and-white sides followed by arranging them according to a pattern formed by examiner or shown on a card [83].

6.3.1.4 Psychometric hepatic encephalopathy score (PHES)

It consists of five paper-pencil tests: NCT-A/B, line tracing time (LTT), digit symbol test, and serial-dotting test (SDOT). This battery measures psychomotor speed and precision, visual perception, visuospatial orientation, visual construction, concentration, attention, and memory and can be completed in less than 20 minutes [68]. The results of PHES can be affected by age and education status of patients. A score is defined as the number of standard deviations of the difference between the two values for each test. MHE was diagnosed with the sum of all scores less than or equal to −4 points. Score < −4 suggests the presence of MHE [1, 84]. A simplified form of PHES, developed using only three of the original five tests, can be as good as the PHES in diagnosing [84]. For illiterate patients, the figure connection test has been used as a subtest instead of the number connection test [1]. PHES has a prognostic value for the occurrence of attacks of overt HE and mortality in cirrhotic patients [42, 43].

6.3.1.5 The animal naming test (ANT)

The ANT (maximum number of animals listed in 1 minute) has recently been developed to predict OHE. ANT is an easy test that has all the required characteristics of simplicity, speed, no cost, and relationship with clinical events to be used routinely for rapid investigation of HE in patients with cirrhosis at the office and at the bedside [85].

6.3.2 Computer-aided psychometric tests

Numerous current studies have showed that, computerization of psychometric tests could lead to simplification and easy administration in the clinic within a few minutes [10, 86, 87].

6.3.2.1 The critical flicker frequency (CFF)

CFF test is a psychophysiological tool that studies the frequency at which a fused light (presented from 60 Hz downward) appears to be flickering to the observer. Similarly, the general arousal of the patient is measured. Earlier studies have shown a reduction in its performance with worsening cognition and improvement after therapy. The CFF test needs numerous trials, intact binocular vision, absence of red-green blindness, and specialized equipment [15]. CFF predicts the first episode of OHE in cirrhotic patients who had never experienced OHE, and predicts mortality risk [88]. CFF test has many advantages, for example, easy administration, application by a non-specialist personal, and results that are independent of numeracy, literacy, and age [89].

6.3.2.2 Continuous reaction time (CRT) test

This test assesses the motor reaction time by having the patient press a button in response to auditory stimuli (through headphones). The most important test result is the CRT index, which measures the stability of the reaction times. The test result can differentiate between organic and metabolic brain impairment. The test is not affected by the patient's age, gender with no learning or tiring impact [90, 91].

6.3.2.3 The inhibitory control test (ICT)

It is a computerized test of response inhibition and working. The ICT requires highly functional patients (**Figure 6**). The ICT can be done using a laptop and is analyzed using an automatic computerized system that significantly improves the

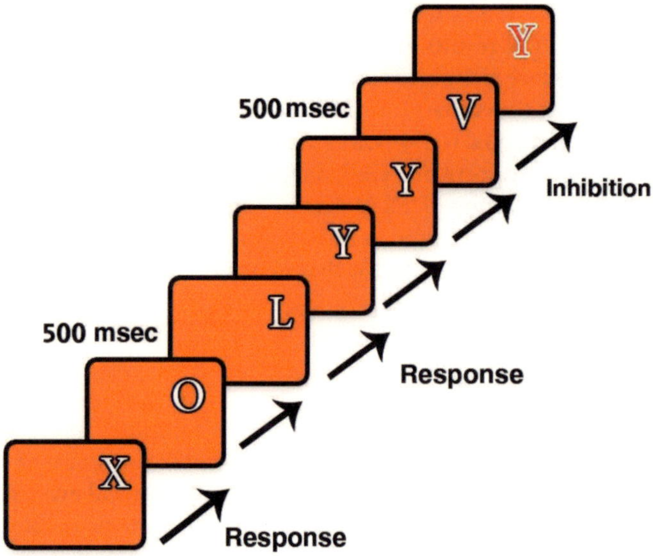

Figure 6.
Inhibitory control test. A continuous sequence of letters is displayed on the computer screen every 500 ms. The patient is educated to respond only if an X is preceded by a Y, or a Y is preceded by an X, but responses must be inhibited if an X is followed by an X, or a Y is followed by a Y.

convenience and flexibility of using this test in the clinical situation [92]. It has been validated for the diagnosis and follow-up of MHE in the USA. It was found that the ICT is simple to administer and has higher sensitivity/specificity for screening MHE than the standard psychometric test (SPT). On the other side, Taneja et al. found that the ICT is not as useful as the PHES in diagnosing MHE in patients with cirrhosis [93].

6.3.2.4 The Stroop test

In 2013, Bajaj et al. developed an application, the EncephalApp-Stroop App, for screening MHE that is operated by the iOS system on the iPhone and iPad. The core of this innovative application is the Stroop test, which assesses psychomotor speed and cognitive alertness by measuring the time required to correctly identify a series of symbols and printed words with different colors [86]. The Stroop test evaluates psychomotor speed and cognitive flexibility by the interference between recognition reaction time to a colored field and a written color name. [86]. In a multicenter study that compared the EncephalApp-Stroop App to the PHES and ICT, the EncephalApp-Stroop App had good sensitivity (70–80%) for MHE screening and was predictive of the progression to OHE [94].

6.3.2.5 The SCAN test

It is a computerized test that measures the patient's speed and accuracy to perform a digit recognition memory task of increasing complexity [40, 95]. It is done by randomly displaying a series of 72 sorted pairs of numbers for 3 s on a computer screen. Patients are instructed to press the appropriate number on a keyboard if they identify a common digit in the sequence of numbers presented. The mean reaction times and the percentage of errors are recorded, and the results are evaluated using the reaction times weighted by the number of errors [96].

6.3.2.6 Cognitive drug research (CDR) assessment battery

It is a computerized battery of cognitive tests designed by the Cognitive Drug Research Ltd. (Goring-on-Thames, UK). The test contains five psychometric subsets that test attention power, attention continuity, speed of memory, and quality of episodic and working memory. It measures reaction time, memory, and recognition. The task stimuli are existing on a laptop, and patients provide the correct response using the "YES" and "NO" buttons on a two-button response box, which records both accuracy and reaction time. The sensitivity and specificity of the CDR assessment battery for screening MHE are 86.4 and 81%, respectively [10].

6.3.3 Electroencephalography examination (EEG)

EEG can discover changes in cortical cerebral activity across the spectrum of HE without patient cooperation or risk of a learning effect [97]. Newly, an-economy friendly device has been found to produce similar results compared with a standard EEG machine across the HE spectrum [97].

7. Treatment

Treatment of minimal hepatic encephalopathy with lactulose, probiotics, or L-ornithine-L-aspartate was seen to be effective in reducing abnormal tests and delay or eradicating risky motor car accident [47, 98–103]. It is therefore rational, especially if the patients or their family/caregivers report symptoms/signs compatible with MHE, to introduce treatment specially in patients who are at particular risk of the consequences of MHE, such as falls, impaired, and driving ability.

7.1 Rifaximin

Rifaximin is an orally administered, non-absorbable, semi-synthetic antibiotic with a broad spectrum of effect on both Gram-positive and Gram-negative bacteria [11, , 104]. It was found that patients with MHE treated with rifaximin for an 8-week period showed significantly greater improvements in driving and cognitive performance and in the psychosocial dimension of the Sickness Impact Profile than those given a placebo [67]. Recently, a randomized controlled trial compared the efficacy of rifaximin with lactulose in reversal of MHE and improvement in HRQoL in cirrhotic patients with MHE. The study concluded that both drugs improve HRQoL equally well, in cirrhotic patients with MHE [105].

7.2 Non-absorbable disaccharides

The recommended standard of care for people with hepatic encephalopathy includes use of the non-absorbable disaccharides (lactulose and lactitol) [106, 107]. It was found that cirrhotic patients with MHE had improvement in health-related quality of life and psychometric performance after lactulose therapy [108]. Lactulose and lactitol, both, have effects on gut flora and are regarded as intestinal prebiotics. Adding lactulose to food can produce a bifidogenic effect connected to a favorable effect on colonic ammonia metabolism [109]. However, a recent meta-analysis evaluating the role of non-absorbable disaccharides in patients with MHE failed to show clear evidence in improving cognitive function and HRQoL [110].

7.3 LOLA (L-ornithine-L-aspartate)

Ammonia scavengers, including L-ornithine-L-aspartate, are agents that reduce blood ammonia concentration by enhancing the metabolism of ammonia to glutamine [111–113]. Bai et al. assessed eight RCTs (646 total patients, 46% diagnosed with MHE), evaluating the efficacy of LOLA compared to placebo in patients with cirrhosis. He found that treatment with LOLA diminished serum ammonia levels [114]. Evidence of important benefit of LOLA was also described in RCTs of patients with MHE assessed by psychometric testing or critical flicker frequency analysis. The oral formulation of LOLA was determined to be particularly effective for the treatment of OHE or MHE [115].

7.4 Probiotics

Prebiotics are non-digestible food ingredients that selectively stimulate the growth and/or activity of the bacteria in the colon. Probiotics are live microbes that alter the intestinal balance of the microflora. The combination of prebiotics and probiotics is named synbiotics. The meta-analysis of nine studies showed substantial evidence for the efficacy of prebiotics, probiotics, and synbiotics in the treatment of MHE [116]. A Cochrane Review examining the use of probiotics in the treatment of HE included seven trials and presented an advantage of probiotics to no treatment in all-cause mortality, number of adverse events, and QoL. Findings included reduced plasma concentrations of ammonia [117].

7.5 Zinc

Zinc, considered as a cofactor of urea cycle enzymes, is deficient in patients with cirrhosis, especially with malnutrition or encephalopathy [118]. Zinc is essential for the synthesis of coenzymes that mediate biogenic amine synthesis and metabolism [14]. Zinc deficiency also leads to change of neurotransmitters like γ aminobutyric acid and norepinephrine [119]. A recent RCT revealed that zinc supplementation can improve MHE in patients with liver cirrhosis associated with significant improvement in neuropsychometric tests and significantly decreased arterial ammonia level [76].

8. Conclusion

The prevalence of MHE is high in liver cirrhosis. MHE is characterized by subtle motor and cognitive deficits, and impairs health-related quality of life. Detection of MHE and subsequent treatment could substantially reduce societal costs by preventing motor vehicle accident.

Conflict of interest

The authors declare that there is no conflict of interest.

Funding

This research received no specific grant from any funding agency in the public, commercial, or not for-profit sectors.

Author details

Gamal Shiha[1,2] and Nasser Mousa[3]*

1 Internal Medicine Department, Mansoura University, Egypt

2 Egyptian Liver Research Institute and Hospital (ELRIH), El-Mansoura, Egypt

3 Tropical Medicine Department, Mansoura University, Egypt

*Address all correspondence to: mousa_medic@yahoo.com

IntechOpen

© 2019 The Author(s). Licensee IntechOpen. This chapter is distributed under the terms of the Creative Commons Attribution License (http://creativecommons.org/licenses/by/3.0), which permits unrestricted use, distribution, and reproduction in any medium, provided the original work is properly cited.

References

[1] Mullen KD, Prakash RK. New perspectives in hepatic encephalopathy. Clinics in Liver Disease. 2012;**16**:1-5

[2] Romero-Gómez M, Boza F, García-Valdecasas MS, García E, Aguilar-Reina J. Subclinical hepatic encephalopathy predicts the development of overt hepatic encephalopathy. The American Journal of Gastroenterology. 2001;**96**:2718-2723

[3] Vilstrup H, Amodio P, Bajaj J, Cordoba J, Ferenci P, Mullen KD, et al. Hepatic encephalopathy in chronic liver disease: 2014 Practice Guideline by the American Association for the Study of Liver Diseases and the European Association for the Study of the Liver. Hepatology. 2014;**60**:715-735

[4] Ferenci P, Lockwood A, Mullen K, Tarter R, Weissenborn K, Blei AT. Hepatic encephalopathy definition, nomenclature, diagnosis, and quantification: Final report of the working party at the 11th World Congresses of Gastroenterology, Vienna, 1998. Hepatology. 2002;**35**:716-721

[5] Labenz C, Worns MA, Schattenberg JM, Huber Y, Galle PR, Labenz J, et al. Epidemiology of hepatic encephalopathy in german hospitals—The EpHE study. Zeitschrift für Gastroenterologie. 2017;**55**:741-747

[6] Dhiman RK, Chawla YK. Minimal hepatic encephalopathy. Indian Journal of Gastroenterology. 2009;**28**(1):5-16

[7] Bajaj JS, Heuman DM, Bell DE, White M, Gilles H, Luketic VA, et al. Burden of cirrhosis and hepatic encephalopathy on patients and caregivers. Hepatology. 2010;**410A**:52

[8] Das A, Dhiman RK, Saraswat VA, Verma M, Naik SR. Prevalence and natural history of subclinical hepatic encephalopathy in cirrhosis. Journal of Gastroenterology and Hepatology. 2001;**16**:531-535

[9] Waghray A, Waghray N, Mullen K. Management of covert hepatic encephalopathy. Journal of Clinical and Experimental Hepatology. 2015;**5**:S75-S81

[10] Bajaj JS, Saeian K, Verber MD, Hischke D, Hoffmann RG, Franco J, et al. Inhibitory control test is a simple method to diagnose minimal hepatic encephalopathy and predict development of overt hepatic encephalopathy. The American Journal of Gastroenterology. 2007;**102**:754-760

[11] Ford JM, Gray M, Whitfield SL, Turken AU, Glover G, Faustman WO, et al. Acquiring and inhibiting prepotent responses in schizophrenia: Event-related brain potentials and functional magnetic resonance imaging. Archives of General Psychiatry. 2004;**61**:119-129

[12] Bajaj JS. Management options for minimal hepatic encephalopathy. Expert Review of Gastroenterology & Hepatology. 2008;**2**:785-790

[13] Schomerus H, Hamster W. Quality of life in cirrhotic with minimal hepatic encephalopathy. Metabolic Brain Disease. 2001;**16**:37-41

[14] Sharma P, Sharma BC, Puri V, Sarin SK. Critical flicker frequency: Diagnostic tool for minimal hepatic encephalopathy. Journal of Hepatology. 2007;**47**:67-73

[15] Romero-Gómez M, Córdoba J, Jover R, del Olmo JA, Ramírez M, Rey R, et al. Value of the critical flicker frequency in patients with minimal hepatic encephalopathy. Hepatology. 2007;**45**:879-885

[16] Cordoba J, Alonso J, Rovira A, Jacas C, Sanpedro F, Castells L, et al.

The development of low-grade cerebral edema in cirrhosis is supported by the evolution of (1) H-magnetic resonance abnormalities after liver transplantation. Journal of Hepatology. 2001;**35**:598-604

[17] Tapper EB, Jiang ZG, Patwardhan VR. Refining the ammonia hypothesis: A physiology-driven approach to the treatment of hepatic encephalopathy. Mayo Clinic Proceedings. 2015;**90**:646-658

[18] Patidar KR, Bajaj JS. Covert and overt hepatic encephalopathy: Diagnosis and management. Clinical Gastroenterology and Hepatology. 2015;**13**(12):2048-2061

[19] Brusilow SW. Hyperammonemic encephalopathy. Medicine (Baltimore). 2002;**81**(3):240-249

[20] Chatauret N, Butterworth RF. Effects of liver failure on inter-organ trafficking of ammonia: Implications for the treatment of hepatic encephalopathy. Journal of Gastroenterology and Hepatology. 2004;**19**:S219-S223

[21] Cichoż-Lach H, Michalak A. Current pathogenetic aspects of hepatic encephalopathy and non cirrhotic hyperammonemic encephalopathy. World Journal of Gastroenterology. 2013;**19**:26-34

[22] Cooper AJ, Plum F. Biochemistry and physiology of brain ammonia. Physiological Reviews. 1987;**67**:440-519

[23] Wijdicks EF. Hepatic encephalopathy. The New England Journal of Medicine. 2016;**375**: 1660-1670

[24] Schomerus H, Hamster W. Neuropsychological aspects of portal-systemic encephalopathy. Metabolic Brain Disease. 1998;**13**:361-377

[25] Szerb JC, Butterworth RF. Effect of ammonium ions on synaptic transmission in the mammalian central nervous system. Progress in Neurobiology. 1992;**39**:135-153

[26] Luo M, Guo JY, Cao WK. Inflammation: A novel target of current therapies for hepatic encephalopathy in liver cirrhosis. World Journal of Gastroenterology. 2015;**21**(41):11815-11824

[27] Shawcross DL, Davies NA, Williams R, Jalan R. Systemic inflammatory response exacerbates the neuropsychological effects of induced hyperammonemia in cirrhosis. Journal of Hepatology. 2004;**40**:247-254

[28] Shawcross DL, Wright G, Olde Damink SW, Jalan R. Role of ammonia and inflammation in minimal hepatic encephalopathy. Metabolic Brain Disease. 2007;**22**:125-138

[29] Aldridgea DR, Tranaha EJ, Shawcross DL. Pathogenesis of hepatic encephalopathy: Role of ammonia and systemic inflammation. Journal of Clinical and Experimental Hepatology. 2015;**5**:S7-S20

[30] Seyan AS, Hughes RD, Shawcross DL. Changing face of hepatic encephalopathy: Role of inflammation and oxidative stress. World Journal of Gastroenterology. 2010;**16**:3347-3357

[31] Bémeur C, Butterworth R. Liver-brain proinflammatory signalling in acute liver failure: Role in the pathogenesis of hepatic encephalopathy and brain edema. Metabolic Brain Disease. 2013;**28**:145-150

[32] Schnabl B, Brenner DA. Interactions between the intestinal microbiome and liver diseases. Gastroenterology. 2014;**146**(6):1513-1524

[33] Bajaj JS, Betrapally NS, Hylemon PB, Heuman DM, Daita K,

White MB, et al. Salivary microbiota reflects changes in gut microbiota in cirrhosis with hepatic encephalopathy. Hepatology. 2015;**62**(4):1260-1271

[34] Zhang Z, Zhai H, Geng J, Yu R, Ren H, Fan H, et al. Large-scale survey of gut microbiota associated with MHE via 16S rRNA-based pyrosequencing. The American Journal of Gastroenterology. 2013;**108**:1601-1611

[35] Bajaj JS, Heuman DM, Hylemon PB, et al. Altered profile of human gut microbiome is associated with cirrhosis and its complications. Journal of Hepatology. 2014;**60**(5):940-947

[36] Patidar KR, Thacker LR, Wade JB, et al. Covert hepatic encephalopathy is independently associated with poor survival and increased risk of hospitalization. The American Journal of Gastroenterology. 2014;**109**:1757-1763

[37] Hartmann IJ, Groeneweg M, Quero JC, Beijeman SJ, de Man RA, Hop WC, et al. The prognostic significance of subclinical hepatic encephalopathy. The American Journal of Gastroenterology. 2000;**95**(8):2029-2034

[38] Das A, Dhiman RK, Saraswat VA, Verma M, Naik SR. Prevalence and natural history of subclinical hepatic encephalopathy incirrhosis. Journal of Gastroenterology and Hepatology. 2001;**16**:531-533

[39] Lockwood AH. "What's in a name?" improving the care of cirrhotics. Journal of Hepatology. 2000;**32**:859-861

[40] Amodio P, del Piccolo F, Marchetti P, Angeli P, Iemmolo R, Caregaro L, et al. Clinical features and survival of cirrhotic patients with subclinical cognitive alterations detected by the number connection test and computerized psychometric tests. Hepatology. 1999;**29**:1662-1667

[41] Romero-Gómez M, Grande L, Camacho I, Benitez S, Irles JA, Castro M. Altered response to oral glutamine challenge as prognostic factor for overt episodes in patients with minimal hepatic encephalopathy. Journal of Hepatology. 2002;**37**(6):781-787

[42] Dhiman RK, Kurmi R, Thumburu KK, Venkataramarao SH, Agarwal R, Duseja A, et al. Diagnosis and prognostic significance of minimal hepatic encephalopathy inpatients with cirrhosis of liver. Digestive Diseases and Sciences. 2010;**55**(8):2381-2390

[43] Romero-Gómez M, Córdoba J, Jover R, et al. Value of the critica flicker frequency in patients with minimal hepatic encephalopathy. Hepatology. 2007;**45**:879-885

[44] Wein C, Koch H, Popp B, Oehler G, Schauder P. Minimal hepatic encephalopathy impairs fitness to drive. Hepatology. 2004;**39**:739-745

[45] Watanabe A, Tuchida T, Yata Y, Kuwabara Y. Evaluation of neuropsychological function inpatients with liver cirrhosis with special reference to their driving ability. Metabolic Brain Disease. 1995;**10**:239-248

[46] Bajaj JS, Hafeezullah M, Hoffmann RG, Varma RR, Franco J, Binion DG, et al. Navigation skill impairment: Another dimension of the driving difficulties in minimal hepaticencephalopathy. Hepatology. 2008;**47**:596-604

[47] Dhiman RK, Sawhney MS, Chawla YK, Das G, Ram S, Dilawari JB. Efficacy of lactulose in cirrhotic patients with subclinical hepatic encephalopathy. Digestive Diseases and Sciences. 2000;**45**:1549-1552

[48] Groeneweg M, Quero JC, De Bruijn I, Hartmann IJ, Essink-bot

ML, Hop WC, et al. Subclinical hepatic encephalopathy impairs daily functioning. Hepatology. 1998;**28**:45-49

[49] Roman E, Cordoba J, Torrens M, Torras X, Villanueva C, Vargas V, et al. Minimal hepatic encephalopathy is associated with falls. The American Journal of Gastroenterology. 2011;**106**:476-482.49

[50] Zhou YQ, Chen SY, Jiang LD, Guo CY, Shen ZY, Huang PX, et al. Development and evaluation of the quality of life instrument in chronic liver disease patients with minimal hepatic encephalopathy. Journal of Gastroenterology and Hepatology. 2009;**24**:408-415

[51] Bajaj JS, Etemadian A, Hafeezullah M, Saeian K. Testing for minimal hepatic encephalopathy in the United States: An AASLD survey. Hepatology. 2007;**45**:833-834

[52] Prasad S, Dhiman RK, Duseja A, Chawla YK, Sharma A, Agarwal R. Lactulose improves cognitive functions and health-relatedquality of life in patients with cirrhosis who have minimal hepaticencephalopathy. Hepatology. 2007;**45**:549-559

[53] Arguedas MR, DeLawrence TG, McGuire BM. Influence of hepatic encephalopathy on health-related quality of life in patients withcirrhosis. Digestive Diseases and Sciences. 2003;**48**:1622-1626

[54] Bao ZJ, Qiu DK, Ma X, Fan ZP, Zhang GS, Huang YQ, et al. Assessment of health-related quality of life in Chinese patients with minimal hepatic encephalopathy. World Journal of Gastroenterology. 2007;**13**:3003-3008

[55] Sidhu SS, Goyal O, Mishra BP, Sood A, Chhina RS, Soni RK. Rifaximin improves psychometric performance and health-relatedquality of life in patients with minimal hepatic encephalopathy (the RIME Trial). The American Journal of Gastroenterology. 2011;**106**:307-316

[56] Marchesini G, Bianchi G, Amodio P, Salerno F, Merli M, Panella C, et al. Italian Study Group for quality of life in cirrhosis. Factors associated with poor health-relatedquality of life of patients with cirrhosis. Gastroenterology. 2001;**120**:170-178

[57] Arguedas MR, DeLawrence TG, McGuire BM. Influence of hepatic encephalopathy on health-related quality of life in patients with cirrhosis. Digestive Diseases and Sciences. 2003;**48**:1622-1626

[58] Kim WR, Brown RS Jr, Terrault NA, El-Serag H. Burden of liver disease in the United States: Summary of a workshop. Hepatology. 2002;**36**:227-242

[59] Qadri AM, Ogunwale BO, Mullen KD. Can we ignore minimal hepatic encephalopathy any longer? Hepatology. 2007;**45**:547-548

[60] Soriano G, Román E, Córdoba J, Torrens M, Poca M, Torras X, et al. Cognitive dysfunction in cirrhosis is associated with falls: A prospective study. Hepatology. 2012;**55**:1922-1930

[61] Urios A, Mangas-Losada A, Gimenez-Garzó C, González-López O, Giner-Durán R, Serra MA, et al. Altered postural control and stability in cirrhotic patients with minimal hepatic encephalopathy correlate with cognitive deficits. Liver International. 2017;**37**:1013-1022

[62] Yildirim M. Falls in patients with liver cirrhosis. Gastroenterology Nursing. 2017;**40**(4):306-310

[63] Gad Y, Zaher A, Mousa N, El-desoky A, Al-Adarosy A. Screening for minimal hepatic encephalopathy in asymptomatic drivers with

liver cirrhosis. Arab Journal of Gastroenterology. 2011;**12**(2):58-61

[64] Bajaj JS, Pinkerton SD, Sanyal AJ, Heuman DM. Diagnosis and treatment of minimal hepatic encephalopathy to prevent motor vehicle accidents: A cost-effectiveness analysis. Hepatology. 2012;**55**:1164-1171

[65] Iwasa M, Sugimoto R, Mifuji-Moroka R, Hara N, Yoshikawa K, Tanaka H. Factors contributing to the development of overt encephalopathy in liver cirrhosis patients. Metabolic Brain Disease. 2016;**31**:1151-1156

[66] Wang AJ, Peng AP, Li BM, Gan N, Pei L, Zheng XL, et al. Natural history of covert hepatic encephalopathy: An observational study of 366 cirrhotic patients. World Journal of Gastroenterology. 2017;**23**(34):6321-6329

[67] Thomsen KL, Macnaughtan J, Tritto G, Mookerjee RP, Jalan R. Clinical and pathophysiological characteristics of cirrhotic patients with grade 1 and minimal hepatic encephalopathy. PLoS One. 2016;**11**:e0146076

[68] Weissenborn K, Ennen JC, Schomerus H, Ruckert N, Hecker H. Neuropsychological characterization of hepatic encephalopathy. Journal of Hepatology. 2001;**34**:768-773

[69] Weissenborn K, Giewekemeyer K, Heidenreich S, Bokemeyer M, Berding G, Ahl B. Attention, memory, and cognitive function in hepatic encephalopathy. Metabolic Brain Disease. 2005;**20**:359-367

[70] Montagnese S, Amodio P, Morgan MY. Methods for diagnosing hepatic encephalopathy in patients with cirrhosis: A multidimensional approach. Metabolic Brain Disease. 2004;**19**:281-312

[71] Prakash R, Mullen KD. Mechanisms, diagnosis and management of hepatic encephalopathy. Nature Reviews. Gastroenterology & Hepatology. 2010;**7**:515-525

[72] Guerit JM, Amantini A, Fischer C, Kaplan PW, Mecarelli O, Schnitzler A, et al. Neurophysiological investigations of hepatic encephalopathy: ISHEN practice guidelines. Liver International. 2009;**29**:789-796

[73] Hilsabeck RC, Perry W, Hassanein TI. Neuropsychological impairment in patients with chronic hepatitis C. Hepatology. 2002;**35**:440-446

[74] Ortiz M, Cordoba J, Alonso J, Rovira A, Quiroga S, Jacas C, et al. Oral glutamine challenge and magnetic resonance spectroscopy in three patients with congenital portosystemic shunts. Journal of Hepatology. 2004;**40**:552-557

[75] Sharma P, Sharma BC, Puri V, Sarin SK. An open-label randomized controlled trial of lactulose and probiotics in the treatment of minimal hepatic encephalopathy. European Journal of Gastroenterology & Hepatology. 2008;**20**:506-511

[76] Mousa N, Abdel-Razik A, Zaher A, Hamed M, Shiha G, Effat N, et al. The role of antioxidants and zinc in minimal hepatic encephalopathy: A randomized trial. Therapeutic Advances in Gastroenterology. 2016;**9**(5):684-691

[77] Dhiman RK, Saraswat VA, Verma M, Naik SR. Figure connection test: A modified number connection test for the objective assessment of mental state in illiterates. Journal of Gastroenterology and Hepatology. 1995;**10**:14-23

[78] Schomerus H, Hamster W. Neuropsychological aspects of portalsystemic encephalopathy. Metabolic Brain Disease. 1998;**13**:361-377

[79] Randolph C, Hilsabeck R, Kato A, Kharbanda P, Li YY, Mapelli D, et al. Neuropsychological assessment of hepatic encephalopathy: ISHEN practice guidelines. Liver International. 2009;**29**(5):629-635

[80] Wuensch T, Ruether DF, Zöllner C, Mueller T, Jung T, Kaffarnik M, et al. Performance characterization of a novel electronic number connection test to detect minimal hepatic encephalopathy in cirrhotic patients. European Journal of Gastroenterology & Hepatology. 2017;**29**(4):456-463

[81] Sharma P, Sharma BC, Puri V, Sarin SK. Natural history of minimal hepatic encephalopathy in patients with extrahepatic portal vein obstruction. The American Journal of Gastroenterology. 2009;**104**:885-890

[82] Kügler CF, Petter J, Taghavy A, Lotterer E, Wensing G, Hahn EG, et al. Dynamics of cognitive brain dysfunction in patients with cirrhotic liver disease: An event-related P300 potential perspective. Electroencephalography and Clinical Neurophysiology. 1994;**91**:33-41

[83] Meyer T, Eshelman A, Abouljoud M. Neuropsychological changes in a large sample of liver transplant candidates. Transplantation Proceedings. 2006;**38**:3559-3660

[84] Riggio O, Ridola L, Pasquale C, Pentassuglio I, Nardelli S, Moscucci F, et al. A simplified psychometric evaluation for the diagnosis of minimal hepatic encephalopathy. Clinical Gastroenterology and Hepatology. 2011;**9**:613-616.e1

[85] Campagna F, Montagnese S, Ridola L, Senzolo M, Schiff S, De Rui M, et al. The animal naming test: An easy tool for the assessment of hepatic encephalopathy. Hepatology. 2017;**66**(1):198-208

[86] Bajaj JS, Thacker LR, Heumann DM, Fuchs M, Sterling RK, Sanyal AJ, et al. The Stroop smartphone application is a short and valid method to screen for minimal hepatic encephalopathy. Hepatology. 2013;**58**:1122-1132

[87] Mardini H, Saxby BK, Record CO. Computerized psychometric testing in minimal encephalopathy and modulation by nitrogen challenge and liver transplant. Gastroenterology. 2008;**135**:1582-1590

[88] Barone M, Shahini E, Iannone A, Viggiani MT, Corvace V, et al. Critical flicker frequency test predicts overt hepatic encephalopathy and survival in patients with liver cirrhosis. Digestive and Liver Disease. 2018;**50**(5):496-500

[89] Coşkun B, Özen M. Critical flicker frequency test for diagnosing minimal hepatic encephalopathy in patients with cirrhosis. The Turkish Journal of Gastroenterology. 2017;**28**:191-196

[90] Lauridsen MM, Gronbaek H, Naeser EB, Leth ST, Vilstrup H. Gender and age effects on the continuous reaction times method in volunteers and patients with cirrhosis. Metabolic Brain Disease. 2012;**27**:559-565

[91] Lauridsen MM, Thiele M, Kimer N, Vilstrup H. The continuous reaction times method for diagnosing, grading, and monitoring minimal/covert hepatic encephalopathy. Metabolic Brain Disease. 2013;**28**:231-234

[92] Bajaj JS, Hafeezullah M, Franco J, Varma RR, Hoffmann RG, Knox JF, et al. Inhibitory control test for the diagnosis of minimal hepatic encephalopathy. Gastroenterology. 2008;**135**:1591-1600.e1591

[93] Taneja S, Dhiman RK, Khatri A, Goyal S, Thumbru K, Agarwal R, et al. Inhibitory control test for the detection of minimal hepatic encephalopathy in patients with cirrhosis of liver.

Journal of Clinical and Experimental Hepatology. 2012;**2**:306-314

[94] Allampati S, Duarte-Rojo A, Thacker LR, Patidar KR, White MB, Klair JS, et al. Diagnosis of minimal hepatic encephalopathy using Stroop EncephalApp: A multicenter US-based, norm-based study. The American Journal of Gastroenterology. 2015;**111**:78-86

[95] Montagnese S, Schiff S, Turco M, Bonato CA, Ridola L, Gatta A, et al. Simple tools for complex syndromes: A three-level difficulty test for hepatic encephalopathy. Digestive and Liver Disease. 2012;**44**:957-960

[96] Amodio P, Marchetti P, Del Piccolo F, Rizzo C, Iemmolo RM, Caregaro L, et al. Study on the Sternberg paradigm in cirrhotic patients without overt hepatic encephalopathy. Metabolic Brain Disease. 1998;**13**:159-172

[97] Schiff S, Casa M, Di Caro V, Aprile D, Spinelli G, De Rui M, et al. A low-cost, user-friendly electroencephalographic recording system for the assessment of hepatic encephalopathy. Hepatology. 2016;**63**(5):1651-1659

[98] Zucker DM, Redulla R. Lactulose management of minimal hepatic encephalopathy: A systematic review. Gastroenterology Nursing. 2019;**42**(1):84-94

[99] Watanabe A, Sakai T, Sato S, Imai F, Ohto M, Arakawa Y, et al. Clinical efficacy of lactulose in cirrhotic patients with and without subclinical hepatic encephalopathy. Hepatology. 1997;**26**(6):1410-1414

[100] Cao Q, Yu CB, Yang SG, Cao HC, Chen P, Deng M, et al. Effect of probiotic treatment on cirrhotic patients with minimal hepatic encephalopathy: A meta-analysis. Hepatobiliary & Pancreatic Diseases International. 2018;**17**(1):9-16

[101] Gluud LL, Dam G, Les I, Marchesini G, Borre M, Aagaard NK, et al. Branched-chain amino acids for people with hepatic encephalopathy. Cochrane Database of Systematic Reviews. 2017;**5**:CD001939

[102] Horsmans Y, Solbreux PM, Daenens C, Desager JP, Geubel AP. Lactulose improves psychometric testing in cirrhotic patients with subclinical encephalopathy. Alimentary Pharmacology & Therapeutics. 1997;**11**(1):165-170

[103] Sidhu SS, Goyal O, Mishra BP, Sood A, Chhina RS, Soni RK. Rifaxim improves psychometric performance and health-related quality of life in patients with minimal hepatic encephalopathy (the RIME Trial). The American Journal of Gastroenterology. 2011;**106**(2):307-316

[104] Kimer N, Krag A, Gluud LL. Safety, efficacy, and patient acceptability of rifaximin for hepatic encephalopathy. Patient Preference and Adherence. 2014;**8**:331

[105] Sidhu SS, Goyal O, Parker RA, Kishore H, Sood A. Rifaximin vs. lactulose in treatment of minimal hepatic encephalopathy. Liver International. 2016;**36**:378-385

[106] Johanson JF. Review of the treatment options for chronic constipation. Medscape General Medicine. 2007;**9**(2):25

[107] Jain L, Sharma BC, Srivastava S, Puri SK, Sharma P, Sarin S. Serum endotoxin, inflammatory mediators, and magnetic resonance spectroscopy before and after treatment in patients with minimal hepatic encephalopathy. Journal of Gastroenterology and Hepatology. 2013;**28**:1187-1193

[108] Prasad S, Dhiman RK, Duseja A, Chawla YK, Sharma A, Agarwal R, et al. Lactulose improves cognitive functions and health-related quality of life in patients with cirrhosis who have minimal hepatic encephallopathy. Hepatology. 2007;**45**(3):549-559

[109] Bouhnik Y, Attar A, Joly FA, Riottot M, Dyard F, Flourié B, et al. Lactulose ingestion increases Faecal bifidobacterial counts: A randomised double-blind study in healthy humans. European Journal of Clinical Nutrition. 2004;**58**:462-466

[110] Gluud LL, Vilstrup H, Morgan MY. Non-absorbable disaccharides versus placebo/no intervention and lactulose versus lactitol for the prevention and treatment of hepatic encephalopathy in people with cirrhosis. Cochrane Database of Systematic Reviews. 2016;**5**:CD003044

[111] Blanco Vela CI, Poo Ramirez JL. Efficacy of oral L-ornithine L-aspartate in cirrhotic patients with hyperammonemic hepatic encephalopathy. Annals of Hepatology. 2011;**10**(Suppl 2):S55-S59

[112] Rahimi RS, Rockey DC. Hepatic encephalopathy: Pharmacological therapies targeting ammonia. Seminars in Liver Disease. 2016;**36**(1):48-55

[113] De Las Heras J, Aldamiz-Echevarria L, Martinez-Chantar ML, Delgado TC. An update on the use of benzoate, phenylacetate and phenylbutyrate ammonia scavengers for interrogating and modifying liver nitrogen metabolism and its implications in urea cycle disorders and liver disease. Expert Opinion on Drug Metabolism & Toxicology. 2017;**13**(4):439-448

[114] Bai M, Yang Z, Qi X, Fan D, Han G. L-ornithine-L-aspartate for hepatic encephalopathy in patients with cirrhosis: A meta-analysis of randomized controlled trials. Journal of Gastroenterology and Hepatology. 2013;**28**:783-792

[115] Butterworth RF, McPhail MJW. L-ornithine L-aspartate (LOLA) for hepatic encephalopathy in cirrhosis: Results of randomized controlled trials and meta-analyses. Drugs. 2019;**79**(Suppl 1):31-37

[116] Shukla S, Shukla A, Mehboob S, Guha S. Meta-analysis: The effects of gut flora modulation using prebiotics, probiotics andsynbiotics on inimal hepatic encephalopathy. Alimentary Pharmacology & Therapeutics. 2011;**33**:662-671

[117] McGee RG, Bakens A, Wiley K, et al. Probiotics for patients with hepatic encephalopathy. Cochrane Database of Systematic Reviews. 2011;**11**:CD008716

[118] Blei A, Córdoba J, Practice Parameters Committee of the American College of Gastroenterology. Hepatic encephalopathy. American Journal of Gastroenterology. 2001;**96**:1968-1976

[119] Chetri K, Choudhuri G. Role of trace elements in hepatic encephalopathy: Zinc and manganese. Indian Journal of Gastroenterology. 2003;**22**(Suppl 2):S28-S30

Chapter 2

Ammonia

Edwin Jin Su Lee and Jonathan C. Huang

Abstract

Ammonia is a compound that is thought to be central to the pathogenesis of hepatic encephalopathy. It is an important biomarker and may also serve as a prognostic indicator in acute liver disease where ammonia levels may be predictive of cerebral edema and herniation. In this chapter, we aim to review and discuss its role in hepatic encephalopathy to include: the cycle within the human body, appropriate measurement and collection, confounding factors and differential diagnosis, the correlation between levels and development of encephalopathy, the physiopathology and increased morbidity-mortality with the incremental rise, clinical utility of sequential measurement, and lastly, an overview of novel treatments and the tight interconnections with ammonia.

Keywords: ammonia, hepatic encephalopathy, role, pathogenesis, novel treatment

1. Introduction

Ammonia, a colorless gas with a unique odor is thought to be central to the pathogenesis of hepatic encephalopathy (HE). It is an important biomarker and may also serve as a prognostic indicator in acute liver disease where ammonia levels may be predictive of cerebral edema and herniation. In this chapter, we aim to review and discuss its role in HE understanding its rise and fall as part of the urea cycle, appropriate measurement and collection, and examine the paradigms differentiating acute liver failure with chronic liver disease. We want to recognize other diseases that may elevate ammonia levels and discuss how different treatments target its reduction.

2. The ammonia cycle within the human body

The homeostasis of ammonia is a multi-organ process involving the brain, gastrointestinal tract, muscles, adipose tissue, kidneys, and mainly the liver. A study involving patients with end-stage liver disease, revealed that branched-chain amino acids (BCAAs) (**Figure 1**) are not metabolized in the liver but rather by muscle, kidney, adipose, and brain tissue. This is in contrast to the aromatic amino acids (tyrosine, phenylalanine, methionine), which are metabolized and deaminated solely by the liver. BCAA supplementation leads to reductions in hyperammonemia as a result of the metabolism of BCAAs by skeletal muscle. The metabolism of BCAAs supplied carbon skeletons for the formation of α-ketoglutarate which combined with two ammonia molecules to form glutamine [1]. In a 1-year double-blind study of 174 patients with advanced cirrhosis who were randomized to receive BCAAs or equicaloric amounts of lactoalbumin, the group given BCAAs had a significantly decreased incidence of the combined endpoint of death and liver decompensation, as well as hospital admissions, compared with lactoalbumin [2]. In addition, a multi-center randomized study of 646

IntechOpen

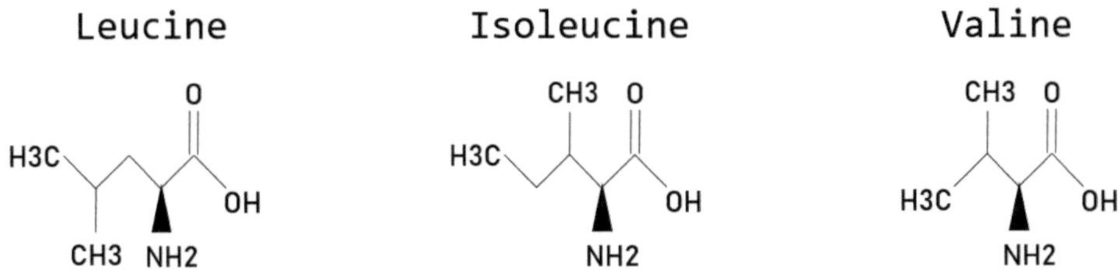

Figure 1.
Branched-chain amino acids.

patients with cirrhosis who were given 12 g of BCAAs per day for 2 years, compared with diet therapy and a defined food intake, found a significant decrease in HE and refractory ascites in the treatment group [3]. Because of their poor palatability and high cost, BCAAs are not routinely recommended, but they were important tools in the proof of concept of liver's importance in ammonia homeostasis.

The mechanism of how the liver processes the ammonia has been described and involves the following steps: ammonia is produced by the enterocytes from glutamine and by colonic bacterial catabolism of nitrogenous sources, such as ingested protein and secreted urea. It then enters the circulation through the portal vein where the liver metabolizes the majority of the ammonia converting it into urea or glutamine and preventing entry into the systemic circulation. These were demonstrated through careful studies of the urea cycle and its disorders [4].

The increase in blood ammonia levels in advanced liver disease is a consequence of impaired liver function and of shunting of blood around/away from the liver. Muscle wasting, a common occurrence in these patients, also may contribute since muscle is also an important site for extrahepatic ammonia removal.

3. Appropriate measurement and collection

The measurement serum ammonia concentration in patients suspected of having HE remains controversial. While it is well known that venous ammonia levels vary immensely and are not useful for screening or following HE [5], arterial ammonia concentrations more accurately correlate with HE as it is further discussed in this chapter. Furthermore, the grade of HE seems to be more closely related to the partial pressure of gaseous ammonia (pNH3) than the total arterial ammonia concentration, since gaseous ammonia readily enters the brain [6]. This can be easily calculated with ammonia levels when correlating with pH.

The accuracy of ammonia determination is influenced by many factors, such as fist clenching, use of a tourniquet, and whether the sample was placed on ice [7]. It is largely recommended that it is tested within an hour of collection, though some agents (sodium borate/l-serine) could potentially stabilize for up to 12 h [8].

Thus, ammonia should be collected in an extremity without trauma with arterial blood, collected in chilled tubes with ammonia-free sodium heparin (green top) or ethylenediaminetetraacetic acid (EDTA; purple top), placed on ice, and delivered rapidly to the laboratory (within an hour). Some chemicals could stabilize for posterior measurement, but more studies are needed to confirm that these agents will not influence in other reactions and measurements.

4. Correlation of levels and development encephalopathy

Normal values for ammonia concentration may differ depending on age groups. It can be often higher in newborns, with the upper limit of normal of ammonia concentration of healthy term infants at birth of 80 to 90 μmol/L, while normal values in children older than 1 month and adults are less than 50 and 30 μmol/L, respectively [9].

Early studies had shown a correlation of levels of ammonia and worsening HE up to two times the upper limit of normality [6]. Further studies have not only cemented this correlation but have shown a more intricate relationship [10, 11]. It can predict the risk and frequency of HE episodes [12].

5. The physiopathology and increased morbidity-mortality with the incremental rise of ammonia

Proof of the role of ammonia in pathogenesis of HE has come from the efficacy of therapies aimed to lower plasma ammonia in improving its symptoms. The mechanisms causing brain dysfunction in liver disease are still not known to the full extent. In coma of models of acute liver failure, the effects of ammonia are present in brain swelling, impaired cerebral perfusion, and reversible impairment of neurotransmitter systems [13].

Stemming from this proof of concept, several studies have tried to elucidate the effects of hyperammonemia. First, ammonia is believed to be a direct neurotoxin potentialized by other toxins, such as mercaptans and short-chain fatty acids [14]. Second, it impairs the blood–brain barrier by changing the protein transport [15]. Third, it increases the intracellular osmolality of astrocytes leading to edema and extreme cases, herniation [13, 16]. Lastly, it increases oxidative stress. In one study, oxidative stress markers in the brain of patients with cirrhosis with severe hepatic encephalopathy included elevated levels of protein tyrosine-nitrated proteins, heat shock protein-27, and 8-hydroxyguanosine as a marker for RNA oxidation [17].

In a recent study of patients with cirrhosis, there was significant evidence that ammonia levels correlate with not only the severity of hepatic encephalopathy but also the failure of other organs in cirrhosis and is an independent risk factor for 28-day mortality. This data provided evidence that the ammonia level has a clinically relevant utility in providing important prognostic information, signifying its potential role as a biomarker in identifying patients at high risk of mortality. A reduction in ammonia level was associated with improved survival, confirming it as a potential therapeutic target. Classically in urea cycle disorders ammonia levels above 200 μmol/L were considered a poor prognostic factor [18], but in this study in cirrhotics even ≥79.5 μmol/L was associated with increased mortality, indicating an additional role of ammonia in dictating clinical outcomes [11].

Classically, there was a clear distinction of the harmful effects of the ammonia in acute liver failure due to the osmotic component [13] and in lesser degree in chronic liver disease, stating that ammonia in cirrhosis increased morbidity and not mortality. But newer studies and prospective analysis shows that it can be harmful in similar way, increasing mortality [11]. Further studies are needed to corroborate both the utility and prognostic value of ammonia in the setting of chronic liver disease.

6. Confounding factors and differential diagnosis

Ammonia levels may rise due to reasons other than acute or chronic liver disease. This may include increased urea absorption/production, decreased extra-hepatic removal, and reduced participation of liver (**Table 1**).

Processes that increase urea absorption/production are the main conditions that make up the differential diagnosis. These conditions include gastrointestinal bleeding, renal disease, urinary tract infection with a urease-producing organism (e.g.,

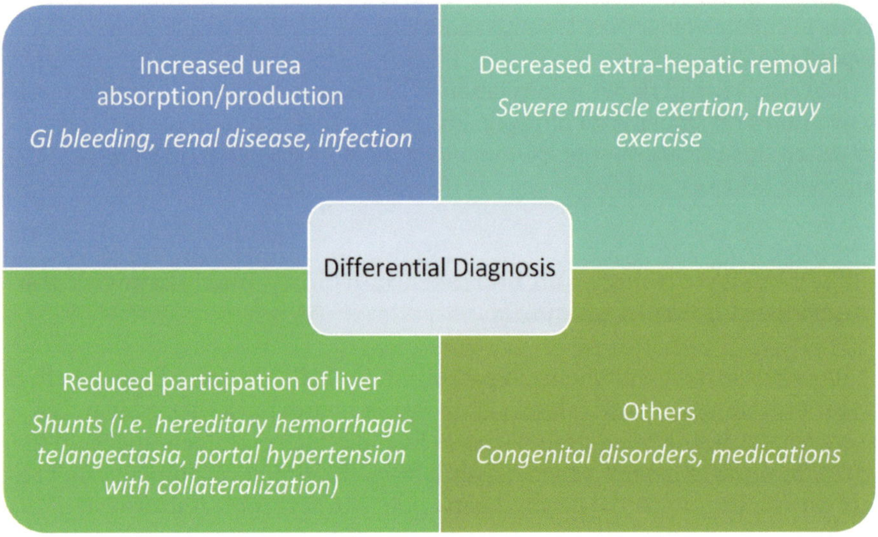

Table 1.
Differential diagnosis for elevated ammonia levels.

Proteus mirabilis), ureterosigmoidostomy, parenteral nutrition, high-dose chemotherapy, and systemic *Mycoplasma hominis* or *Ureasplasma* spp. infection in lung transplant recipients.

Within the conditions that decrease extrahepatic removal of ammonia, diseases affecting the muscles such as severe muscle exertion/heavy exercise are worth noting.

Reduced participation of liver in the removal of ammonia may occur in any cause of portosystemic shunting of blood, such as in hereditary hemorrhagic telangiectasia (Osler-Weber-Rendu disease) and portal hypertension with collateral formation.

Two other groups of conditions are considered controversial in their role in the development of hyperammonemia: congenital disorders (certain inborn errors of metabolism such as urea cycle defects and organic acidemia) and medication induced (valproic acid, barbiturates, narcotics, diuretics, alcohol, and salicylate-Reye syndrome). Some authors classify both as a cause for hyperammonemia while others would englobe in subgroups of liver diseases as they are believed to have similar pathophysiology [19, 20].

7. Overview on treatments

The treatment HE resonates around decreasing ammonia. It can be achieved through three major mechanisms: decreasing ammoniagenic substrates, inhibiting ammonia production, and metabolic removal of ammonia (**Table 2**).

7.1 Decreasing ammoniagenic substrates: enemas

Enemas are the main treatment of this category. These are administered to patients at increased risk of aspiration. Different agents have been used, including

DOI: http://dx.doi.org/10.5772/intechopen.88044

Decreasing ammoniagenic substrates	• Enemas
Inhibiting ammonia production	• Antibiotics • Laxatives • Modification of flora
Metabolic removal of ammonia	• Ornithine-aspartate/Zinc • Sodium Benzoate • Dialysis

Table 2.
Mechanisms used in treatment of hyperammonemia.

tap water, milk/molasses, and lactulose. The efficacy of enema administration has not been evaluated [19].

7.2 Inhibiting ammonia production: antibiotics (neomycin, paromomycin, metronidazole, rifaximin, and vancomycin), laxatives (disaccharides-lactulose/lactitol, polyethylene glycol), and modification of flora (Lactobacillus SF68, acarbose)

The use of laxatives, especially non-absorbable disaccharides, has been the cornerstone of the treatment HE. Oral lactulose or lactitol (the latter is not available in the United States) are thought to have an *in vitro* benefit over other laxatives. This is due their multi-mechanistic properties. Not only do they cause catharsis but they convert ammonia to ammonium and also reduce intestinal pH, thereby reducing ammonia absorption. These agents improve symptoms in patients with acute and chronic encephalopathy when compared with placebo but do not improve psychometric test performance or mortality. Side effects are common and include abdominal cramping, bloating, flatulence, and electrolyte imbalance.

Oral antibiotics have been used with the aim of modifying the intestinal flora and lowering stool pH to enhance the excretion of ammonia. Antibiotics are generally used as second-line agents after lactulose or in patients who are intolerant of non-absorbable disaccharides. Rifaximin given orally in a dose of 550 mg twice daily was approved in 2010 for the treatment of chronic hepatic encephalopathy and reduction in the risk of recurrence of overt encephalopathy in patients with advanced liver disease. The tolerability and side-effect profile of rifaximin are superior to those of lactulose, albeit at greater financial cost. Other antibiotics, including neomycin, paromomycin, metronidazole, and vancomycin, have been studied in small trials and case series, but some may have an increased side effect profile and the effectiveness of others are not well established.

Agents that may modify intestinal flora and modulate the generation or intestinal absorption of ammonia have been evaluated as potential treatments. Acarbose, an intestinal α-glucosidase inhibitor used to treat type 2 diabetes mellitus, inhibits the intestinal absorption of carbohydrates and glucose and results in their enhanced delivery to the colon. As a result, the ratio of saccharolytic to proteolytic bacterial flora is increased and blood ammonia levels are decreased. A randomized controlled double-blind crossover trial has demonstrated that acarbose improves mild hepatic encephalopathy in patients with cirrhosis and adult-onset diabetes mellitus. Similarly, probiotic regimens (such as *Lactobacillus* SF68) have been used to modify intestinal flora and diminish ammonia generation. Several studies have suggested that these agents may be beneficial in humans with mild encephalopathy. A Cochrane Database review in 2011 was unable to conclude that probiotics improve clinically relevant outcomes [19].

7.3 Metabolic removal of ammonia: ornithine-aspartate (ornithine-transcarbamylase/zinc), sodium benzoate (phenylbutyrate, phenylacetate), and dialysis

Sodium benzoate, sodium phenylbutyrate, and sodium phenylacetate, all of which increase ammonia excretion in urine, are approved by the FDA for the treatment of hyperammonemia resulting from urea cycle enzyme defects and may improve HE in patients with cirrhosis. Administration of sodium benzoate, however, results in a high sodium load, and the efficacy of this agent is not clearly established [21].

Administration of zinc, which has been used because zinc deficiency is common in patients with cirrhosis. Furthermore, because it increases the activity of ornithine transcarbamylase, an enzyme in the urea cycle, it may also improve HE; however, clear efficacy has not been established. L-ornithine–l-aspartate (LOLA), a salt of the amino acids ornithine and aspartic acid that activates the urea cycle and enhances ammonia clearance, has been shown in several randomized controlled studies to improve HE compared with lactulose; however, this agent is not available in the United States.

Extracorporeal albumin dialysis using the molecular adsorbent recirculating system (MARS) has resulted in a reduction in blood ammonia levels and improvement in severe encephalopathy in patients with acute-on-chronic liver failure. Further studies are needed to clarify whether albumin dialysis has a role in treatment of HE [19].

7.4 Treatments on the horizon

Fecal microbiota transplant is being studied prospectively in a few centers in North America. As an established treatment in *C. difficile* colitis, this treatment aims to modify the intestinal flora, as it happens with use of antibiotics, such as rifaximin.

Studies are currently underway comparing different formulations of rifaximin, evaluating the difference between the immediate release against the sustained extended release.

Other antibiotics, cheaper and with safer profiles are being studied prospectively to compare with the current gold standard, rifaximin. One such antibiotic notably is nitazoxanide.

Data regarding dialysis as a treatment modality has not been satisfactory in order to justify its regular use in the setting of HE. There are prospective studies evaluating other exchange therapies such as plasmapheresis as viable alternative treatment options especially in the setting of refractory HE.

AST-120, an oral spherical carbonaceous adsorbent approved and used in chronic kidney disease to decrease uremia by decreasing intestinal indole absorption and consequently indoxyl sulfate production [23] has been extrapolated to HE with promising results, but still in initial phases and further studies are needed to better characterize its role in the treatment of HE.

8. Conclusions

Our understanding of the interactive physiology between ammonia and HE has greatly increased since its first proposition by Hippocrates of Kos B.C. and its first description in 1860 by von Frerichs [22]. There are multiple effective treatments available and yet others in the horizon. However, there is still much more to be understood about the role of ammonia in HE and other factors may still be involved in the pathophysiology of portosystemic encephalopathy. The future of HE appears bright and future treatment options will hopefully improve the quality of life of patients with this potentially debilitating disease.

Conflict of interest

The authors declare no conflict of interest.

Appendices and nomenclature

BCAAs	branched-chain amino acids
BC	before Christ
EDTA	ethylenediaminetetraacetic acid
FMT	fecal microbiota transplant
HE	hepatic encephalopathy
HHT	hereditary hemorrhagic telangiectasia
LOLA	l-ornithine–l-aspartate
MARS	molecular adsorbent recirculating system
pNH3	partial pressure of gaseous ammonia
PSE	portosystemic encephalopathy

Author details

Edwin Jin Su Lee and Jonathan C. Huang*
University of Rochester, Rochester, NY, USA

*Address all correspondence to: jonathan_huang@urmc.rochester.edu

IntechOpen

© 2019 The Author(s). Licensee IntechOpen. This chapter is distributed under the terms of the Creative Commons Attribution License (http://creativecommons.org/licenses/by/3.0), which permits unrestricted use, distribution, and reproduction in any medium, provided the original work is properly cited.

References

[1] Dam G, Ott P, Aagaard NK, et al. Branched-chain amino acids and muscle ammonia detoxification in cirrhosis. Metabolic Brain Disease. 2013;**28**: 217-220. DOI: 10.1007/s11011-013-9377-3

[2] Marchesini G, Bianchi G, Merli M, et al. Nutritional supplementation with branched-chain amino acids in advanced cirrhosis: A double-blind, randomized trial. Gastroenterology. 2003;**124**:1792-1801

[3] Muto Y, Sato S, Watanabe A, et al. Effects of oral branchedchain amino acid granules on event-free survival in patients with liver cirrhosis. Clinical Gastroenterology and Hepatology. 2005; **3**:705-713

[4] Braissant O. Current concepts in the pathogenesis of urea cycle disorders. Molecular Genetics and Metabolism. 2010;**100**(Suppl 1):S3. DOI: 10.1016/j.ymgme.2010.02.010

[5] Stahl J. Studies of the blood ammonia in liver disease. Its diagnostic, prognostic, and therapeutic significance. Annals of Internal Medicine. 1963;**58**:1

[6] Kramer L, Tribl B, Gendo A, et al. Partial pressure of ammonia versus ammonia in hepatic encephalopathy. Hepatology. 2000;**31**:30. DOI: 10.1002/hep.510310107

[7] Nikolac N et al. The evidence based practice for optimal sample quality for ammonia measurement. Clinical Biochemistry. 2014;**47**(12):991-995. DOI: 10.1016/j.clinbiochem.2014.05.068

[8] Gifford JL et al. Stabilizing specimens for routine ammonia testing in the clinical laboratory. Clinica Chimica Acta. 2018 Mar;**478**:37-43. DOI: 10.1016/j.cca.2017.12.022

[9] Usmani SS, Cavaliere T, Casatelli J, Harper RG. Plasma ammonia levels in very low birth weight preterm infants. The Journal of Pediatrics. 1993;**123**:797

[10] Ong JP, Aggarwal A, Krieger D, et al. Correlation between ammonia levels and the severity of hepatic encephalopathy. The American Journal of Medicine. 2003;**114**:188

[11] Shalimar et al. Prognostic role of ammonia in patients with cirrhosis. Hepatology. 2019;**70**:982-994. DOI: 10.1002/hep.30534

[12] Vierling JM, Mokhtarani M, Brown RS Jr, Mantry P, Rockey DC, Ghabril M, et al. Fasting blood ammonia predicts risk and frequency of hepatic encephalopathy episodes in patients with cirrhosis. Clinical Gastroenterology and Hepatology. 2016;**14**:903-906

[13] Clemmesen JO, Larsen FS, Kondrup J, Hansen BA, Ott P. Cerebral herniation in patients with acute liver failure is correlated with arterial ammonia concentration. Hepatology. 1999;**29**:648-653

[14] Zieve L, Doizaki WM, Zieve J. Synergism between mercaptans and ammonia or fatty acids in the production of coma: A possible role for mercaptans in the pathogenesis of hepatic coma. The Journal of Laboratory and Clinical Medicine. 1974;**83**:16

[15] Grippon P, Le Poncin Lafitte M, Boschat M, et al. Evidence for the role of ammonia in the intracerebral transfer and metabolism of tryptophan. Hepatology. 1986;**6**:682

[16] Vogels BA, van Steynen B, Maas MA, et al. The effects of ammonia and portal-systemic shunting on brain metabolism, neurotransmission and intracranial hypertension in

hyperammonaemia-induced encephalopathy. Journal of Hepatology. 1997;**26**:387

[17] Görg B, Qvartskhava N, Bidmon HJ, et al. Oxidative stress markers in the brain of patients with cirrhosis and hepatic encephalopathy. Hepatology. 2010;**52**:256

[18] Enns G, Berry S, Berry G, et al. Survival after treatment with phenylacetate and benzoate for urea-cycle disorders. The New England Journal of Medicine. 2007;**356**: 2282-2292

[19] Feldman M, Friedman L, Brandt L. Sleisenger and Fordtran's – Gastrointestinal and Liver Disease. 10th ed. Saunders: Elsevier; 2016. pp. 1577-1580

[20] Lemberg A et al. Reyes's syndrome, encephalopathy, hyperammonemia and acetyl salicylic acid ingestion in a city hospital of Buenos Aires, Argentina. Current Drug Safety. 2009;**4**(1):17-21

[21] Efrati C, Masini A, Merli M, et al. Effect of sodium benzoate on blood ammonia response to oral glutamine challenge in cirrhotic patients: A note of caution. The American Journal of Gastroenterology. 2000;**95**:3574-3578

[22] Wijdicks EF et al. Hepatic encephalopathy. The New England Journal of Medicine. 2016;**375**(17): 1660-1670. DOI: 10.1056/NEJMra1600561

[23] Yamaguchi J et al. Effect of AST-120 in chronic kidney disease treatment: Still a controversy? Nephron. 2017;**135**(3): 201-206. DOI: 10.1159/000453673

Chapter 3

The Neurobiology of Hepatic Encephalopathy

Daniel Simplicio Torres, Jefferson Abrantes and Carlos Eduardo Brandão-Mello

Abstract

Despite significant recent breakthroughs, with rapid discoveries provided by the twentieth century, hepatic encephalopathy remains an ancestral enigma that accompanies the history of mankind. Much of this is due to the reductionist view that a single process would have primacy over others, with the emphasis on hyperammonemic theory being its greatest example. Since other factors, such as the intestinal microbiota composition, the synergism with neuroinflammation, and the role of glutamatergic and GABAergic tonus balance have been discovered, it has become clear that the traditional and linear view of scientific research allows the understanding of the initial state of multiple dysfunctional systems, but is unable to predict the overall behavior of the disease. As consequence, there is a lack of innovative interventions for controlled clinical trials, making its therapeutic management very limited. The objective of this chapter is to provide a general theoretical overview of the most relevant hypotheses and findings in the neurobiology of hepatic encephalopathy, and how its toxic, metabolic and immunological alterations affect the cellular metabolism and neurotransmission dynamics, causing its characteristic cognitive and motor manifestations.

Keywords: cirrhosis, hepatic encephalopathy, cognition, minimal hepatic encephalopathy, motor, neurotransmission

1. Introduction

Since ancient Babylonian times (1894–1595 B.C.), people have been aware of the influence of liver dysfunction on cognition [1]. In the Ancient Orient, the liver was considered the center of life and mental activity. Hippocrates (460–370 B.C.) and Celsus (25 B.C.–50 A.D.) were pioneers in the description of behavioral disorders associated with the hepatic failure. In the *Corpus Hippocraticum*, there is the report of a patient with jaundice who "barked like a dog, could not be contained, and said nothing understandable" [2]. Galenus (129–199 A.D.), physician of the Roman centurions, considered the liver responsible, alongside the heart and the brain, for the triple control of the natural, animal and vital spirits. In his theory, he imagined that these spirits were derived from food processing and routed through the bloodstream to the cerebral ventricles [3]. In the Modern Age, especially in the eighteenth century, several records of neuropsychiatric disorders in cirrhotic patients have been described. It is from that time that Giovanni Battista Morgagni (1682–1771 A.D.) detailed the progressive nature of the disease in the famous *De Sedibus et Causis*

IntechOpen

Morborum Per Anatomen Indagatis (1761). In the Contemporary Age, Friedrich Theodor von Frerichs (1819–1885 A.D.) carried out an extensive documentation of the cognitive and motor changes found in cirrhosis [2]. In the twentieth century, especially since the 1930s, several publications have enumerated the typical alterations in the disorder known as hepatic encephalopathy, with particular emphasis on the hypothesis that its pathophysiology would be caused, in some way, by the reduction of ammonia clearance produced in the gut [4].

The mechanisms of hepatic encephalopathy, however, remain far from being fully elucidated. No significant breakthrough occurred simultaneously in clinical and basic research in the second half of the twentieth century. Indeed, up to the present moment, in the twenty-first century, it seems unlikely that any new paradigm will emerge in a short term. In consequence, there is a lack of innovative interventions for controlled clinical trials, making its therapeutic management very limited [5].

The American and European Associations for the Study of the Liver (AASLD and EASL) define hepatic encephalopathy as "a brain dysfunction caused by liver insufficiency and/or portosystemic shunt" and add that "it manifests as a wide spectrum of neurological or psychiatric abnormalities ranging from subclinical alterations to coma" [6]. Such a definition encompasses the need for detection, quantification, and differentiation of other conditions that affect cognition, regardless of insufficiency and shunt. Unfortunately, little attention has been paid to the importance of the differential diagnosis of secondary causes of cognitive deficits in patients with cirrhosis [5]. In the practice of a reference unit in Brazil, 84% of the studied population had a concomitant condition that justified or aggravated the cognitive dysfunction, such as interferon use, major psychiatric illness (mainly depression), diabetes mellitus, neoplastic disease, use of psychotropic drugs, hypothyroidism, visual impairment, use of illicit drugs, chronic obstructive pulmonary disease, heart failure, HIV seropositivity, and vitamin B12 deficiency [7].

Approximately 30–50% of patients with chronic liver diseases, such as cirrhosis, have minimal hepatic encephalopathy, with decreased information processing speed, attention deficits, and motor incoordination. There is evidence that even minimal cognitive deficits can have a major impact on quality of life, with decreased learning and driving ability, as well as increased caregiver overload [5]. The 2014 Practice Guideline on Hepatic Encephalopathy describes minimal hepatic encephalopathy as a condition in which there are "psychometric or neuropsychological alterations of tests exploring psychomotor speed/executive functions or neurophysiological alterations without clinical evidence of mental change" [6]. This definition has a primary requisite that patients do not present any clinically evident manifestations of cerebral dysfunction in the clinical evaluation. The Guideline Development Group suggests that the operational criterion for the diagnosis of this condition should be "abnormal results of psychometric and neuropsychological tests without any clinical manifestations", although it is clear that there are no universal diagnostic criteria and that, therefore, local testing standards are necessary [8].

To overcome all difficulties related to the understanding of hepatic encephalopathy, it is essential to establish a common language among the several research areas related to the disease. The aim of this chapter is to provide a general theoretical overview of the most relevant hypotheses and findings in the neurobiology of hepatic encephalopathy, in order to contribute to the construction of an integrated approach to the subject.

2. The role of intestinal microbiota and enterocytes

Since the 1930s, ammonia has been known to play an important role in the pathophysiology of hepatic encephalopathy [4]. However, hyperammonemia can be found in patients without hepatic encephalopathy, and normal levels of ammonia can be seen in patients with advanced hepatic encephalopathy [9]. Serum ammonia dosage is also not a good parameter for evaluating the severity of the disease [10]. In addition, studies have demonstrated that hyperammonemia is not a sufficient condition to produce cognitive deficits in minimal hepatic encephalopathy [11].

Ammonia is produced in the body from the metabolism of intermediate amino acids, and its concentration is increased by the action of intestinal bacteria. In adults, approximately 1000 mmol (17 g) of ammonia is produced per day [12]. In cirrhotics, its serum concentration increases two to three times, an increase that is also exacerbated by the induction of glutaminase expression by enterocytes, which hydrolyzes the amino acid glutamine into glutamate and ammonia to obtain energy [9]. At least one haplotype of the glutaminase gene appears to be related to a higher propensity to develop clinically symptomatic encephalopathy, demonstrating that the constitutive activity of this enzyme undergoes genetic variations [13].

The small and large intestines are colonized by a massive variety of microorganisms, collectively known as microbiota. About two-thirds of the gut microbiota is unique to each individual, being composed of more than a thousand species of bacteria, although less than 170 commensals predominate, such as *Bacteroides* and *Firmicutes* [14]. Some studies have shown that the composition of the intestinal microbiota affects the severity of hepatic encephalopathy by modulating its toxicological profile [15].

Recently, the concept of intestinal dysbiosis has been highlighted as a risk factor for the development of hepatic encephalopathy [5]. It refers to changes in bacterial composition, with a decrease in the rate of potentially beneficial autochthons and an increase in the rate of pathogens such as *Staphylococcaceae*, *Enterobacteriaceae*, and *Enterococcaceae* [9]. Such alterations potentiate ammonia synthesis and a proinflammatory systemic environment, contributing to neuroinflammation [14]. One of the major obstacles in assessing the impact of these changes, however, is that the composition of the microbiota varies according to geographic differences, making it practically impossible to compare individuals from different cultures and environments [9].

The use of non-absorbable disaccharides (e.g., lactulose and lactitol) remains the mainstay for the treatment and secondary prevention of hepatic encephalopathy. Although widely known for their laxative properties and their capacity to inhibit glutaminase activity, they have the ability to modify positively the intestinal microbiota, inducing the growth of commensal microorganisms. The 2014 Guideline on hepatic encephalopathy does not recommend its use for the treatment of minimal hepatic encephalopathy, but states that exceptions can be made on a case-by-case basis if there is impairment in driving ability, work performance, or quality of life [16].

3. The role of hepatocytes and endothelial cells

Ammonia reaches the liver through the portal circulation and is purified by periportal hepatocytes, which incorporate it into urea synthesis, or by perivenular hepatocytes, which catalyze the condensation of glutamate and ammonia into glutamine by the action of glutamine synthetase [9]. The ammonia concentration in the portal vein ranges from 300 to 600 μmol, dropping to 20–60 μmol in the hepatic veins [12]. The liver, thus, plays a central role in the regulation of its levels and, in healthy individuals, removes it almost completely: small amounts of escaping ammonia are metabolized in the skeletal muscle (which also expresses glutamine synthetase), and in the kidneys (where more than 70% of it is reabsorbed). In case of hepatic failure and portosystemic shunt, ammonia escapes this detoxification process, increasing its serum concentration [9]. This leads the skeletal muscle to play an important role in its clearance, but this metabolic pathway is not sufficient to eliminate it from the body and there is a loss of muscle mass in about 40–76% of those with cirrhosis [17]. Moreover, it is common for such patients to have concomitant zinc deficiency, an important cofactor for glutamine synthetase, which may aggravate its elimination [9].

In cirrhosis, hepatic gluconeogenesis is impaired. The amino acid precursors of glucose synthesis, such as alanine, threonine, glycine, and aspartate, are increased, whereas peripheral anaerobic glycolysis increases lactate and pyruvate levels [18]. Of particular importance, studies demonstrate that glycine may be an ammoniagenic amino acid, causing increased ammonia synthesis in the gut and brain through induction of a reaction mediated by glycine oxidase [19]. This has been explored as a potential therapeutic target, since the reaction is bi-directional and the removal of glycine can lead to the use of ammonia to replenish its stocks, lowering its levels [20].

On the other hand, the low systemic availability of glucose causes hepatocytes to produce more ketone bodies from fatty acids, for the energetic metabolism of nervous and muscular tissues. However, it is hypothesized that in situations like this, hepatocytes prioritize the production of energy for its own subsistence rather than synthesizing products destined for exportation to other tissues [18]. Thus, ketogenesis would also be impaired, which is corroborated by significantly decreased beta-hydroxybutyrate and acetoacetate levels, resulting in a precarious energy metabolism in the central nervous system in the advanced stages of the disease [18, 21].

Given its location and abundant vascular supply, with immense exposure to antigens absorbed by the intestine, the liver regulates important immune functions [9]. In cirrhosis, intestinal bacterial overgrowth associated with hepatocellular failure triggers a systemic immune reaction, bypassing endotoxins such as membrane lipopolysaccharides, flagellins, and peptidoglycans for arterial circulation [15, 22]. Circulating cytokines, such as tumor necrosis factor alpha (TNFα), interleukin 1b (IL-1b) and interleukin 6, induce the synthesis of nitric oxide and prostanoids in endothelial cells, triggering a state of inflammatory hyperemia that facilitates the uptake of ammonia by the central nervous system [9]. In addition, the proinflammatory cytokines generated by the vascular endothelium activate the cells of the immune system in the brain parenchyma and the microglia, contributing indirectly to neuroinflammation [11].

4. The role of astrocytes

Astrocytes are part of the blood-brain barrier and protect neurons from the toxic effects of ammonia [12]. Its perivascular extensions are rich in aquaporin 4, a protein constituent of water channels. Astrocytes are among the cells with the highest glycolytic activity of the central nervous system and are estimated to be responsible for 30% of its metabolism. They are believed to be particularly susceptible to the development of edema because they are part of the glymphatic system [23], a paravascular system discovered in 2012, which receives continuous influx of periarterial cerebrospinal fluid and has a leakage network through the perivascular spaces into the cerebral veins [24].

Liver failure can result in an uncontrollable rise in ammonia levels, which penetrate virtually all organs. Although the central nervous system is partially protected by the blood-brain barrier, which remains relatively intact until advanced stages of the disease, excessive amounts of ammonia can overtake it [12, 25]. Therefore, concentrations that normally range from 0.2 to 0.3 μmol in normal subjects can reach the mark of 3 to 5 mmol in patients with hepatic encephalopathy [4]. However, along with perivenular hepatocytes and skeletal muscle, astrocytes express glutamine synthetase and have the ability to convert ammonia into glutamine [4, 9].

The accumulation of glutamine in astrocytes, although not directly toxic, drastically affects its functioning [26]. Firstly, glutamine has an osmotic action, inducing predominantly cytotoxic and slightly vasogenic edema [25]. Generally, any form of edema increases the distance for diffusion of oxygen and metabolites in the brain parenchyma, exposing microareas of borderline irrigation to hypoxia [23]. This phenomenon is more pronounced in acute hepatic failure, in which the counterregulatory mechanisms do not have time to act, but can also be detected in the magnetic resonance imaging (MRI) of patients with chronic liver failure [9, 26]. Secondly, exceeding glutamine is transported to the mitochondria, where, by glutaminase action, it is hydrolyzed back into glutamate and ammonia. The passage of the latter to the interior of the mitochondria causes oxidative stress and modifies the internal mitochondrial membrane diffusivity, through the opening of permeability transition pore, causing water accumulation in the mitochondrial matrix, low capacity of oxidative phosphorylation, and low adenosine triphosphate (ATP) production [11, 12]. This results in a vicious cycle of formation of reactive oxygen and nitrogen species (free radicals) with mitochondrial damage [9].

Studies with cultures of astrocytes and neurons show that only the former increase the production of free radicals when exposed to glutamine [12] and that's why astrocytes can be considered the basic morphofunctional unit of hepatic encephalopathy: the histopathological milestone of the disease is the swelling of astrocytes, both in the cytoplasm and in the nucleus, with chromatin marginalization, prominent nucleoli and glycogen accumulation, accompanied by little neuronal alteration [4, 27].

The effects of chronic hyperammonemia and astrocytic edema can be verified in specific sequences of brain MRI. In the spectroscopy of the basal ganglia, the Glx/ creatine ratio is increased and myo-inositol/ creatine and choline/ creatine ratios are decreased [14, 22]. Creatine is a constitutive marker of neurons and astrocytes. The increase of Glx demonstrates the accumulation of glutamine and glutamate [22]. This increase, however, seems to present large interindividual variations, and within a same animal model, there are forms in which there is a gradual increase, a strong increase followed by a plateau or only by a late rise [21]. Choline is a marker for the turnover of membrane phospholipids, and its decrease reflects reduction of basal metabolism of neurons and glial cells [22]. Furthermore, due to the osmotic imbalance generated by the accumulation of glutamine and glutamate, astrocytes export choline and myo-inositol, its main osmolyte, to the extracellular space, which leads to a reduction in the levels of the later, in an attempt to counterbalance the intracellular edema. This mechanism is known as regulatory volume decrease [11, 21, 23]. The diffusion-weighted imaging, in turn, shows interstitial edema resulting from the exportation of osmolytes from the astrocytes into the extracellular space, both in the white and gray matters. Because of that, multiple sites in the brain have an increase in mean diffusivity, including the frontal, temporal, inferior parietal, and insular lobes, as well as the corpus callosum, putamen, thalamus, and pons [22, 27]. The diffusion of water molecules, however, is not free; it reflects interactions with macromolecules, fibers, and membranes. It is important to emphasize that the diffusion-weighted sequences only show changes in the intra- and extracellular volume, and do not allow a definitive conclusion about the total amount of water present in the brain parenchyma [23].

5. The role of microglial cells

The activity of astrocytes and neurons can be modulated by microglia. The microglial cells are innate of the immune system, have phagocytic function and perform active surveillance of the brain parenchyma. In the absence of inflammatory stimuli, they remain quiescent and have an aspect endowed with ramifications (resting phenotype). When an inflammatory stimulus occurs, they become reactive and acquire an ameboid aspect (active phenotype), migrating to the injured site, where they proliferate and produce neurotoxic and neurotrophic factors that control tissue damage and regeneration. In hepatic encephalopathy, molecules such as ammonia, glutamate, and some locally produced neuroactive steroids (neurosteroids) may trigger the transition from the resting phenotype to the active phenotype [11].

Neuroinflammation modulates glutamatergic activity. Studies have shown that microglial activation in the cerebellum of rats exposed to chronic hyperammonemia promotes an increase in the production of proinflammatory cytokines, such as TNFα and IL-1b, in addition to an increase in the expression of TNFα receptors. Of particular importance, TNFα receptors are also expressed on the surface of astrocytes and their stimulation induces increased glutaminase, contributing to the increase of glutamate synthesis [28]. There is also evidence that excess glutamate causes microglial activation, resulting in an intercellular vicious cycle [11].

Another important neurotransmission system affected by neuroinflammation includes a class of peripheral gamma-aminobutyric acid (GABA) receptor, known as translocator protein (TSPO), which is expressed in the outer mitochondrial membrane of neurons. Although poorly present under normal conditions, microglial activation strongly increases its concentration, which can be seen in cirrhotic patients through studies with positron emission tomography and carbon 11-labeled radiotracer that specifically bind to it [11]. It is known that TSPO mediates the synthesis of neurosteroids from cholesterol, and its increased expression provides an important link between neuroinflammation and increased GABAergic activity [12].

Like hyperammonemia, neuroinflammation is not sufficient to produce minimal hepatic encephalopathy: evidence of this is the fact that microglial proliferation can also be found in cirrhosis without encephalopathy, suggesting that it plays a role much more associated with neuroprotection than production of tissue damage [11]. Current knowledge supports the theory that there is the necessity of the coexistence of hyperammonemia and neuroinflammation, interacting synergistically, for the occurrence of neuropsychiatric disorders [10, 26]. In addition, at least one experimental study demonstrates that it is possible to produce cognitive deficits with the combination of these two factors, even in the absence of underlying liver disease [11].

6. The role of neurons

Hepatic encephalopathy has traditionally been assumed to be a metabolic disorder that affects glial cells but maintains the neuronal architecture preserved. However, this belief is easily contradicted by the presence of neuronal loss in its most extreme form: hepatocerebral degeneration. Such disorder is characterized by chronic manifestations (ataxia, dysarthria, apraxia, and parkinsonian symptoms), often associated with repeated and prolonged episodes of hepatic encephalopathy. Its anatomopathological study demonstrates not only astrocytic changes, but also neuronal loss in the basal ganglia, cerebral cortex, and cerebellum [15].

Most patients who develop episodes of hepatic encephalopathy demonstrate some degree of brain injury. Studies have shown that previous episodes of hepatic encephalopathy are risk factors for the development of cognitive impairment, which persists even after hepatic transplantation. In MRI, these findings are related to the fall of N-acetylaspartate in spectroscopy, a marker of neuronal density. This loss may be greater in some brain areas, such as the basal ganglia, which are particularly sensitive to oxidative stress injury, which explains some of its more prominent clinical manifestations, such as movement disorders [15].

It is known that in normal individuals, nitric oxide acts as a retrograde neurotransmitter to the neurons, activating the guanylate cyclase, with consequent increase of the cyclic GMP (cGMP) and decrease of the intracellular influx of chlorine in the glycine receptors. The resulting electrochemical imbalance decreases the threshold of neuronal depolarization, facilitating the generation of action potentials, with subsequent intracellular influx of calcium through ionotropic channels, which amplifies the phosphorylating cascade of the calcium-calmodulin complex, in a process that culminates with learning [29].

Hyperammonemia induces an increased expression of nitric oxide synthase in astrocytes, promoting the formation of excessive amounts of nitric oxide, which diffuses into the extracellular environment. Prolonged hyperexposure of neurons adjacent to nitric oxide depletes the formation of cGMP, but the activity of nitric oxide synthase remains unchanged. The result is a high intraneuronal calcium influx and subsequent activation of NADPH oxidase, leading to the formation of superoxide. Superoxide and nitric oxide then combine to form the free radical peroxynitrite, in another vicious cycle that results in apoptosis [12]. In addition, neuronal ATP depletion is observed because of low nucleotide synthesis and high degradation rate, although its levels do not appear to correlate linearly with the concentration of glutamine and ammonia in the brain parenchyma [21].

Cyclic GMP also plays an important role in the reduction of neuroinflammation and microglial activation. It is known that this reduction is associated with an increase in the concentration of IL-1b and TNFα receptors [28]. The fact that chronic hyperammonemia promotes decreased cGMP production has been explored as a potential target for drug-based experimental treatments that increase the concentration of cGMP by inhibiting its degradation (e.g., sildenafil and zaprinast). One of the major obstacles to this strategy, however, is the fact that cGMP seems to act within narrow concentration limits, above which its accumulation becomes equally counterproductive to neuronal activity [29].

Under normal conditions, glutamine and glutamate synthesized by astrocytes are transferred to neurons, which internalize them via excitatory amino acid transporters 1 and 2 (EEAT1 and EEAT2). In neurons and astrocytes, the storage process of glutamate within presynaptic vesicles depends on the activity of vesicular glutamate transporters (VGLUT), which have three isoforms (VGLUT1–3). The VGLUT3 isoform, expressed mainly by astrocytes, is easier to release glutamate than the VGLUT1 and VGLUT2 isoforms found in neurons, which depend on intracellular calcium variations. That is the reason why astrocytes are more likely to release accumulated vesicular glutamate than neurons [4, 12]. Moreover, glutamate is able to donate amines for the synthesis of serine, a precursor amino acid of glycine, increasing its synthesis and, consequently, of ammonia in the brain parenchyma [19]. Hyperammonemia, on the other hand, reduces the expression of EEAT1 and 2 on the neuronal surface, impairing its capacity of uptake. The result is the extracellular accumulation of glutamate, with consequent hyperactivation of adjacent receptors. This sequence of events seems to be the key in the pathophysiology of hepatic encephalopathy [4, 12].

7. Effects on neural networks

Cognitive functions—attention, executive functions, memory, visuospatial skills, language, and social cognition—are the emerging results of neurotransmission [26]. They depend on the cooperation of multiple cortical areas, connected to each other through the white matter by bundles and fascicles of axonal fibers, in circuits known as neural networks. Changes in the synchronization of the activity of these different regions contribute to the appearance of neurological deficits. This synchronization depends on the integrity of the white matter, which modulates the information processing speed [30].

During the progression of hepatic encephalopathy, the diffusion-weighted imaging on MRI demonstrates cumulative abnormalities in the white matter. In addition to interstitial edema, there may be macroscopic atrophy of the white matter and damage to the microstructural integrity of bundles and fascicles. Studies in patients with cirrhosis have shown that these changes correlate with the incidence of attention deficit, executive dysfunction, and increase in the number of falls [30]. The largest reductions appear to occur in the frontal white matter and in the globus pallidus [27]. In addition, cortical thickness decreases in several regions, such as the lateral superior temporal gyrus and the precuneus, which may also present correlations, respectively, with attention and visuospatial deficits [30].

The final result of the accumulation of toxic, metabolic, cellular, and immunological alterations produced by liver failure and portosystemic shunt is the occurrence of dysfunction in the main axes of neurotransmission [31]. It is important to emphasize, however, that a same system may be involved with more than one cognitive function and that the mechanisms that lead to cognitive impairment are different from those involved in motor impairment [26]. **Table 1** summarizes the main changes found in neurotransmission. The most known repercussions for each neural system will be discussed below.

Neurotransmission changes in hepatic encephalopathy		
Increased synthesis of neurotransmitters at presynaptic terminals	↑ Glutamate	[28]
	↑ Glycine	[19]
	↑ Histamine	[31]
Increased release of neurotransmitters at presynaptic terminals	↑ Glutamate (VGLUT3)	[4]
Decreased reuptake of neurotransmitters at presynaptic terminals	↑ Glutamate (↓ EEAT1 and 2)	[4]
	↑ GABA (reversal of GAT3)	[32]
Increased degradation of neurotransmitters in the synaptic cleft	↑ GABAergic modulatory neurosteroids	[33]
	↓ Acetylcholine (↑ acetylcholinesterase and butyrylcholinesterase)	[34]
	↓ Serotonin (↑ MAO-A)	[35]
Modulation of receptor activity at postsynaptic terminals	↑ GABAergic modulatory neurosteroids	[12, 26]
	↑ Activity of metabotropic and ionotropic glutamatergic receptors (AMPA)	[26]
	↓ Activity of adenosinergic receptors	[36]
Changes in signal transduction cascade at postsynaptic terminals	↑ Intracellular calcium	[12]
	↑ cGMP	[28]
Increased synthesis of retrograde neurotransmitters at postsynaptic terminals	↑ Nitric oxide	[29]

Table 1.
Main alterations found in neurotransmission in hepatic encephalopathy.

8. Effects on the glutamatergic system

Glutamate is the main excitatory neurotransmitter of the central nervous system [31]. Two glutamatergic circuits are particularly important in the pathophysiology of hepatic encephalopathy: (1) an yet unproven hypothetic pathway that would descend from the frontal lobe and (2) the perforant pathway originated in the entorhinal cortex.

It is believed that the frontal descending pathway (**Figure 1**) originates in layer V pyramidal neurons and projects to the centers of other neurotransmitters in the brainstem. There, it performs synapses with dopaminergic neurons of the ventral tegmental area and the substantia nigra, the serotonergic neurons of raphe nuclei and noradrenergic neurons of the locus coeruleus, influencing their activity [37]. If this hypothesis is correct, glutamatergic hyperactivity would act as a final pathway common to the changes induced by hyperammonemia and neuroinflammation, disturbing other neurotransmission systems, in steps that would invoke neuropsychiatric symptoms, and, in more severe cases, cause coma [4]. In addition, the frontal descending pathway would act as a "brake" for the dopaminergic pathway that leaves the ventral tegmental area toward the accumbens nucleus (located between the putamen and the caudate nucleus), influencing its activity through inhibitory GABAergic interneurons in the brainstem. This would result in tonic inhibition of dopamine release, with important consequences for executive and motor functions [37].

The perforant pathway (**Figure 2**) originates in the medial portion of the temporal cortex, called the entorhinal cortex, and projects to the granular cells of the dentate gyrus. The axons of these cells form a pathway of mossy fibers, which goes to the *Cornu Ammonis* (CA) or Ammon's horn, more precisely to the pyramidal cells of the CA3 region. Then, the pyramidal cells emit excitatory collaterals, the Schaffer collaterals, that go to the pyramidal cells of the CA1 region. A brief discharge of high-frequency stimuli in any of these three components of the perforant pathway increases the excitatory postsynaptic potentials in hippocampal neurons, which can last for hours, days, or even weeks. This facilitation is called long-term potentiation and, in addition to the hippocampus, also occurs in the amygdala, striatum (putamen and caudate nucleus), and cerebellar Purkinje cells, being essential for the formation of new traces of memory and learning [29, 32].

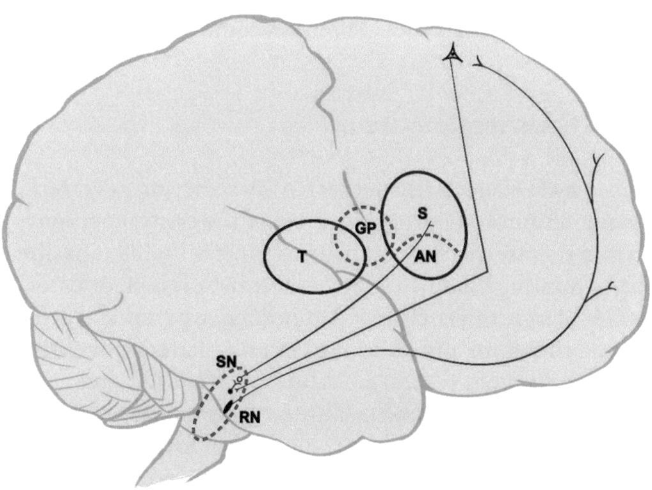

Figure 1.
The frontal descending pathway would originate in the frontal cortex and influence directly or indirectly (through inhibitory interneurons) the activity of the neurotransmitter centers of the brainstem. AN: accumbens nucleus, GP: globus pallidus, RN: raphe nucleus, S: striatum, SN: substantia nigra, and T: thalamus.

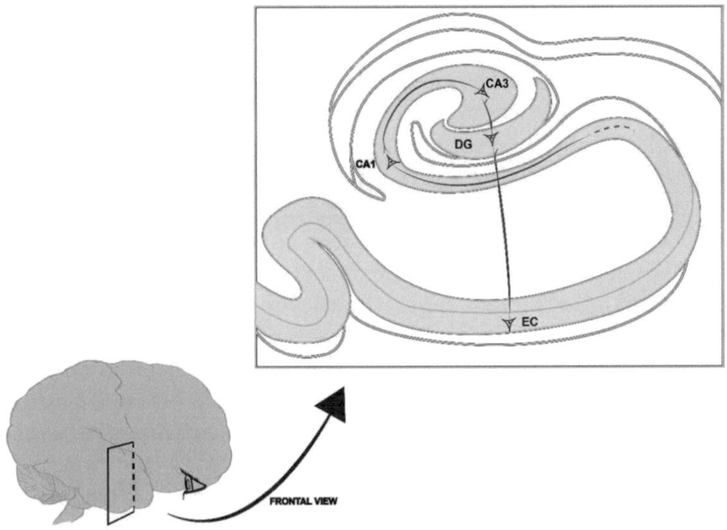

Figure 2.
The perforant pathway originates in the entorhinal cortex (EC) and extends to the dentate gyrus (DG), from which neurons establish synapses with the CA3 and CA1 regions of the hippocampus, being involved with memory formation.

Glutamate receptors are classified as metabotropic (coupled to G protein) and ionotropic (bound to ion channels). There are at least eight subtypes of metabotropic receptors and three classes of ionotropic receptors named according to agonists that selectively bind to them: NMDA (N-methyl-D-aspartate), AMPA (α-hydroxy-5-methyl-4-isoxazolepropionic acid), and kainate [37]. The first two have a particular relevance in hepatic encephalopathy, since the accumulation of glutamate in the synaptic clefts causes its hyperactivation, with excessive calcium influx [12]. This constant opening (tonic) of the ionotropic channels results in greater production of free radicals, with consequent neuronal apoptosis [26, 31]. The development of this process in the perforant pathway is a possible explanation for the episodic memory deficits presented by cirrhotics [12, 32]. Ammonia also induces apoptosis as a result of overproduction of nitric oxide [12], and this could explain why in some individuals such deficits become irreversible.

9. Effects on the GABAergic system

Cortical neurons are also modulated by GABA-secreting neighboring interneurons, the main inhibitory neurotransmitter of the central nervous system [31]. Such cells organize themselves so that they can project their axons directly onto pyramidal cells, inhibiting glutamatergic neurotransmission, or extending their axons to other GABAergic interneurons that influence pyramidal cells, inhibiting the inhibition (and therefore, disinhibiting) of glutamatergic activity.

There are three main types ($GABA_A$, $GABA_B$, and $GABA_C$) and numerous subtypes of GABA receptors. $GABA_A$ and $GABA_C$ receptors are ionic channels sensitive to ligands and are part of a macromolecular complex that forms an inhibitory chlorine channel, whereas $GABA_B$ receptors are members of a different class, bound to protein G (metabotropic receptors). Depending on the composition of their subunits, $GABA_A$ receptors may be sensitive to benzodiazepines [37]. Nonbenzodiazepine-sensitive subtypes are located outside the synapses, capturing not only GABA that diffuses beyond it but also locally released neuroactive steroids as a consequence of microglial activation [31]. Nonbenzodiazepine-sensitive extrasynaptic $GABA_A$ receptors promote tonic inhibition of postsynaptic neurons, as opposed to phasic inhibition induced by benzodiazepine-sensitive $GABA_A$ receptors. In addition, $GABA_A$ receptors bind effectively to other modulators, such as alcohol and neurosteroids, in a different location than GABA agonists, the so-called allosteric sites [37].

Experimental studies have shown that, in chronic hepatic encephalopathy, increased GABAergic tone in the cerebellar cortex results in motor incoordination [28, 32]. Several theories have been proposed throughout the history to explain the elevation of the activity of this neurotransmission pathway: (1) increased GABA synthesis, (2) increased expression of $GABA_A$ receptors in postsynaptic terminals, (3) modulation of $GABA_A$ receptors by neuroactive steroids, and (4) reversion of the action of astrocytic GABA transporters [26, 28]. Most studies, however, show with confidence that: (1) although glutamine is a precursor for GABA, GABA synthesis is not increased in hepatic encephalopathy and (2) $GABA_A$ receptor expression does not change in chronic liver insufficiency [12, 21, 26]. Therefore, hypotheses (3) and (4) regarding the modulation of $GABA_A$ receptors by neurosteroids and reversion of the action of astrocytic transporters are those that require greater considerations.

Experimental studies with acute hepatic failure demonstrate that neurosteroids synthesized locally by microglial cells from cholesterol participate in the modulation of $GABA_A$ receptor activity. Such neuroactive steroids may have an inhibitory effect (e.g., pregnenolone), functioning as positive allosteric modulators of $GABA_A$, or excitatory receptors (e.g., allopregnanolone and tetrahydrodeoxycorticosterone), functioning as negative allosteric modulators of $GABA_A$. It is believed that under the influence of hyperammonemia, both have their synthesis increased, but it is difficult to understand what emerges from the elevation of these two classes of hormones, which have antagonic actions [26]. However, the current body of evidence supports the exploration of $GABA_A$ receptors as potential treatment targets (e.g., pregnenolone sulfate and bicuculline) in chronic hepatic encephalopathy [29].

On the other hand, some of the effects of GABA are terminated by the action of the GABA transporter (GAT), which acts reuptaking it at the presynaptic neuron terminal [37]. Although there is disagreement over the exact location of the four subtypes of GABA transporters (GAT1–4) in pre- and postsynaptic neurons and glial cells, it is clear that a key transporter in hepatic encephalopathy is GAT3 [38]. It is found on the surface of astrocytes and microglial cells, and its action can be reversed both in the presence of chronic hyperammonemia and/or glutamatergic hyperactivity, increasing the availability of GABA in the synaptic cleft and, consequently, the GABAergic tone [28].

10. Effects on the dopaminergic system

The main dopaminergic projections originate predominantly in the neurotransmission centers of the brainstem, especially the ventral tegmental area and substantia nigra. They are modulated by glutamatergic and GABAergic neurons and, among other functions, regulate movements, reward, and cognition [37]. Three dopaminergic circuits are particularly important in the pathophysiology of chronic hepatic encephalopathy: (1) the mesocortical pathway, (2) the striatal-thalamic-cortical pathway, and (3) the nigrostriatal pathway.

The mesocortical pathway (**Figure 3**) originates in the cellular bodies of the ventral tegmental area and extends to the prefrontal cortex, where it regulates executive functions [37]. The latter correspond to a set of abilities that, in an integrated way, allow the individual to direct behaviors to goals, to evaluate the efficiency and

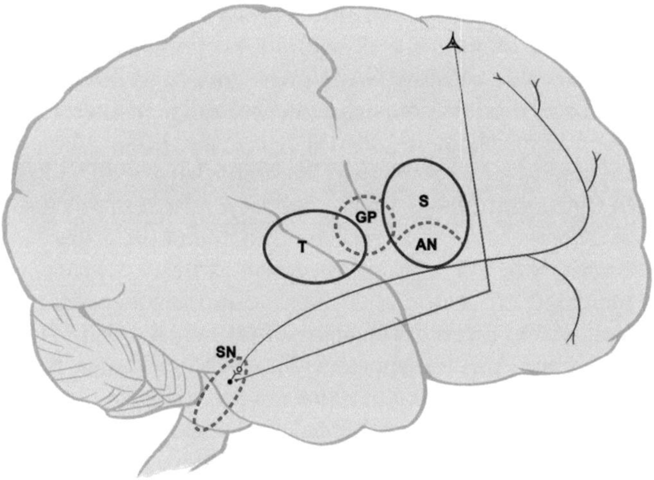

Figure 3.
The mesocortical pathway originates in the dopaminergic neurons in the ventral tegmental area and extends to the prefrontal cortex, where it regulates the executive functions. It is influenced by the activity of the frontal glutamatergic cells through GABAergic inhibitory interneurons. AN: accumbens nucleus, GP: globus pallidus, S: striatum, SN: substantia nigra, and T: thalamus.

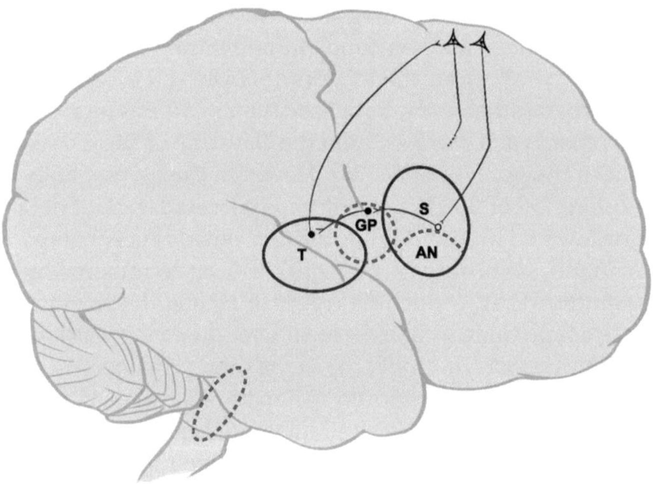

Figure 4.
The striatal-thalamic-cortical pathway originates in the dopaminergic neurons in the accumbens nucleus (AN) and extends to the globus pallidus (GP), where it regulates GABAergic interneurons that inhibit the activity of GABAergic interneurons in the thalamus (T), disinhibiting frontal glutamatergic activity. S: striatum.

adequacy of these behaviors; to abandon ineffective strategies in favor of others more efficient; and, thus, solve immediate, medium, and long-term problems [3]. It is hypothesized that the dopaminergic neurons of the ventral tegmental area are influenced by the glutamatergic neurons of the frontal descending pathway [37]. Moreover, in chronic hepatic encephalopathy, there is an increase in the activity of the enzyme monoamine oxidase B (MAO-B), with increased dopamine degradation, contributing to the development of a dysexecutive syndrome [33].

Experimental research demonstrates that the striatal-thalamic-cortical pathway (**Figure 4**) originates in the nucleus accumbens and projects to the internal globus pallidus, having an important role in the regulation of motor activity. It is believed that it is also influenced by the glutamatergic neurons from the frontal lobes, which would excite inhibitory GABAergic interneurons. This would lead, in physiological circumstances, to a decrease in dopaminergic activity that extends from the accumbens nucleus to the internal globus pallidus, disinhibiting GABAergic interneurons that extend from the internal globus pallidus to the thalamus, where another group of GABAergic interneurons is located, with inhibitory projections to cortical glutamatergic cells. If the circuit is normofunctioning, very little dopamine is released from the accumbens nucleus, increasing the inhibitory activity that the internal globus pallidus exerts on the thalamus and preventing the latter from restricting the release of glutamate by the cortical neurons. The result is an increase in frontal glutamatergic activity, responsible for motor function. In rats submitted to a portosystemic shunt, it is observed that hyperammonemia causes greater activation of glutamatergic metabotropic receptors in the accumbens nucleus, from which results a greater release of glutamate in the frontal region, a mechanism involved in the appearance of mini-asterixis [26]. It is also hypothesized that the portosystemic shunt can promote a cerebral deposition of manganese, which characteristically generates a hypersignal in the globus pallidus in T1-weighted sequence on MRI [9]. Moreover, manganese also has a predilection for deposition in substantia nigra, with a profound toxic action on the dopaminergic neurons, which could induce or aggravate the parkinsonian symptoms of hepatic encephalopathy [10]. Human studies, however, do not demonstrate a correlation between the hyperintensity of the globus pallidus and the severity of motor symptoms [27].

The nigrostriatal pathway (**Figure 5**) extends from the dopaminergic cell bodies of the substantia nigra to the striatum, forming part of the extrapyramidal system. It is modulated by the glutamatergic pathway and the accumbens nucleus, both being connected to it through inhibitory GABAergic interneurons. In rats submitted to a portosystemic shunt, hyperammonemia causes activation of glutamatergic ionotropic AMPA receptors in the accumbens nucleus [26], and neuroinflammation decreases the expression of glutamatergic transporters EEAT1 and VGLUT1, increasing the availability of glutamate in substantia nigra [11]. The result of this glutamatergic hyperactivity is an increase in inhibition of the nigrostriatal pathway [26], whose deficiency in dopaminergic release leads to the onset of parkinsonian symptoms such as stiffness, bradykinesia, and tremor [37]. Interestingly, experimental studies show

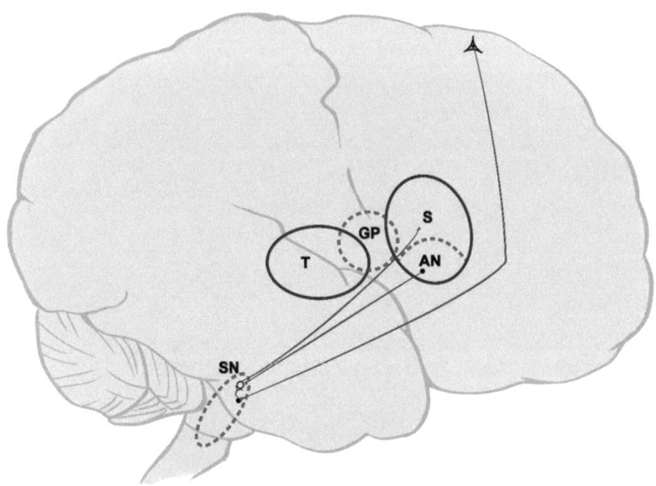

Figure 5.
The nigrostriatal dopaminergic pathway originates from the substantia nigra (SN) and extends to the striatum (S), where it regulates the extrapyramidal system. It is inhibited by GABAergic interneurons in the accumbens nucleus (AN) or brainstem, the latter being modulated by frontal glutamatergic cells. GP: globus pallidus and T: thalamus.

that the activation of glutamatergic metabotropic receptors in the substantia nigra can also cause a decrease in the locomotion of rodents, since the substantia nigra has a second pathway of GABAergic neurons that extends into the thalamus, where a group of GABAergic interneurons inhibit motor cells, resulting in hypokinesia [26].

11. Effects on the cholinergic system

Acetylcholine is a neurotransmitter and modulator that, when bound to nicotinic receptors, favors neuronal excitability, and when bound to muscarinic receptors (mainly of the M2 subtype), inhibits the inhibitory activity triggered by the activation of $GABA_A$ receptors, i.e., disinhibits the postsynaptic terminal [31]. Two cholinergic pathways are particularly important in the pathophysiology of hepatic encephalopathy (**Figure 6**): (1) those originating from the ascending activating reticular system in the brainstem (particularly the laterodorsal tegmental nuclei and pedunculopontine nuclei) and (2) those originating from the basal forebrain, an area that includes the nucleus basalis of Meynert, the medial septal nucleus, and the diagonal band of Broca [37].

The projections of acetylcholine that originate in the ascending reticular activating system extend to the prefrontal cortex, basal forebrain, thalamus, hypothalamus, amygdala, and hippocampus; they are considered to be involved in vigilance (sustained attention) [39]. Cholinergic neurons that originate in the basal forebrain extend to the prefrontal cortex, hippocampus, and amygdala; they are involved with the formation of episodic memory [37].

The effects of acetylcholine are terminated by two enzymes, acetylcholinesterase and butyrylcholinesterase. Both convert acetylcholine to choline, which is then transported back to the presynaptic terminal for further synthesis of this neurotransmitter [37]. Cirrhosis is associated with an increase of approximately 30% in acetylcholinesterase activity in humans, which contributes to a decrease in acetylcholine levels and a consequent potentiation of the effects of GABAergic tonus [34]. Little is known about how chronic hyperammonemia and neuroinflammation induce changes in the cholinergic system [31]. There is no correlation, for example, between serum ammonia levels and acetylcholinesterase activity [34]. However, experimental studies have shown that the increased availability of acetylcholine in

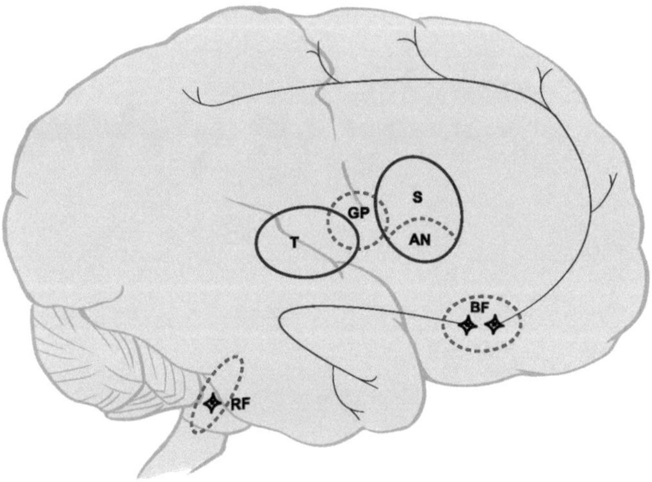

Figure 6.
The cholinergic pathways originate in the basal forebrain (BF) and reticular formation (RF). They extend to the prefrontal cortex and medial portion of the temporal cortex. AN: accumbens nucleus, GP: globus pallidus, S: striatum, and T: thalamus.

the synaptic cleft, either by direct administration or by inhibition of its degradation, is related to the reduction in glutamate neurotoxicity and improvement in the severity of hepatic encephalopathy [31].

12. Effects on the serotonergic system

Serotonin is a neurotransmitter and modulator that favors the excitability of cortical neurons; a decrease in serotonergic tonus potentiates the effects of increased GABAergic tone [31]. Serotonergic neurons have both ascending and descending projections (**Figure 7**). The ascending projections originate in the raphe nuclei in the brainstem and extend to the cerebellum, hypothalamus, thalamus, amygdala, hippocampus, striatum, accumbens nucleus, basal forebrain, and prefrontal cortex [37]. They are related to the regulation of mood, hunger, impulsivity, and circadian rhythm [35]. The descending projections extend to the lower portions of the brainstem and spinal cord, being important for pain regulation [37].

The dysfunction of the serotonergic system has been widely documented in both minimal hepatic encephalopathy and overt hepatic encephalopathy: it underlies several early neuropsychiatric disorders in the disease, such as mood and sleep disorders. Serotonin levels correlate with the severity of cirrhosis and the degree of portosystemic shunt [35]. There is an increase in the circulation of l-tryptophan, the precursor amino acid of this neurotransmitter, in blood and cerebrospinal fluid. It is hypothesized that hyperammonemia not only stimulates serotonin synthesis, but also its degradation by the enzyme monoamine oxidase A (MAO-A), which is shown by the concomitant increase of the main product of its metabolism, 5-hydroxyindoleacetic acid [31, 33, 35].

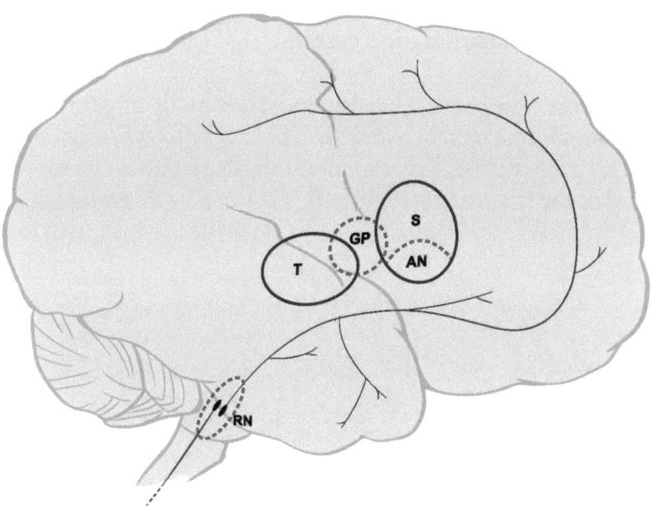

Figure 7.
The ascending serotonergic pathway originates in the raphe nucleus (RN) and extends to the medial portion of the temporal cortex and prefrontal cortex, while the descending pathway modulates the activity of the spinal cord. AN: accumbens nucleus, GP: globus pallidus, S: striatum, and T: thalamus.

13. Effects on the histaminergic system

Histamine acts in conjunction with serotonin to regulate the circadian rhythm [31]. Histaminergic neurons originate in the tuberomammillary nucleus of the hypothalamus and make extensive projection throughout the central nervous system, including the spinal cord (**Figure 8**) [37]. Significant increase in histamine

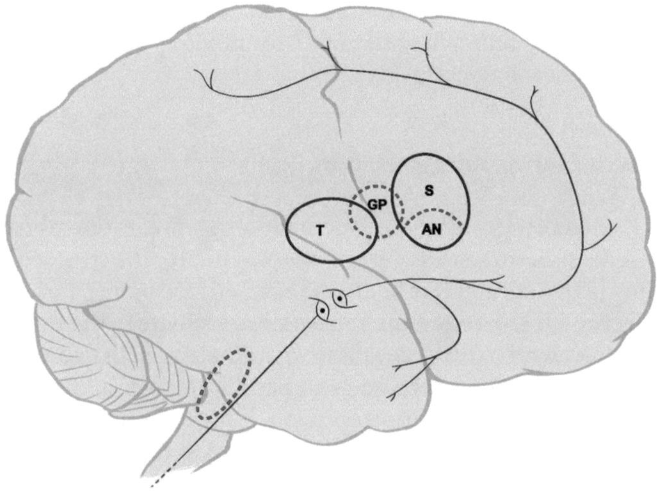

Figure 8.
The ascending histaminergic pathway originates in the hypothalamus and extends to the medial portion of the temporal cortex and prefrontal cortex, while the descending pathway modulates the activity of the spinal cord. AN: accumbens nucleus, GP: globus pallidus, S: striatum, and T: thalamus.

levels have been documented in patients with hepatic encephalopathy [31]. Histamine is produced from the amino acid histidine [37]; hyperammonemia increases both the concentration of histidine and the activity of its membrane transporter into the histaminergic neurons, stimulating the synthesis of histamine [31].

14. Effects on the noradrenergic system

In the 1970s, it was believed that hepatic encephalopathy might reflect a disturbance in catecholaminergic metabolism [31]. The main projections of noradrenaline originate in the locus coeruleus, although there are also some in the laterodorsal tegmental nuclei of the brainstem (**Figure 9**). They can be ascending or descending.

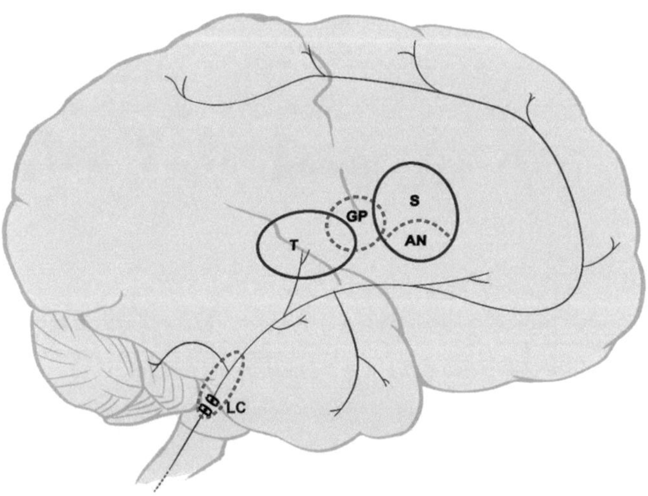

Figure 9.
The ascending noradrenergic pathway originates in the locus coeruleus (LC) and extends to the thalamus (T), medial portion of the temporal cortex, and prefrontal cortex, while the descending pathway modulates the activity of the spinal cord. AN: accumbens nucleus, GP: globus pallidus, and S: striatum.

Ascending projections regulate vigilance and mood: they end diffusely throughout the brain, including many of the same sites for which serotoninergic pathways extend, although there are few noradrenergic extensions to the striatum and accumbens nucleus. The descending projections extend to the spinal cord and regulate pain [37].

Currently, it is widely accepted that changes in catecholaminergic metabolism do not precipitate hepatic coma [31]. Studies have shown that, in patients with cirrhosis, there is no decrease in norepinephrine concentration in most brain regions, with the maintenance of α1 and α2 receptor density. However, it is assumed that more subtle chronic changes may coexist with some neuropsychiatric symptoms, such as depression and anxiety [31, 33].

15. Effects on the adenosinergic system

Adenosine is a modulator of neuronal excitability, which inhibits postsynaptic potentials generated by classical neurotransmitters, such as glutamate, GABA, dopamine, and serotonin. Since 1960s, studies have shown reduced expression of adenosinergic receptors in the striatum and cortex of patients with mild hepatic encephalopathy [31].

Although the mechanisms through which adenosine exerts its function are still not fully understood [36], it is known that the decrease in the expression of its receptors occurs in the early stages of the disease and contributes to an increase in glutamatergic activity, potentializing its excitotoxic effects, while increasing GABAergic tone, also potentializing its inhibitory effects [31].

16. Final Considerations

The twentieth century provided the greatest scope of information on the neurobiology of hepatic encephalopathy throughout history, but failed to create an integrated theory that would allow the adoption of more effective intervention strategies. This was due to the reductionist view that a single process would have primacy over the others, with the emphasis on hyperammonemic theory being its greatest example. As other factors such as the composition of the intestinal microbiota, synergism with neuroinflammation, and the role of glutamatergic and GABAergic tonus balance were discovered, it became clear that this traditional and linear view of scientific research allows the understanding of the initial state of multiple dysfunctional systems, but is not able to predict the overall behavior of the disease. As twenty-first century progresses, it is imperative to incorporate concepts such as convergence, emergency, and complexity into research related to the theme, both in diachronic and synchronic processes, for the construction of a true dynamic and integrated vision that allows more effective therapeutic interventions, in a total hermeneutical cycle.

Author details

Daniel Simplicio Torres[1*], Jefferson Abrantes[2*] and Carlos Eduardo Brandão-Mello[2*]

1 Rio de Janeiro State University (UERJ), RJ, Brazil

2 Federal University of the State of Rio de Janeiro (UNIRIO), RJ, Brazil

*Address all correspondence to: daniel.simplicio@hotmail.com, jeffabrantes@uol.com.br and cedubrandao@gmail.com

IntechOpen

© 2019 The Author(s). Licensee IntechOpen. This chapter is distributed under the terms of the Creative Commons Attribution License (http://creativecommons.org/licenses/by/3.0), which permits unrestricted use, distribution, and reproduction in any medium, provided the original work is properly cited.

References

[1] Osler W. The Evolution of Modern Medicine. Fairford: Echo Library; 2009. pp. 20-26

[2] Dooley JS, Lok A, Burroughs AK, Heathcote J. Sherlock's Diseases of the Liver and Biliary Systems. 12th ed. West Sussex: Wiley-Blackwell; 2011

[3] Fuentes F, Malloy-Diniz LF, Ciancio A, Sacco A. Neuropsicologia: Teoria e Prática. 2nd ed. Porto Alegre: Artmed; 2014

[4] Montana V, Verhrastsky A, Parpura V. Pathological role for exocytotic glutamate release from astrocytes in hepatic encephalopathy. Current Neuropharmacology. 2014;**12**(4):324-333

[5] Amodio P, Montagnese S, Mullen K, Orr JG, Vilstrup H. Where are we going? Translational research in hepatic encephalopathy. Metabolic Brain Disease. 2016;**31**(6):1231-1237

[6] Vilstrup H, Amodio P, Bajaj J, Cordoba J, Ferenci P, Mullen KD, et al. Hepatic encephalopathy in chronic liver disease: 2014 practice guideline by the American Association for the Study of Liver Diseases and the European Association for the Study of the Liver. Hepatology. 2014;**60**(2):715-735

[7] Torres DS, Abrantes J, Brandão-Mello CE. Cognitive assessment of patients with minimal hepatic encephalopathy in Brazil. Metabolic Brain Disease. 2013;**28**(3):473-483

[8] Morgan MY, Amodio P, Cook NA, Jackson CD, Kircheis G, Lauridsen MM, et al. Qualifying and quantifying minimal hepatic encephalopathy. Metabolic Brain Disease. 2016;**31**(6):1217-1229

[9] Patel VC, White H, Stoy S, Bajaj JS, Shawcross DL. Clinical science workshop: Targeting the gut-liver-bain axis. Metabolic Brain Disease. 2016;**31**(6):1327-1337

[10] Butterworth RF. Pathogenesis of hepatic encephalopathy in cirrhosis: The concept of synergism revisited. Metabolic Brain Disease. 2016;**31**(6):1211-1215

[11] Su YY, Yang GF, Lu GM, WU S, Zhang LJ. PET and MRI imaging of neuroinflammation in hepatic encephalopathy. Metabolic Brain Disease. 2015;**30**(1):31-45

[12] Oja SS, Saransaari P, Korpi ER. Neurotoxicity of ammonia. Neurochemical Research. 2017;**42**(3): 713-720

[13] Baker L, Lanz B, Andreola F, Apuero J, Wijeyesekera A, Holmes E, et al. New technologies—New insights into the pathogenesis of hepatic encephalopathy. Metabolic Brain Disease. 2016;**31**(6):1259-1267

[14] Ahluwalia V, Betrapally NS, Hylemon PB, White MB, Gillevet PM, Unser AB, et al. Impaired gut-liver-brain axis in patients with cirrhosis. Scientific Reports. 2016;**6**:26800

[15] Milewski K, Oriua M. What we know: The inflammatory basis of hepatic encephalopathy. Metabolic Brain Disease. 2016;**31**(6):1239-1247

[16] Morgan MY. Current state of knowledge of hepatic encephalopathy (part III): Non-absorbable dissacharides. Metabolic Brain Disease. 2016;**31**(6):1361-1364

[17] Merli M, Iebba V, Giusto M. What is new about diet in hepatic encephalopathy. Metabolic Brain Disease. 2016;**31**(6):1289-1294

[18] Dabos KJ, Parkinson JA, Sadler IH, Plevris JN, Hayes PC. 1H nuclear

magnetic resonance spectroscopy-based metabonomic study in patients with cirrhosis and hepatic encephalopathy. World Journal of Hepatology. 2015;**7**(12):1701-1707

[19] Kristiansen RG, Rose CF, Ytrebo LM. Glycine and hyperammonemia: Potential target for the treatment of hepatic encephalopathy. Metabolic Brain Disease. 2016;**31**(6):1269-1273

[20] Kristiansen RG. Current state of knowledge of hepatic encephalopathy (part I): Newer treatment strategies for hyperammonemia in liver failure. Metabolic Brain Disease. 2016;**31**(6):1357-1358

[21] Rakayova V, Braissant O, Mclin VA, Berset C, Lanz B, Cudalbu C. 1H and 31P magnetic resonance spectroscopy in a rat model of chronic hepatic encephalopathy: In vivo longitudinal measurements of brain energy metabolism. Metabolic Brain Disease. 2016;**31**(6):1303-1314

[22] Yadav SK, Goel A, Saraswat VA, Thomas MA, Wang E, Marincola FM, et al. Evaluation of cognitivity, proinflamatory cytokines, and brain magnetic resonance imaging in minimal hepatic encephalopathy induced by cirrhosis and extrahepatic portal vein obstruction. Journal of Gastroenterology and Hepatology. 2016;**131**(12):1986-1994

[23] Bémeur C, Cudalbu C, Dam G, Thrane AS, Cooper AJL, Rose CF. Brain edema: A valid endpoint for measuring hepatic encephalopathy? Metabolic Brain Disease. 2016;**31**(6):1249-1258

[24] Jessen NA, Munk ASF, Lundgaard I, Nedergaard M. The glymphatic system—A beginner's guide. Neurochemical Research. 2016;**40**(12):2583-2599

[25] Wright G, Swain M, Annane D, Saliba F, Samuel D, Arroyo V, et al. Neuroinflammation in liver disease: Sessional talks from ISHEN. Metabolic Brain Disease. 2016;**31**(6):1339-1354

[26] Cauli O, Rodrigo R, Llansola M, Montoliu C, Monfort P, Piedrafita B, et al. Glutamatergic and GABAergic neurotransmission and neuronal circuits in hepatic encephalopathy. Metabolic Brain Disease. 2009;**24**(1):69-80

[27] Grover VPB, Crossey MME, Fitzpatrick JA, Saxby BK, Shaw R, Waldman AD, et al. Quantitative magnetic resonance imaging in patients with cirrhosis: A cross-sectional study. Metabolic Brain Disease. 2016;**31**(6):1315-1325

[28] Cabrera-Pastor A, Balzano T, Hernández-Rabaza V, Malarguanera M, Llansola M, Felipo V. Increasing extracellular cGMP in cerebellum in vivo reduces neuroinflamation, GABAergic tone and motor in-coordination in hyperammonemic rats. Brain, Behavior, and Immunity. 2018;**69**:386-398

[29] Cabrera-Pastor A, Malarguanera M, Taoro-Gonzales L, Llansola M, Felipo V. Extracellular cGMP modulates learning biphasically by modulating glycine receptors, CAMKII and glutamate-nitric oxide-cGMP pathway. Scientific Reports. 2016;**6**:33124

[30] Montoliu C, Felippo V. Current state of knowledge of hepatic encephalopathy (part II): Changes in brain white matter tracts integrity are associated with cognitive deficits in minimal hepatic encephalopathy. Metabolic Brain Disease. 2016;**31**(6):1359-1360

[31] Palomero-Gallagher N, Zilles K. Neurotransmitter receptor alterations in hepatic encephalopathy: A review. Archives of Biochemistry and Biophysics. 2013;**536**(2):109-121

[32] Hérnandez-Rabaza V, Cabrera-Pastor A, Taoro-González L, Malaguarnera M, Agustí A, Llansola M, et al. Hyperammonemia induces glial

activation, neuroinflammation and alters neurotransmitter receptors in hippocampus, impairing spatial learning: Reversal by sulforaphane. Journal of Neuroinflammation. 2016a;**13**:41-52

[33] Dhanba S, Sandhir R. Role of dopaminergic and serotoninergic neurotransmitters in behavioral alterations observed in rodent model of hepatic encephalopathy. Behavioural Brain Research. 2015;**286**(1):222-235

[34] García-Ayllón MS, Cauli O, Silveyra MX, Rodrigo R, Candela A, Compañ A, et al. Brain cholinergic impairment in liver failure. Brain. 2008;**131**(11):2946-2956

[35] Lozeva-Thomas V. Serotonin brain circuits with a focus on hepatic encephalopathy. Metabolic Brain Disease. 2004;**19**(3-4):413-420

[36] Palomero-Gallagher N, Bidmon HJ, Cremer M, Schleicher G, Kircheis G, Reifenberger G, et al. Neurotransmitter receptor imbalances in motor cortex and basal ganglia in hepatic encephalopathy. Cellular Physiology and Biochemistry. 2009;**24**(3-4):291-306

[37] Stahl SM. Stahl's Essential Psychopharmacology Neuroscientific Basis and Practical Application. 4th ed. New York: Cambridge University Press; 2013

[38] Hérnandez-Rabaza V, Cabrera-Pastor A, Taoro-González L, Gonzalez-Usano A, Agustí A, Balzano T, et al. Neuroinflammation increases GABAergic tone and impairs cognitive and motor function in hyperammonemia by increasing GAT3 membrane expression. Reversal by sulforaphane by promoting M2 polarization of microglia. Journal of Neuroinflammation. 2016b;**13**:83-96

[39] Karczmar AG. Exploring the Vertebrate Central Cholinergic Nervous System. New York: Springer; 2007. pp. 34-36

Chapter 4

Non-alcoholic Fatty Liver Disease and Surgery

Monjur Ahmed

Abstract

There is an epidemic of nonalcoholic fatty liver disease (NAFLD) paralleling the epidemic of obesity and metabolic syndrome. NAFLD is the most common cause of abnormal liver function test and chronic liver disease in the Western world. NAFLD can progress to nonalcoholic steatohepatitis, cirrhosis of the liver, and hepatocellular carcinoma. Most patients with NAFLD die from cardiovascular disease and malignancy. Medical therapy for NAFLD is not very effective at the present time. Treatment of NAFLD starts with weight loss. Bariatric surgery is able to cause significant and sustained weight loss. There are different models of bariatric surgery. Commonly performed ones are Roux-en-Y gastric bypass (RYGB), sleeve gastrectomy, and laparoscopic adjustable gastric banding (LAGB). They can improve steatosis, steatohepatitis, and fibrosis in non-cirrhotic and compensated cirrhotic patients. Each of them has benefits and risks. The bariatric surgical procedures need to be individualized according to the patient's condition.

Keywords: nonalcoholic fatty liver disease, bariatric surgery, role of surgery in NAFLD, liver transplantation and NAFLD

1. Introduction

There is a tremendous rise in the prevalence of nonalcoholic fatty liver disease (NAFLD) throughout the world [1]. About 20% of the world population suffer from NAFLD [2]. NAFLD is the most common cause of chronic liver disease in the developed countries. In the United States, it is the second most common indication of liver transplantation. It affects all age groups and ethnicities [3]. The epidemic of NAFLD parallels the epidemic of obesity and metabolic syndrome in the world. In fact, most (80%) of the patients suffering from NAFLD are overweight [4], and 85% of morbidly obese individuals with body mass index (BMI) >40 have NAFLD [5]. As the disease is related to insulin resistance, 70% of non-insulin-dependent diabetic patients suffer from NAFLD [6]. The disease starts with benign reversible macrovesicular steatosis affecting more than 5% of the hepatocytes. Then it progresses to nonalcoholic steatohepatitis (NASH), steatofibrosis, cirrhosis of the liver, liver failure, and hepatocellular carcinoma [7]. Weight loss, pharmacological intervention, and bariatric surgery are the three main modes of therapy of NAFLD. Weight loss by diet, exercise, and lifestyle modification is the first-line treatment of NAFLD. There are few pharmacologic agents available for the treatment of NAFLD. But as it is difficult to lose weight and maintain targeted body weight by lifestyle modifications, and pharmacological interventions are not that successful, there is a potential role of bariatric surgery in the treatment of NAFLD. In this chapter, we will be discussing the indications and types of bariatric surgery as well as their benefits and risks.

At the present time, bariatric surgery is indicated only for morbidly obese individuals. The American Society for Metabolic and Bariatric Surgery (ASMBS) recommends bariatric surgery for individuals who have BMI of ≥40 or ≥35 plus at least one or more obesity-related complications (type II diabetes mellitus, hypertension, hyperlipidemia, obstructive sleep apnea, nonalcoholic fatty liver disease, gastrointestinal disorders, osteoarthritis, heart disease) and have failed to achieve targeted weight loss despite diet and exercise [8]. The American Association for the Study of Liver Diseases (AASLD) recommends to consider bariatric surgery in otherwise obese individuals with NALFD or NASH.

Bariatric surgery is able to achieve severe (40–71%) weight loss and improve insulin resistance and obesity-related metabolic complications [9]. There are many studies showing the benefits of weight loss in NAFLD following bariatric surgery. But at the present time, there is no large randomized control trial evaluating the effects of bariatric surgery in NAFLD.

Bariatric surgical procedures are classified into three broad categories on the basis of their mechanism of action [10]:

1. Restrictive procedures: The size of the stomach is surgically reduced, and as a result, the food intake is diminished. These procedures include sleeve gastrectomy, laparoscopic adjustable gastric banding (LAGB), and vertical band gastroplasty (not done anymore because of high complication rate and difficulty in maintaining weight loss). In sleeve gastrectomy (**Figure 1**), the gastric fundus and greater curvature of the stomach are resected vertically (>80% of the stomach is removed) making the stomach tubular (like a banana) with less capacity (initial filling volume of <100 ml) and less stretchy with rapid gastric emptying. Feeling of hunger is reduced because of resection of fundus containing ghrelinergic cells [11]. In LAGB (**Figure 2**), an adjustable and inflatable silicone band is placed around the upper stomach dividing the stomach into two compartments: a proximal small gastric pouch (20–30 ml volume) and

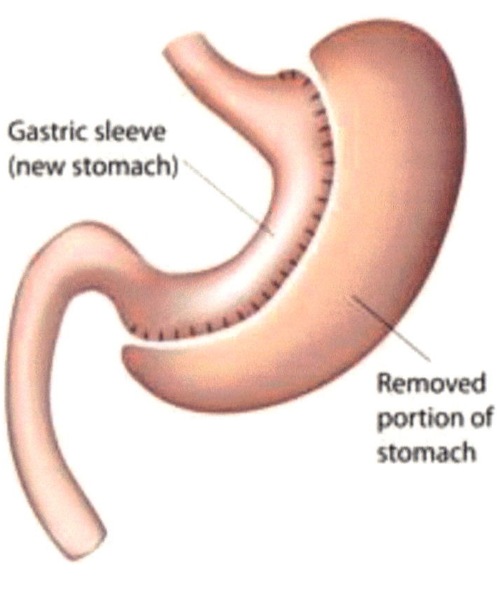

Figure 1.
Sleeve gastrectomy.

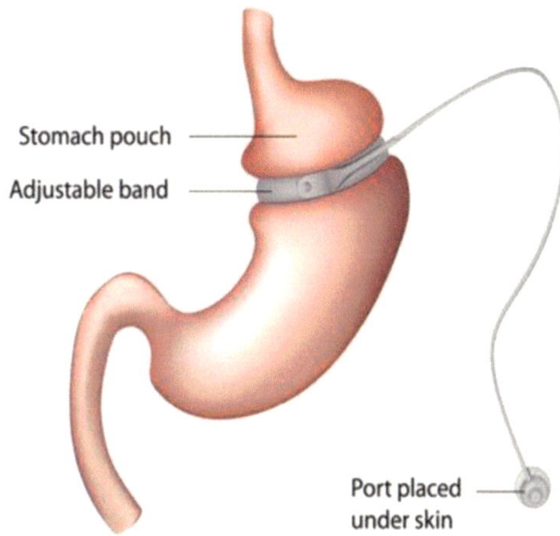

Figure 2.
LAGB.

a distal larger residual stomach. The size of the opening between the gastric pouch and the residual stomach can be adjusted as the band is connected to a subcutaneous infusion port [12].

2. Malabsorptive procedures: A long segment of the small intestine is bypassed, and as a result, the digestive juices digest the food in the distal part of the small intestine, and malabsorption of food occurs. These procedures include biliopancreatic diversion with duodenal switch (**Figure 3**) and biliopancreatic diversion (**Figure 4**).

In biliopancreatic diversion (BPD) with duodenal switch (DS), the stomach size is first reduced by doing a partial sleeve gastrectomy and preserving the pylorus. Then the first part of the duodenum is divided distal to the pylorus. The distal

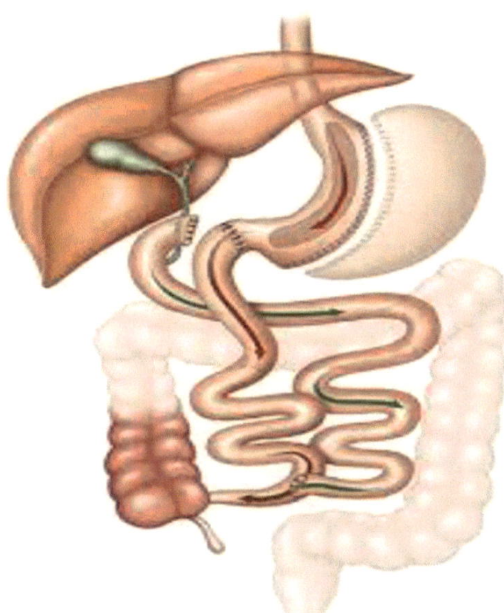

Figure 3.
BPD with duodenal switch.

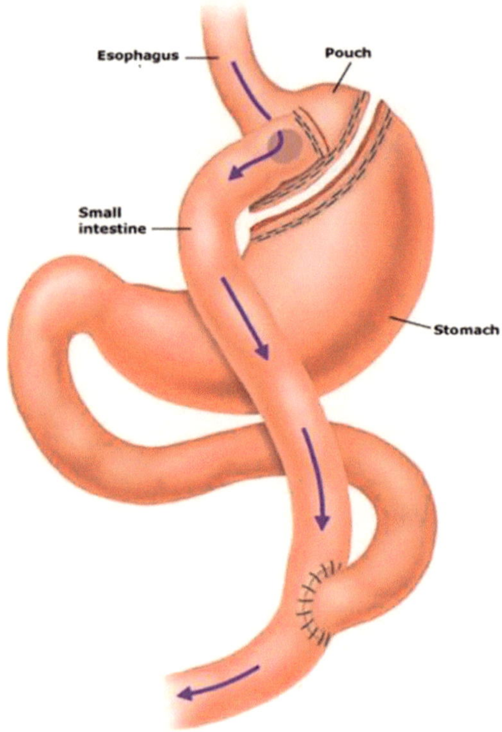

Figure 4.
Biliopancreatic diversion (BPD).

end of the duodenum is closed. The jejunum is then divided 250 cm proximal to the ileocecal valve. The distal end of the jejunum is then anastomosed to the proximal end of the duodenum creating a duodenojejunostomy (duodenal switch). The proximal end of the jejunum is then attached to the ileum 100 cm proximal to the ileocecal valve. As a result, there is restriction of food intake due to gastric sleeve, and most of the small intestine is bypassed leading to malabsorption of nutrients. The biliary pancreatic limb carries biliary and pancreatic secretions into the distal part of the ileum (biliary pancreatic diversion).

In biliopancreatic diversion (BPD), the lower and middle third of the stomach is resected leaving a small gastric pouch. The upper end of the duodenum is closed. The distal jejunum is divided. The distal end of the jejunum is then anastomosed to the gastric pouch. The proximal end of the jejunum is then anastomosed to the distal ileum forming a short common channel in which biliary and pancreatic juices mix with food prior to proceeding into the colon [13].

3. Hybrid procedures: There is combination of restriction of food intake and malabsorption of food. The typical example is Roux-en-Y gastric bypass (RYGB). This procedure divides the upper part of the stomach to create a small gastric pouch with a capacity of 20–30 ml (**Figure 5**). The proximal jejunum is divided 50 cm beyond the ligament of Treitz. The distal jejunal end is then connected to the gastric pouch. The proximal jejunal end of the small bowel is sutured to the jejunum (75–150 cm from the gastric pouch) to form the so-called Roux-en-Y reconstruction. The small gastric pouch (restrictive component) causes early satiety and helps in decreasing food intake. The Roux or alimentary limb (typically 75–150 cm long) extends from the gastric pouch to the

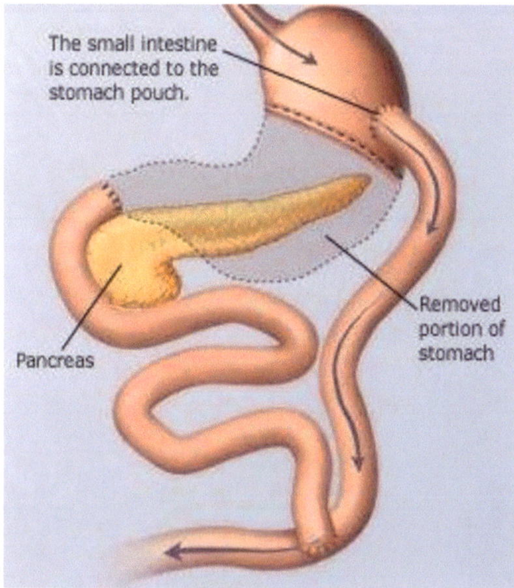

Figure 5.
RYGB.

jejunojejunostomy site and carries ingested food. The proximal biliopancreatic limb (30–60 cm long) containing excluded stomach, duodenum, and proximal jejunum transfers biliary and pancreatic secretions to the jejunojejunostomy site. Most of the digestion and absorption occur in the common channel which extends from the jejunojejunostomy site to the ileocecal valve.

A schematic diagram of different bariatric surgeries is shown below.

2. Benefits and risks of bariatric surgery on NAFLD

Sleeve gastrectomy: Different studies were done to find out the effect of sleeve gastrectomy on NAFLD. Algooneh et al. observed that 56% of total 84 transabdominal ultrasonographically diagnosed NAFLD patients showed complete resolution of hepatic steatosis 3.3 years (average) after isolated sleeve gastrectomy [14]. Karcz et al. found that there was significant reduction (>50%) of transaminases in NASH patients within 6 months of isolated sleeve gastrectomy [15]. Parveen-Raj et al. did a prospective observational trial and found that surgically induced weight loss improved NAFLD histology significantly 6 months after isolated sleeve gastrectomy in morbidly obese patients [16].

LAGB: There have been several studies showing the effects of LAGB on NAFLD. Most of the studies reported improvement of hepatic steatosis, steatohepatitis, and fibrosis, but some studies showed mild increase in fibrosis.

Few LAGB studies with their effects on NAFLD are mentioned in **Table 1**.

Biliopancreatic diversion (BPD) and biliopancreatic diversion with duodenal switch (BPD with DS): Both procedures produce long-term malabsorption and severe weight loss. They are not widely done. Their effects on NAFLD are summarized in two studies in **Table 2**.

In patients with BPD with DS, the transient deterioration of transaminases and steatohepatitis seen in the first 6 months postoperatively was possibly due to rapid weight loss. Transaminases became normalized by 12 months. Then there

Study	Outcome	Sample size	Follow-up
Luyckx et al. [17]	↓ Steatosis ↑ Mild hepatitis	69	27 ± 15 months
Busetto et al. [18]	↓ Steatosis	6	24 weeks
Stratopoulas et al. [19]	↓ Steatosis ↓ Steatohepatitis ↓ Fibrosis	51	17 months
Jaskiewicz et al. [20]	↓ Steatosis ↓ Steatohepatitis	87	41 months
Phillips et al. [21]	↓ Steatosis ↓ Gamma-glutamyl transferase	29	3 months
Dixon et al. [22]	↓ Steatosis ↓ Steatohepatitis ↓ Fibrosis	60	29.5 ± 10 months
Mathurin et al. [23]	↓ Steatosis ↓ Fibrosis	381	60 months

Table 1.
Summary of LAGB studies showing effects on NAFLD.

Study	Type of surgery	Outcome	Sample size	Follow-up
Keshishian et al. [24]	BPD with DS	Transaminases and NASH worsened at 6 months Steatosis and NASH decreased after 6 months	78	36 months
Kral et al. [25]	BPD	Severe fibrosis decreased in 27% and mild fibrosis appeared in 40%: 41 ± 25 months after BPD	104	41 ± 25 months

Table 2.
Summary of effects of BPD and BPD with DS on NAFLD.

Study	Outcome	Sample size	Follow-up
Mottin et al. [26]	↓ Steatosis	90	12 months
Matter et al. [27]	↓ Steatosis ↓ Fibrosis	90	12 months
Clark et al. [28]	↓ Steatosis ↓ Steatohepatitis ↓ Fibrosis	16	305 ± 131 days
Silverman et al. [29]	↓ Steatosis ↓ Fibrosis	91	18.4 months
Lie et al. [30]	↓ Steatosis ↓ Steatohepatitis ↓ Fibrosis	39	18 months
Barker et al. [31]	↓ Steatosis ↓ Steatohepatitis ↓ Fibrosis	19	21.4 months
Klein et al. [32]	↓ Steatosis	7	12 months

Study	Outcome	Sample size	Follow-up
Furuya et al. [33]	↓ Steatosis ↓ Fibrosis	18	24 months
Weiner et al. [34]	↓ Steatosis ↓ Steatohepatitis ↓ Fibrosis	116	18.6 ± 8.3 months
De Almeida et al. [35]	↓ Steatosis ↓ Steatohepatitis ↓ Fibrosis	16	23.5 ± 8.4 months

Table 3.
Summary of effects of RYGB on NAFLD.

was progressive improvement of steatosis and steatohepatitis up to 3 years. In patients who had BPD, the appearance of mild fibrosis was possibly related to severe diarrhea, hypoalbuminemia, some intake of alcohol, and postmenopausal status.

Roux-en-Y gastric bypass (RYGB): Effects of RYGB have been studied extensively in different studies. Most of the studies showed improvement of steatosis, steatohepatitis, and hepatic fibrosis. Summary of some of the RYGB studies are mentioned in **Table 3**.

3. How does bariatric surgery help NAFLD?

1. By achieving weight loss: Weight loss is the key in the treatment of NAFLD [36]. Seven to ten percent of weight loss by lifestyle modification has been shown to improve hepatic steatosis and steatohepatitis [37]. Significant and sustained weight loss is common after bariatric surgery.

2. By improving insulin resistance: Obesity is associated with insulin resistance, i.e., insulin receptors fail to work. How does this happen? Adipose tissue works as a metabolically active endocrine organ and produces proinflammatory cytokines—TNF-α, IL-1, IL-6, IL-8, IL-18, and C-reactive protein [38]. In obesity, excessive production of these cytokines occurs leading to a proinflammatory state which is associated with insulin resistance. Adiponectin is a fat cell hormone produced in the white adipose tissue. It plays an important role in the regulation of glucose and fat metabolism in insulin-sensitive tissues. It increases fatty acid oxidation and decreases de novo synthesis of fatty acid. In diet-induced obesity, the circulating level of adiponectin is paradoxically decreased [39]. Hypoadiponectinemia in obesity is associated with insulin resistance [40]. In obesity, excessive intraperitoneal fat promotes free fatty acid (FFA) reflux directly into the hepatocytes via the portal vein [41]. FFA metabolites (long-chain acyl-CoAs and diacylglycerol) then transfer cytoplasmic protein kinase Cs to the cell membrane. Subsequently, intracellular portions of insulin receptors are phosphorylated by protein kinase C leading to insulin resistance.

As a result of insulin resistance, lipolysis occurs in the adipose tissue with increased levels of plasma FFA and excessive influx of FFA into the hepatocytes. In the hepatocytes, fatty acid oxidation is inhibited, and de novo synthesis of fatty acid occurs leading to triglyceride synthesis and hepatic steatosis.

Bariatric surgery reduces insulin resistance by decreasing production of proinflammatory cytokines and improving the adiponectin level.

3. By improving dyslipidemia: NAFLD is associated with increased levels of serum triglyceride (TG) and low-density lipoprotein (LDL) and decreased level of high-density lipoprotein (HDL). As they are the main risk factors for the development atherosclerosis and coronary artery disease, cardiovascular disease is the main cause of mortality in NAFLD patients [42]. Bariatric surgery significantly improves the dyslipidemic state, and most of the patients do not need anymore lipid-lowering agents [43].

4. By improving the metabolic hormone profile: Gastrointestinal hormones play important roles in the success of weight loss and thus improve manifestations of metabolic syndrome following bariatric surgery. Ghrelin is the hunger hormone (orexigenic) mainly produced in oxyntic glands of gastric fundus [44]. Ghrelin also increases gastrointestinal motility and decreases insulin secretion [45]. In patients with Roux-en-Y gastric bypass, sleeve gastrectomy, and BPD with DS, ghrelin levels are profoundly low, and this may explain loss of hunger sensation and rapid weight loss in these patients [46, 47]. Glucagon-like peptide-1 (GLP-1) is secreted by the L cells in the distal ileum and colon. It promotes glucose-dependent insulin secretion, inhibits glucagon secretion, delays gastric emptying, inhibits gastric acid secretion, and reduces hunger sensation. Peptide tyrosine-tyrosine (PYY) is co-secreted with GLP-1 by the L cells of the distal ileum and colon after ingestion of food. It reduces hunger [48], delays gastric emptying, and decreases gastric acid secretion [49]. Serum levels of GLP-1 and PYY are high in post-RYGB patients because of rapid delivery of nutrients to the distal gut. As a result, the post-RYGB patients experience early satiety, their blood glucose and triglyceride levels decrease, and HDL level increases. The metabolic improvement can be seen as early as 2 days after surgery and do not correlate with the degree of weight loss. Many patients' diabetes mellitus, hypertension, and dyslipidemia either disappear or get under control. The improvement of components of metabolic syndrome has positive effects on NAFLD.

4. Bariatric surgery and cirrhosis of the liver

Bariatric surgery carries an increased risk of morbidity and mortality in patients with cirrhosis of the liver due to NAFLD. Risk assessment should be done by evaluating the severity of liver disease and presence of hepatic reserve. The Child-Turcotte-Pugh (CTP) score and the Model for End-Stage Liver Disease (MELD) score can predict postoperative mortality. The presence of portal hypertension (HVPG >10 mm Hg) indicates worse outcome. Clinically patients may have gastroesophageal varices, ascites, and splenomegaly with thrombocytopenia [50]. Transjugular intrahepatic portosystemic shunt (TIPS) placement is an option for these patients to reduce postoperative complications [51]. There has been no randomized clinical trial of doing bariatric surgery on cirrhotic patients due to NAFLD. Most of the studies were done on unsuspected compensated cirrhotic patients. Brolin et al. published a study in 1998 on unsuspected cirrhotic patients discovered during surgery. Four percent of patients died in the perioperative period, and 8% died late due to liver disease [52]. Mosko et al. reviewed nationwide data collection of patients who had bariatric surgery in the United States between 1998 and 2007 [53]. Non-cirrhotic patients had less mortality and shorter length of hospital stay in comparison with compensated and decompensated cirrhotic patients (mortality 0.3 vs. 0.9 and 16.3%, respectively, and length of stay 3.2 vs. 4.4 and 6.7 days, respectively). The study also found that high-volume centers (performing >100 surgeries per year) had lower mortality rate (0.2 vs. 0.7%; $p < 0.0001$) than low volume centers (performing <50 surgeries per year). Shimizu et al. did a study on 22 Child's A and 1 Child's B cirrhotic patients who underwent laparoscopic RYGB, laparoscopic sleeve gastrectomy, and LAGB between 2004 and 2011. No patient had decompensation of liver disease after surgery [54]. Pestana et al. did a retrospective review on 14 Child's A cirrhotic patients (4 with portal hypertension and 10 without portal hypertension) who had bariatric surgeries (sleeve gastrectomy and gastric bypass) between 2009 and 2011. Significant weight loss with improvement of hepatic steatosis, diabetes mellitus, hypertension, and dyslipidemia occurred. None of them had peri- or postoperative surgical complications or bleeding [55].

From the above studies, it is apparent that bariatric surgeries can be safely performed in high-volume centers with acceptable morbidity and mortality in carefully selected compensated cirrhotic patients. The next question comes: What type of bariatric surgery is suitable for cirrhotic patients? Currently, three types of bariatric surgery are most commonly done. These include laparoscopic RYGB, laparoscopic sleeve gastrectomy, and LAGB. Each type has its own pros and cons which are mentioned in **Table 4**.

Modality of gastric bypass surgery should be individualized according to patients' comorbidities and pros and cons of each type of surgery. Sleeve gastrectomy is becoming more popular. Although bariatric surgery poses significant risks to patients with cirrhosis due to NAFLD, the considerable benefits of significant

Type of surgery	Pros	Cons
Laparoscopic RYGB	Most significant weight loss out of the three procedures	1. Endoscopic access to the excluded stomach is difficult if there is a need to deal with gastroduodenal bleeding, biliary obstruction, pancreatic mass, or cyst when patients may need laparoscopic gastroduodenoscopy [56] or EUS-guided transgastric access for ERCP and EUS/FNA [57, 58] 2. Malabsorption of micronutrients and vitamin may cause progressive liver dysfunction 3. Alteration of anatomy may complicate future liver transplantation
LAGB	Least invasive procedure out of the three	Foreign device implantation may cause infection, particularly in the presence of ascites Currently contraindicated by the FDA to be placed in cirrhosis of the liver [59]
Laparoscopic sleeve gastrectomy	4. Technically less challenging to the surgeon with short operating time 5. Does not cause malabsorption of micronutrients and vitamins 6. No requirement of foreign device implantation	Risk of significant bleeding in patients with gastric varices

EUS, endoscopic ultrasound; ERCP, endoscopic retrograde cholangiopancreatography; FNA, fine needle aspiration.

Table 4.
Pros and cons of different types of bariatric surgery in cirrhosis of the liver.

weight loss (including decreasing the risk of cardiovascular diseases and malignancy) and candidacy for liver transplantation may overweigh the risks. The AASLD guidelines published in January 2018 do not recommend bariatric surgery to patients with cirrhosis of the liver attributed to NAFLD as the type, safety, and efficacy of bariatric surgery are not yet established in this group of patients [60].

5. Bariatric surgery and orthotopic liver transplantation

Some transplant centers have a strict criteria of not performing orthotopic liver transplantation with BMI > 35. Orthotopic liver transplantation in morbidly obese patients is technically difficult and can be associated with increased bleeding, postoperative complications, morbidity, and mortality [61]. The longevity of morbidly obese transplanted patients is also shortened. Pretransplant bariatric surgery is considered in these patients to reach the BMI goal for liver transplantation. Lin et al. did a retrospective study in pretransplant morbidly obese patients and found that laparoscopic sleeve gastrectomy was safe and successful in causing significant weight loss and improving candidacy for liver transplantation [62]. On the other hand, one third of post-liver transplant patients become obese, and some of them become morbidly obese due to increased appetite, increased calorie intake, sedentary lifestyle, and corticosteroid therapy. A proportion of these patients may develop metabolic syndrome and NAFLD in the transplanted liver. Both RYGB and laparoscopic sleeve gastrectomy have been found to be safe and feasible in post-liver transplant morbidly obese patients [63, 64]. Another small study showed combined liver transplantation and sleeve gastrectomy in morbidly obese patients led to effective weight loss and less metabolic complications. There was no mortality or graft loss in those patients [65]. So bariatric surgery has been found to be safe before, during, and after liver transplantation in selected patients in small studies although there is no consensus about the optimal timing yet.

6. Conclusion

With the epidemic of obesity, there will be steep rise in performing bariatric surgery on NAFLD patients. Multiple cohort studies suggest that bariatric surgeries are extremely effective in lowering significant amount of body weight and in improving the metabolic syndrome and histology of NAFLD. Bariatric surgery helps NAFLD in achieving significant and durable weight loss, decreasing insulin resistance, ameliorating dyslipidemia, and improving metabolic hormone profile. As most of the patients with NAFLD die from cardiovascular diseases and malignancy, bariatric surgery should be considered in otherwise obese individuals with NAFLD. The commonly used bariatric surgeries include laparoscopic RYGB, laparoscopic sleeve gastrectomy, and LAGB. According to cohort studies, bariatric surgeries can be performed safely in patients with compensated Child's A cirrhosis attributed to NAFLD. But at the present time, AASLD does not recommend bariatric surgery in patients with cirrhosis attributed to NAFLD because of the lack of randomized controlled trial. Prospective randomized controlled trials are also needed in morbidly obese patients with end-stage liver disease attributed to NAFLD to find out whether performing simultaneous orthotopic liver transplantation and bariatric surgery are safe and effective.

DOI: http://dx.doi.org/10.5772/intechopen.86146

Author details

Monjur Ahmed
Thomas Jefferson University, Philadelphia, PA, USA

*Address all correspondence to: monjur.ahmed@jefferson.edu

IntechOpen

© 2019 The Author(s). Licensee IntechOpen. This chapter is distributed under the terms of the Creative Commons Attribution License (http://creativecommons.org/licenses/by/3.0), which permits unrestricted use, distribution, and reproduction in any medium, provided the original work is properly cited.

References

[1] Sherif ZA, Saeed A, Ghavimi S, Nouraie SM, Laiyemo AO, Brim H, et al. Global epidemiology of nonalcoholic fatty liver disease and perspectives on US minority populations. Digestive Diseases and Sciences. 2016;**61**(5):1214-1225. DOI: 10.1007/s10620-016-4143-0

[2] Sattar N, Forrest E, Preiss D. Non-alcoholic fatty liver disease. British Medical Journal. 2014;**349**:g4596. DOI: 10.1136/bmj.g4596

[3] Adams LA, Angulo P. Treatment of non-alcoholic fatty liver disease. Postgraduate Medical Journal. 2006;**82**(967):315-322. DOI: 10.1136/pgmj.2005.042200

[4] Bellentani S, Tiribelli C. The spectrum of liver disease in the general population: Lesson from the Dionysos study. Journal of Hepatology. 2001;**35**(4):531-537

[5] Fabbrini E, Sullivan S, Klein S. Obesity and nonalcoholic fatty liver disease: Biochemical, metabolic, and clinical implications. Hepatology. 2010;**51**(2):679-689. DOI: 10.1002/hep.23280

[6] Leite NC, Salles GF, Araujo AL, Villela-Nogueira CA, Cardoso CR. Prevalence and associated factors of non-alcoholic fatty liver disease in patients with type-2 diabetes mellitus. Liver International. 2009;**29**(1):113-119. DOI: 10.1111/j.1478-3231.2008.01718.x [Epub Apr 1, 2008]

[7] Goh GB, McCullough AJ. Natural history of nonalcoholic fatty liver disease. Digestive Diseases and Sciences. 2016;**61**(5):1226-1233. DOI: 10.1007/s10620-016-4095-4 [Epub Mar 22, 2016]

[8] Bariatric Surgery Procedures | ASMBS. https://asmbs.org› Treat your Obesity | Patient Learning Center | ASMBS.

[9] Stephen S, Baranova A, Younossi ZM. Nonalcoholic fatty liver disease and bariatric surgery. Expert Review of Gastroenterology & Hepatology. 2012;**6**(2):163-171. DOI: 10.1586/egh.11.97

[10] Runkel N, Colombo-Benkmann M, Hüttl TP, Tigges H, Mann O, Sauerland S. Bariatric surgery. Deutsches Ärzteblatt International. 2011;**108**(20):341-346. DOI: 10.3238/arztebl.2011.0341 [Epub May 20, 2011]

[11] Himpens J, Dapri G, Cadière GB. A prospective randomized study between laparoscopic gastric banding and laparoscopic isolated sleeve gastrectomy: Results after 1 and 3 years. Obesity Surgery. 2006;**16**(11):1450-1456. DOI: 10.1381/096089206778869933

[12] Belachew M, Legrand M, Vincenti VV, Deffechereux T, Jourdan JL, Monami B, et al. Laparoscopic placement of adjustable silicone gastric band in the treatment of morbid obesity: How to do it. Obesity Surgery. 1995;**5**(1):66-70

[13] Biliopancreatic diversion (BPD). Available from: https://medlineplus.gov/ency/imagepages/19499.htm

[14] Algooneh A, Almazeedi S, Al-Sabah S, Ahmed M, Othman F. Non-alcoholic fatty liver disease resolution following sleeve gastrectomy. Surgical Endoscopy. 2016;**30**(5):1983-1987. DOI: 10.1007/s00464-015-4426-0 [Epub Jul 21, 2015]

[15] Karcz WK, Krawczykowski D, Kuesters S, Marjanovic G, Kulemann B, Grobe H, et al. Influence of sleeve gastrectomy on NASH and type 2 diabetes mellitus. Journal of Obesity. 2011;**2011**:765473. DOI: 10.1155/2011/765473 [Epub Dec 26, 2010]

[16] Praveen Raj P, Gomes RM, Kumar S, Senthilnathan P, Karthikeyan P, Shankar A, et al. The effect of surgically induced

weight loss on nonalcoholic fatty liver disease in morbidly obese Indians: "NASHOST" prospective observational trial. Surgical Obesity and Related Diseases. 2015;**11**(6):1315-1322. DOI: 10.1016/j.soard.2015.02.006 [Epub Feb 11, 2015]

[17] Luyckx FH, Desaive C, Thiry A, Dewé W, Scheen AJ, Gielen JE, et al. Liver abnormalities in severely obese subjects: Effect of drastic weight loss after gastroplasty. International Journal of Obesity and Related Metabolic Disorders. 1998;**22**(3):222-226

[18] Busetto L, Tregnaghi A, De Marchi F, Segato G, Foletto M, Sergi G, et al. Liver volume and visceral obesity in women with hepatic steatosis undergoing gastric banding. Obesity Research. 2002;**10**(5):408-411. DOI: 10.1038/oby.2002.56

[19] Stratopoulos C, Papakonstantinou A, Terzis I, Spiliadi C, Dimitriades G, Komesidou V, et al. Changes in liver histology accompanying massive weight loss after gastroplasty for morbid obesity. Obesity Surgery. 2005;**15**(8):1154-1160. DOI: 10.1381/0960892055002239

[20] Jaskiewicz K, Raczynska S, Rzepko R, Sledziński Z. Nonalcoholic fatty liver disease treated by gastroplasty. Digestive Diseases and Sciences. 2006;**51**(1):21-26. DOI: 10.1007/s10620-006-3077-3

[21] Phillips ML, Boase S, Wahlroos S, Dugar M, Kow L, Stahl J, et al. Associates of change in liver fat content in the morbidly obese after laparoscopic gastric banding surgery. Diabetes, Obesity and Metabolism. 2008;**10**(8):661-667 [Epub Oct 17, 2007]. DOI: 10.1111/j.1463-1326.2007.00793.x

[22] Dixon JB, Bhathal PS, O'Brien PE. Weight loss and non-alcoholic fatty liver disease: Falls in gamma-glutamyl transferase concentrations are associated with histologic improvement. Obesity Surgery. 2006;**16**(10):1278-1286. DOI: 10.1381/096089206778663805

[23] Mathurin P, Hollebecque A, Arnalsteen L, Buob D, Leteurtre E, Caiazzo R, et al. Prospective study of the long-term effects of bariatric surgery on liver injury in patients without advanced disease. Gastroenterology. 2009;**137**(2):532-540. DOI: 10.1053/j.gastro.2009.04.052 [Epub May 4, 2009]

[24] Keshishian A, Zahriya K, Willes EB. Duodenal switch has no detrimental effects on hepatic function and improves hepatic steatohepatitis after 6 months. Obesity Surgery. 2005;**15**(10):1418-1423. DOI: 10.1381/096089205774859290

[25] Kral JG, Thung SN, Biron S, Hould FS, Lebel S, Marceau S, et al. Effects of surgical treatment of the metabolic syndrome on liver fibrosis and cirrhosis. Surgery. 2004;**135**(1):48-58. DOI: 10.1016/j.surg.2003.10.003.

[26] Mottin CC, Moretto M, Padoin AV, Kupski C, Swarowsky AM, Glock L, et al. Histological behavior of hepatic steatosis in morbidly obese patients after weight loss induced by bariatric surgery. Obesity Surgery. 2005;**15**(6):788-793. DOI: 10.1381/0960892054222830.

[27] Mattar SG, Velcu LM, Rabinovitz M, Demetris AJ, Krasinskas AM, Barinas-Mitchell E, et al. Surgically-induced weight loss significantly improves nonalcoholic fatty liver disease and the metabolic syndrome. Annals of Surgery. 2005;**242**(4):610-617

[28] Clark JM, Alkhuraishi AR, Solga SF, Alli P, Diehl AM, Magnuson TH. Roux-en-Y gastric bypass improves liver histology in patients with non-alcoholic fatty liver disease. Obesity Surgery. 2005;**13**(7):1180-1186. DOI: 10.1038/oby.2005.140

[29] Silverman EM, Sapala JA, Appelman HD. Regression of hepatic steatosis in morbidly obese persons after gastric bypass. American Journal of Clinical Pathology. 1995;**104**(1):23-31

[30] Liu X, Lazenby AJ, Clements RH, Jhala N, Abrams GA. Resolution of nonalcoholic steatohepatits after gastric bypass surgery. Obesity Surgery. 2007;**17**(4):486-492. DOI: 10.1007/s11695-007-9086-2

[31] Barker KB, Palekar NA, Bowers SP, Goldberg JE, Pulcini JP, Harrison SA. Non-alcoholic steatohepatitis: Effect of Roux-en-Y gastric bypass surgery. The American Journal of Gastroenterology. 2006;**101**(2):368-373. DOI: 10.1111/j.1572 0241.2006.00419.x

[32] Klein S, Mittendorfer B, Eagon JC, Patterson B, Grant L, Feirt N, et al. Gastric bypass surgery improves metabolic and hepatic abnormalities associated with nonalcoholic fatty liver disease. Gastroenterology. 2006;**130**(6):1564-1572. DOI: 10.1053/j.gastro.2006.01.042

[33] Furuya CK Jr, de Oliveira CP, de Mello ES, Faintuch J, Raskovski A, Matsuda M, et al. Effects of bariatric surgery on nonalcoholic fatty liver disease: Preliminary findings after 2 years. Journal of Gastroenterology and Hepatology. 2007;**22**(4):510-514. DOI: 10.1111/j.1440-1746.2007.04833.x

[34] Weiner RA. Surgical treatment of non-alcoholic steatohepatitis and non-alcoholic fatty liver disease. Digestive Diseases. 2010;**28**(1):274-279. DOI: 10.1159/000282102 [Epub May 7, 2010]

[35] de Almeida SR, Rocha PR, Sanches MD, Leite VH, da Silva RA, Diniz MT, et al. Roux-en-Y gastric bypass improves the nonalcoholic steatohepatitis (NASH) of morbid obesity. Obesity Surgery. 2006;**16**(3):270-278

[36] Tilg H, Moschen A. Weight loss: Cornerstone in the treatment of non-alcoholic fatty liver disease. Minerva Gastroenterologica e Dietologica. 2010;**56**:159-167

[37] Promrat K, Kleiner DE, Niemeier HM, Jackvony E, Kearns M, Wands JR, et al. Randomized controlled trial testing the effects of weight loss on nonalcoholic steatohepatitis. Hepatology. 2010;**51**(1):121-129. DOI: 10.1002/hep.23276

[38] Holdstock C, Lind L, Engstrom BE, Ohrvall M, Sundbom M, Larsson A, et al. CRP reduction following gastric bypass surgery is most pronounced in insulin-sensitive subjects. International Journal of Obesity. 2005;**29**(10):1275-1280. DOI: 10.1038/sj.ijo.0803000

[39] Arita Y, Kihara S, Ouchi N, Takahashi M, Maeda K, Miyagawa J, et al. Paradoxical decrease of an adipose-specific protein, adiponectin, in obesity. Biochemical and Biophysical Research Communications. 1999;**257**(1):79-83

[40] Weyer C, Funahashi T, Tanaka S, Hotta K, Matsuzawa Y, Pratley RE, et al. Hypoadiponectinemia in obesity and type 2 diabetes: Close association with insulin resistance and hyperinsulinemia. Journal of Clinical Endocrinology and Metabolism. 2001;**86**(5):1930-1935. DOI: 10.1210/jcem.86.5.7463

[41] Garg A, Misra A. Hepatic steatosis, insulin resistance, and adipose tissue disorders. Journal of Clinical Endocrinology and Metabolism. 2002;**87**:3019-3022. DOI: 10.1210/jcem.87.7.8736

[42] Zhang QQ, Nonalcoholic Fatty LLG. Liver disease: Dyslipidemia, risk for cardiovascular complications, and treatment strategy. Journal of Clinical and Translational Hepatology. 2015;**3**(1):78-84. DOI: 10.14218/JCTH.2014.00037 [Epub Mar 15, 2015]

[43] Jamal M, Wegner R, Heitshusen D, Liao J, Samuel I. Resolution of

hyperlipidemia follows surgical weight loss in patients undergoing Roux-en-Y gastric bypass surgery: A 6-year analysis of data. Surgery for Obesity and Related Diseases. 2011;**7**(4):473-479. DOI: 10.1016/j.soard.2010.08.009 [Epub Aug 26, 2010]

[44] Kojima M, Hosoda H, Date Y, Nakazato M, Matsuo H, Kangawa K. Ghrelin is a growth-hormone-releasing acylated peptide from stomach. Nature. 1999;**402**(6762):656-660. DOI: 10.1038/45230

[45] Beckman LM, Beckman TR, Earthman CP. Changes in gastrointestinal hormones and leptin after Roux-en-Y gastric bypass procedure: A review. Journal of the American Dietetic Association. 2010;**110**(4):571-584. DOI: 10.1016/j.jada.2009.12.023

[46] Lin E, Gletsu N, Fugate K, McClusky D, Gu LH, Zhu JL, et al. The effects of gastric surgery on systemic ghrelin levels in the morbidly obese. Archives of Surgery. 2004;**139**(7):780-784. DOI: 10.1001/archsurg.139.7.780

[47] Pournaras DJ, le Roux CW. Ghrelin and metabolic surgery. International Journal of Peptides. 2010;**2010**:733-743. DOI: 10.1155/2010/217267. pii: 217267 [Epub Jan 27, 2010]

[48] Vincent RP, Ashrafian H, le Roux CW. Mechanisms of disease: The role of gastrointestinal hormones in appetite and obesity. Nature Clinical Practice. Gastroenterology & Hepatology. 2008;**5**(5):268-277. DOI: 10.1038/ncpgasthep1118 [Epub Apr 1, 2008]

[49] le Roux CW, Bloom SR. Peptide YY, appetite and food intake. The Proceedings of the Nutrition Society. 2005;**64**(2):213-216

[50] Goh GB, Schauer PR, McCullough AJ. Considerations for bariatric surgery in patients with cirrhosis. World Journal of Gastroenterology. 2018;**24**(28):3112-3119. DOI: 10.3748/wjg.v24.i28.3112

[51] Kim JJ, Dasika NL, Yu E, Fontana RJ. Cirrhotic patients with a transjugular intrahepatic portosystemic shunt undergoing major extrahepatic surgery. Journal of Clinical Gastroenterology. 2009;**43**(6):574-579. DOI: 10.1097/MCG.0b013e31818738ef

[52] Brolin RE, Bradley LJ, Taliwal RV. Unsuspected cirrhosis discovered during elective obesity operations. Archives of Surgery. 1998;**133**(1):84-88

[53] Mosko JD, Nguyen GC. Increased perioperative mortality following bariatric surgery among patients with cirrhosis. Clinical Gastroenterology and Hepatology. 2011;**9**(10):897-901. DOI: 10.1016/j.cgh.2011.07.007 [Epub Jul 23, 2011]

[54] Shimizu H, Phuong V, Maia M, Kroh M, Chand B, Schauer PR, et al. Bariatric surgery in patients with liver cirrhosis. Surgery for Obesity and Related Diseases. 2013;**9**(1):1-6. DOI: 10.1016/j.soard.2012.07.021 [Epub Sep 11, 2012]

[55] Pestana L, Swain J, Dierkhising R, Kendrick ML, Kamath PS, Watt KD. Bariatric surgery in patients with cirrhosis with and without portal hypertension: A single-center experience. Mayo Clinic Proceedings. 2015;**90**(2):209-215. DOI: 10.1016/j.mayocp.2014.11.012

[56] Issa H, Al-Saif O, Al-Momen S, Bseiso B, Al-Salem A. Bleeding duodenal ulcer after Roux-en-Y gastric bypass surgery: The value of laparoscopic gastroduodenoscopy. Annals of Saudi Medicine. 2010;**30**(1):67-69. DOI: 10.4103/0256-4947.59382

[57] Tyberg A, Nieto J, Salgado S, Weaver K, Kedia P, Sharaiha RZ, et al. Endoscopic ultrasound (EUS)-directed transgastric endoscopic retrograde cholangiopancreatography or EUS:

Mid-term analysis of an emerging procedure. Clinical Endoscopy. 2017;**50**(2):185-190. DOI: 10.5946/ce.2016.030 [Epub Sep 19, 2016]

[58] Sica M, Mutignani M, Alberto T, Manta R. Endoscopic ultrasound-guided drainage of pancreatic pseudocyst after gastrogastric anastomosis in patient with Roux-en-Y gastric bypass: The dream becomes reality! Endoscopic Ultrasound. 2017;**6**(3):215-216. DOI: 10.4103/2303-9027.208176

[59] Food and Drug Administration. 2012. Available from: http://www.accessdata.fda.gov/cdrh_docs/pdf7/P070009b.pdf

[60] Chalasani N, Younossi Z, Lavine JE, Charlton M, Cusi K, Rinella M, et al. Sanyal AJ the diagnosis and management of nonalcoholic fatty liver disease: Practice guidance from the American Association for the Study of Liver Diseases. Hepatology. 2018;**67**(1):328-357. DOI: 10.1002/hep.29367 [Epub Sep 29, 2017]

[61] Pajecki D, Cesconetto DM, Macacari R, Joaquim H, Andraus W, de Cleva R, et al. Bariatric surgery (sleeve gastrectomy) after liver transplantation: Case report. Arquivos Brasileiros de Cirurgia Digestiva. 2014;**27**(Suppl 1):81-83

[62] Lin MY, Tavakol MM, Sarin A, Amirkiai SM, Rogers SJ, Carter JT, et al. Laparoscopic sleeve gastrectomy is safe and efficacious for pretransplant candidates. Surgery for Obesity and Related Diseases. 2013;**9**(5):653-658. DOI: 10.1016/j.soard.2013.02.013 [Epub Mar 21, 2013]

[63] Duchini A, Brunson ME. Roux-en-Y gastric bypass for recurrent nonalcoholic steatohepatitis in liver transplant recipients with morbid obesity. Transplantation. 2001;**72**(1):156-159

[64] Tichansky DS, Madan AK. Laparoscopic Roux-en-Y gastric bypass is safe and feasible after orthotopic liver transplantation. Obesity Surgery. 2005;**15**(10):1481-1486. DOI: 10.1381/096089205774859164

[65] Heimbach JK, Watt KD, Poterucha JJ, Ziller NF, Cecco SD, Charlton MR, et al. Combined liver transplantation and gastric sleeve resection for patients with medically complicated obesity and end-stage liver disease. American Journal of Transplantation. 2013;**13**(2):363-368. DOI: 10.1111/j.1600-6143.2012.04318.x [Epub Nov 8, 2012]

Chapter 5

HCC in Cirrhotic and Non-cirrhotic Liver: Timing to Surgery and Outcome - State of the Art

Stefania Brozzetti, Simone Bini, Chiara D'Alterio, Chiara De Lucia, Leonardo Luca Chiarella, Katia Fazzi and Michele Di Martino

Abstract

In this chapter we aim at presenting the state of the art in liver surgery. After a brief introduction about natural evolution of hepatocellular carcinoma (HCC) either in cirrhotic or non-cirrhotic patients, this manuscript will focus on planning and timing surgery: CT evaluation of the remnant liver; biopsy and ultrasonography (US) evaluation of liver disease; intraoperative US; surgical techniques, such as major and limited hepatectomies and two-stage hepatectomies, each of them in open or mini-invasive approach; and their possible complications. Follow-up and further interventions during expected recurrences will be highlighted. Our chapter will also treat topics such as patient's quality of life, importance of multidisciplinary evaluation and the role of surgeon in it.

Keywords: HCC, liver cirrhosis, liver surgery, open surgery, laparoscopic liver surgery, robotic liver surgery, HCC management, HCC follow up, staged hepatectomy, ALPSS

1. Introduction

Hepatocellular carcinoma (HCC) accounts for about 75–85% of primary liver malignancy. Being the most common histotype of liver cancer, it contributes significantly to global disease and mortality. Liver cancer ranks sixth for worldwide incidence and third for worldwide mortality. In Europe it ranks 14th for incidence and 8th for mortality [1]. In cirrhotic patients it remains one of the major causes of death [2, 3].

HCC incidence is worldwide heterogeneous because of the distribution of its main risk factors: hepatitis B, hepatitis C, alcoholic hepatitis, non-alcoholic fatty liver disease (NAFLD) and steatohepatitis (NASH) (**Table 1**) [4] chronic liver disease is the main background in which HCC arises (70–90% of all patients) [2]. It usually develops in cirrhotic liver, even if 10–20% of cases involve patients not yet cirrhotic [3]. These ones tend to receive a late diagnosis, due to the lack of symptomatology in early stage and/or inadequate surveillance [3].

IntechOpen

Parameter	Mean incidence in cirrhotic liver	Mean incidence in non-cirrhotic liver
HBV	41.65%	30.60%
HCV	44.18%	14.36%
Alcoholic hepatitis	30%	21.77%
NAFLD-NASH	6.48% from a single study	6.45% from a single study

Desai et al. [3].

Table 1.
HCC incidence in cirrhotic and non-cirrhotic patients per risk factor.

Clinical evaluation and multidisciplinary approach are fundamental to submit patients to the most appropriate treatment. Assessment must consider patients' characteristics (general conditions, performance status, physiological age, life expectancy, treatment tolerability), HCC stage, oncological principles and liver status [4].

Several approaches, both surgical and non-surgical, are available for HCC treatment. Surgery is the first-line treatment in terms of overall survival and disease-free survival [5].

Surgical approaches include liver resections (LRs) and liver transplantation (LT).

LR is the gold standard in non-cirrhotic liver, whereas cirrhotic patients should be properly selected because of higher risk of complications [5].

LT allows radical tumor removal (R0) combined with the cure of underlying liver disease [6]. It is the treatment of choice in patients unsuitable for resective surgery that fall within the Milan criteria [5]. LT is indicated in patients ≤65 years (extended to 70 and 70+ patients, in some cases) [7] with severe cirrhosis (MELD > 15). According to the Milan criteria, patients should have a single nodule ≤5 cm or up to three nodules measuring ≤3 cm [8, 9], with no macroscopic vascular invasion nor extrahepatic metastases [5, 9]. After some years of experience, the Milan criteria were extended, developing up-to-seven criteria, in which patients are considered eligible for liver transplant when the sum of the size (in cm) of the largest tumor and the number of lesions is ≤7, in the absence of microscopic vascular invasion [10]. Up-to-seven criteria should be used carefully because overall survival decreases as the number and size of tumor grows [11]. This principle is called "Metro ticket" [12]. Because of organs' low availability, lower recurrence risk patients shall be selected for transplantation in order to optimize organ allocation [12]. Resection and noninvasive therapies could be performed to control lesion progression during waiting period (bridging) or in order to downstage HCC [5, 6]. Liver function in waiting list is commonly evaluated through Child-Pugh (CTP), MELD and MELD-Na scores [13]. The latter is a good predictor of waitlist mortality in cirrhotic patients, so it shall be taken into account to improve organ allocation system [14]. Pretransplant mortality rate in liver malignancy accounts for about 10 deaths per 100 patient years of waiting [15].

Non-surgical approaches include percutaneous radiofrequency thermoablation (RFA), microwave thermoablation (MWA), drug-eluting bead transarterial chemoembolization (DEB-TACE), transarterial radioembolization (TARE), percutaneous ethanol injection (PEI), cryoablation and laser ablation (LA). Except from thermoablations, which are considered curative in small lesion (≤2 cm), non-surgical approaches are commonly palliative [16]. Elderly, very elderly and frail patients, either at presentation or in the case of recurrences, may benefit from these techniques in terms of survival and quality of life [4].

RFA and MWA are the most appropriate treatment in patients with BCLC 0 and A tumors not eligible for surgery [5, 17]. RFA induces coagulative necrosis in tumor cells and in a "safety ring" of peritumoural tissue using frictional heat generated by high-frequency alternating current. Lesions adjacent to the vessels and biliary tree or in subcapsular positions could compromise RFA effectiveness and safety [5, 18, 19]. However, microwave ablation has been recognized as effective in this kind of lesions, due to damage concentration and less heat dispersion [17, 20]. MWA uses electromagnetic energy to induce a larger necrotic area than RFA thanks to faster heating and higher temperature [17]. Overall, RFA and MWA provide similar results in terms of local control and survival rates [17].

DEB-TACE induces tumor necrosis through intraarterial delivery of microspheres fulfilled with chemotherapic drug that may vary in size and chemotherapic agent to treat different types of HCC [21]. This technique profits from the presence of a singular artery feeding the tumor. TACE is a palliative treatment indicated in patients not eligible for surgery or percutaneous ablation, with tumor at stage BCLC B (Child-Pugh ≤ B8; PS < 2). HCC nodule >10 cm, macroscopic vascular invasion, extrahepatic disease, untreatable ascites, jaundice and kidney disfunction strongly contraindicate TACE [4, 5]. Potential adverse effects are liver enzyme abnormalities (18.1%), fever (17.2%), hematological/bone marrow toxicity (13.5%), pain (11%), vomiting (6%) and even death (0.6%) for liver failure [5].

RFA can be used as a complementary technique with TACE, to treat residual neoplastic tissue [22]. Patients with bigger nodules (>3 cm) and with capillary vascularization receive higher benefit from this combination [5, 23].

TARE is also called selective internal radiation therapy (SIRT). It is a palliative brachytherapy that uses radioactive substances (Y^{90}-microspheres) injected into tumor-feeding arteries. This complex procedure is indicated in patients with conserved liver function (Child-Pugh ≤ 8, bilirubin ≤ 2.0 mg/dl, no ascites) and locally advanced HCC, not eligible for surgery or TACE (portal system invasion or unencapsulated large lesions). Pulmonary shunt and other vascular anomalies contraindicate to this technique [4, 5].

PEI induces tumor cell necrosis through dehydration, protein denaturation and small tumor vessel disruption. It is indicated in patients not eligible neither for resection nor for other forms of ablation, especially in HCC nodules ≤3 cm in the hepatic hilum area. The application of this procedure is restricted because it allows only an incomplete necrosis in lesions >3 cm and leads to high recurrence rate [5, 24].

Cryoablation induces tumor cell necrosis using recurring applications of freezing temperature. Despite its good efficacy, this procedure is barely used because it is associated with high risk of life-threatening complications such as cryoshock, cold injury to adjacent organs and massive bleeding [25].

LA induces tissue necrosis through conversion of absorbed light (usually infrared) into heat. It can be used to treat up to five lesions, measuring ≤5 cm, located in the deep parenchyma and distant from the vessels, biliary ducts, bowel or diaphragm, when patients are not eligible for resection [26]. It is rarely used because of difficulties in the technique's management [5].

Surgical and non-surgical treatments, and the possibility of combined approach, should be carefully evaluated aiming for a tailored therapy.

Follow-up is fundamental in HCC patients, both in cirrhotic and non-cirrhotic ones, in order to promptly identify possible recurrences and to treat them in the best way. Intrahepatic recurrences, far from previously treated lesions, are always possible and generated by chronic hepatopathy; therefore, lifelong surveillance is necessary [4, 27].

The aim of this chapter is to illustrate the state of the art in liver surgery to achieve the best treatment for patients suffering from hepatocellular carcinoma.

2. Planning and timing surgery

2.1 Multidisciplinary evaluation

The multidisciplinary unit is a highly specialized and dedicated team, composed of hepatobiliary and transplants surgeons, hepatologists, radiologists, pathologists, oncologists, interventional radiologists and supportive care specialists (**Figure 1**) [28]. The aim of the unit is to discuss complex patients, developing the best possible care plan for every different case. First of all, liver status and disease shall always be evaluated and taken into account, assessing them according to Child-Pugh (CTP), MELD or MELD-Na scores [5, 14, 29]. CTP score seems to have a higher specificity than MELD in patients undergoing resective surgery (**Table 2**) [13]. Other important factors are preoperative platelet count, INR and hepatic venous pressure gradient (HVPG) [5, 30]. Cirrhotic patients eligible for hepatic resection should have ideally HPVG < 10 mmHg and platelet count ≥100,000/ml [5].

In addition to Child-Pugh and MELD scores, in borderline liver function, indocyanine green kinetics and cholinesterase/bilirubin ratio are useful to improve patients selection [5].

Thanks to multidisciplinary discussions in international meetings, many HCC staging systems have been proposed during the years [31]. The Cancer of the Liver Italian Program (CLIP) score and Barcelona Clinic Liver Cancer (BCLC) staging classification are the most comprehensive and commonly used systems to stage HCC patients. They consider the liver status and function, physical status, cancer-related symptoms and number and extension of lesions. Patients are classified in six stages (CLIP score) or five stages (BCLC), each linked with a specific survival rate and treatment algorithm (**Table 3**, **Figure 2**) [32].

According to BCLC criteria, liver resection is indicated in BCLC stage A patients only, but several studies show that it could provide long-term survival with reduced intraoperative mortality in selected BCLC stage B patients (**Figure 3**) [33–36]. Patients having singular large nodule (>5 cm) and/or lateralized multinodular tumor and a very well-preserved liver function are considered

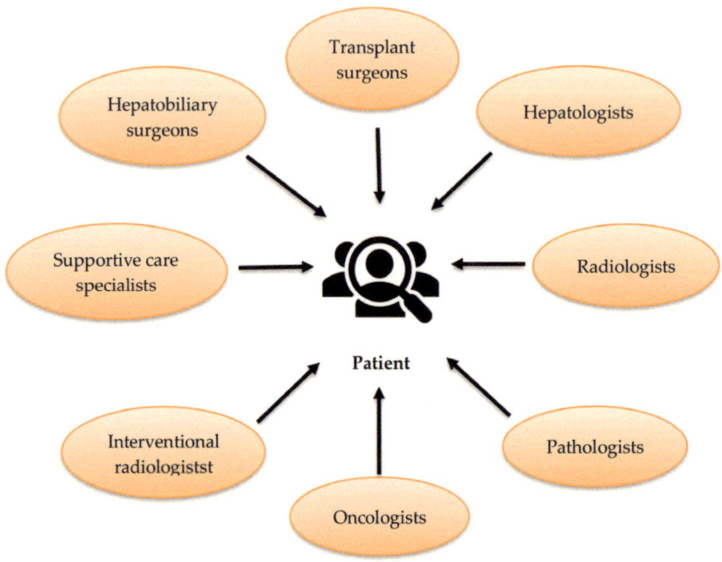

Figure 1.
Composition of liver multidisciplinary units. Source: Siddique et al. [28].

Child-Pugh score Parameters	**Points**		
	1	**2**	**3**
Serum bilirubin (mg/dl)	2.0	2-3	>3.0
Serum albumin (g/dl)	>3.5	2.8-3.5	<2.8
Prothrombin time Seconds prolonged	1-4	4-6	>6
Hepatic encephalopathy	None	Mild to moderate (grade1 or 2)	Severe (grade 3 or 4)
Ascites	None	Mild to moderate (diuretic responsive)	Severe (grade 3 or 4)
5–6 points Child-Pugh A 7–9 points Child-Pugh B 10–15 points Child-Pugh C			

Table 2.
Child-Pugh scoring system.

resectable stage B patients [38]. In order to achieve a parenchyma-sparing surgery, these patients may benefit from combining surgery with intraoperative ablation (RF/MW) [39, 40].

2.2 US evaluation of liver disease

Ultrasonography (US) has a primary role in HCC screening. US sensitivity ranges from 63 (for small lesions) to 94%, whereas specificity from 52 to 98% [41–43].

US is highly operator-dependent. Machine quality, tumor size and localization, liver echotexture and abdomen characteristic influence the diagnostic accuracy of the exam [44].

Six-month US is relevant in detecting early-stage HCC in high-risk patients [45]. US detection of small HCC nodules in cirrhotic livers is arduous due to altered echotexture [46].

If combined with serum marker alpha-fetoprotein (AFP), it allows further unidentified lesions' detection in 6–8% of the cases [47]. AFP alone is a weak screening test (Se 39–64%, Sp 76–91%, cut-off 20 mg/ml) [41], since high AFP levels could be also related to inflammatory status (exacerbation of underlying chronic liver disease or hepatitis), and it is not increased in about 20% of HCC

CLIP score Parameters	**Points**		
	0	**1**	**2**
Tumor morphology	Uninodular and extension ≤ 50%	Multinodular and extension ≤ 50%	Massive or extension > 50%
Child-Pugh score	A	B	C
Alpha-fetoprotein	<400 ng/ml	≥400 ng/ml	—
Portal vein thrombosis	Absent	Present	—
Maida et al. [31].			

Table 3.
CLIP score evaluation system.

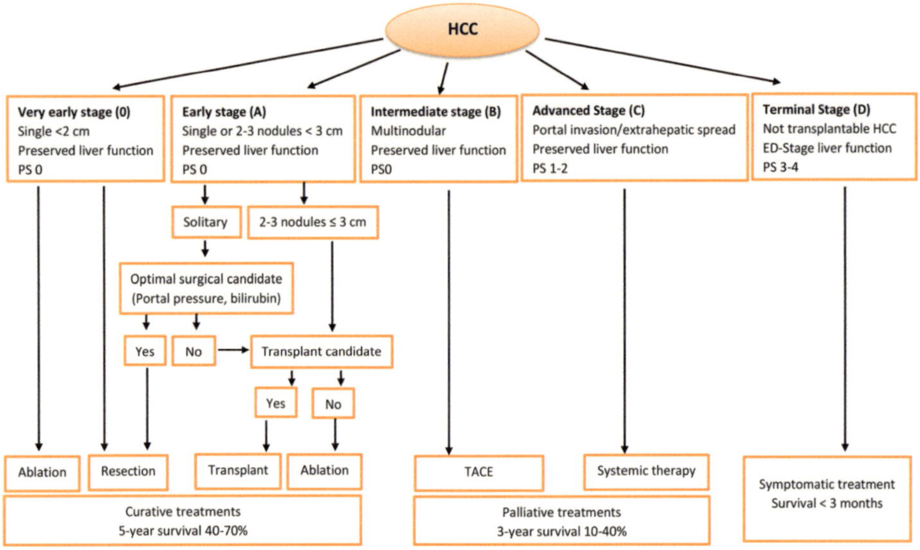

Figure 2.
BCLC staging. Galle et al. [5].

cases, especially in early stages [41]. PIVKA-II is another serum marker still under evaluation in combination with US for screening purposes, even if not enough evidences have been published yet to justify its use [48].

US is useful to evaluate liver status while planning treatment and to identify possible contraindication to surgery, such as portal vein thrombosis [5].

Contrast-enhanced ultrasound (CEUS) uses gas microbubbles as a contrast agent that highlights lesions with well-represented vasculature. Due to pulmonary clearance, it is suitable for patients with reduced renal function or renal failure. It is repeatable, noninvasive and without risks [49].

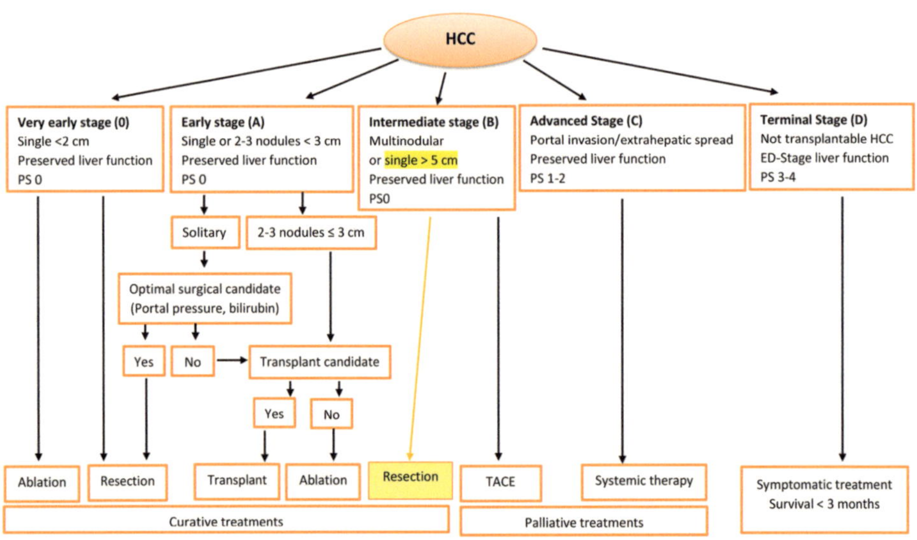

Figure 3.
Modified indications in BCLC staging. Source: Torzilli et al. [35] and Bolondi et al. [37].

DOI: http://dx.doi.org/10.5772/intechopen.86638

Differently from US, CEUS is not indicated for screening but for characterizing known nodules. HCC is characterized by arterial-phase enhancement and low and later wash-out (after at least 60 seconds) on CEUS [50, 51]. It may differentiate HCC from other nodules in cirrhotic liver and distinguish neoplastic portal vein thrombosis from a benignant one [49]. However CEUS does not detect small (<20 mm) and deep-located lesions, and it hardly discriminates between HCC and cholangiocarcinoma (CCC) [5, 45].

CEUS alone is not enough neither for diagnosis nor for staging of HCC, so it shall be considered as a second-line method in patients unfit either for contrast CT (due to chronic kidney disease) or MRI (due to possible vascular metallic devices or claustrophobia) [50].

2.3 CT evaluation

CT is a second-line imaging technique that enables a high diagnostic accuracy, if proper technique and contrast administration are applied. The CT appearance of HCC is extremely variable and depends on growth pattern (solitary, multifocal masses of infiltrating neoplasm), size and histologic composition [52].

Hepatocellular carcinoma (HCC) is most often hypoattenuating on unenhanced scan. After contrast agent injection, HCC is typically hypervascular during the arterial phase: small lesions show more homogeneous enhancement than larger neoplasms that are heterogeneous. During the portal venous phase, HCC becomes iso- to hypoattenuating to the surrounding liver. On delayed phase the tumors wash out more rapidly than the hepatic parenchyma [45].

Based on the guidelines, these diagnostic criteria are sufficient for a noninvasive diagnosis of HCC [5].

HCC could also present atypical findings such as hypervascular lesion without wash-out or hypovascular tumor: hypovascular nodules are not uncommon, and they usually represent early stages like dysplastic nodules with focal HCC or well-differentiated small HCCs [53].

Perfusion CT (PCT) allows quantitative evaluation of tumor-related angiogenesis, tissue perfusion and segmental hepatic function. Higher radiation dose and lower resolution are the main limitations of this method [45].

CT with higher spatial resolution is fundamental in preoperative management: firstly, in detection of vascular or bile ducts anatomical variants and also in calculation of the future remnant liver (FRL) if a major resection is considered [54].

Evaluation of anatomical variation is critic while planning hepatic resections. Hepatic arterial anatomy variations are common (approximately 45%), and different hepatic venous anomalies, such as drainage of segment VIII into the middle hepatic vein, of segments V and VI directly into the inferior vena cava and of accessory middle hepatic vein directly into the inferior vena cava, can impact surgery. Also portal vein variants and biliary anatomy variations should be carefully investigated [55].

The FRL is calculated by dedicated software that analysed the total liver volume, the tumour volume and the liver volume after surgical procedure. The FRL volume of 20–30% is the lowest limit for a safe resection in healthy livers, 40% in elderly, whereas in patients with diffuse liver disease, a volumetric evaluation shall be associated with FRL function assessment (e.g. indocyanine green retention test or liver maximum capacity test) [54, 56, 57].

2.4 MRI

MRI is superior to CT for the diagnosis of HCC [53].

At MR imaging small HCCs have variable signal intensity on T1-weighted pre-contrast imaging: they commonly appear hypointense, but high signal intensity has been reported with a frequency ranging between 34 and 61%. On T2-weighted images, HCC is iso- to hyperintense to the surrounding liver parenchyma. Generally, hyperintense lesions on T1 and isointense in T2 are well-differentiated, due to the presence of fat and or glycoprotein; on the contrary lesions hypointense on T1 and hyper on T2 are moderately/poor differentiated. After contrast agent injection, HCC shows the same imaging patterns described on CT examination [45, 58].

The introduction in clinical practice of liver-specific contrast agents, superparamagnetic as well as paramagnetic, significantly improves the detection and characterization of HCC, in particular for lesions between 1 and 2 cm. With paramagnetic contrast agents, the absence of functional hepatocytes, which is considered a sign of malignancy, is represented as a loss of signal intensity during the hepatobiliary phase. Nevertheless, fewer than 20% of well-differentiated and moderately differentiated HCCs appear iso- or hyperintense on hepatobiliary phase images [45, 58].

HCC can rarely invade biliary ducts, both microscopically and macroscopically [59]. Incidence of biliary duct invasion ranges from 1.2 to 9%. It shall be carefully evaluated while staging patients, in order to choose the best treatment and to assess prognosis. Biliary invasion, in fact, is an independent adverse prognostic factor and is often linked to higher biological aggressiveness and portal vein invasion which make prognosis worse [60].

MR cholangiopancreatography (MRCP) is a noninvasive procedure aimed for evaluating the hepatobiliary and pancreatic systems. This method is helpful in assessing biliary invasion. Biliary duct tumor thrombus appears as an intraluminal soft tissue with arterial-phase enhancement on MRCP, and biliary ducts could be seen dilated because of obstructing tumor fragments [60].

Several studies have shown that biliary ducts invasion in HCC is not a contraindication to surgical resection, even in patients with obstructive jaundice caused by biliary tumor thrombus, as long as R0 resection can be achieved. If jaundice is present, biliary drainage should be performed preoperatively [59, 61–63].

MRI also enables the estimation of fat storage in the liver parenchyma: proton density fat fraction (PDFF) technique is a fast, accurate and easy-to-use MR modality that allows liver fat quantification [52].

2.5 Bioptic evaluation

Biopsy of hepatic lesions is an invasive procedure. Its use is restricted, as a typical pattern in one second-line imaging technique is enough to make an HCC diagnosis, according to the guidelines [64]. In performing liver biopsy, indeed, there is a high risk of bleeding, even higher if the patient has a bleeding disorder due to cirrhosis, and an established possibility of seeding along the needle tract. However, haemorrhagic risk can be reduced with infusion of fresh frozen plasma and platelets before the procedure [51]. Subcapsular and extended tumor and ascites could compromise safe needle insertion too [46].

The procedure allows histological analysis, so it may be used when HCC has atypical growing pattern, so that there is a high suspicion of cholangiocarcinoma (CCC), considering that in such cases bioptic results will impact on therapeutic choice, changing it completely [51].

Furthermore liver parenchyma biopsy is currently the reference procedure for assessing and staging fibrosis and cirrhosis. Stages are classified according to METAVIR score, a histopathologic grading system. Hepatic biopsy has some important limitations: it allows the evaluation of a sample, and not of the entire liver, and, above all, it is an invasive method that could cause minor (temporary pain in 20%

of cases) or major (bleeding, sepsis, pneumothorax and even death in 1.1% of cases) complications [65].

2.6 Intraoperative US

Intraoperative ultrasonography (IOUS) is fundamental while performing hepatic resections. It can give further information about lesions and parenchyma and can determine modifications both in tumor staging and in surgical management as well [66].

IOUS and contrast-enhanced intraoperative ultrasound (CE-IOUS) have higher sensitivity compared to preoperative US and CEUS and allow better detection and characterization of small nodules [66].

Without these intraoperative procedures, surgical inspection and palpation can overlook up to 50% of preoperatively undetected lesions, especially those located in deep parenchyma and in cirrhotic liver [67].

Furthermore, IOUS became a mandatory tool in major hepatic surgery, as it allows visualizing of major vessels, assessing their location in relation to HCC lesion and delimiting resection area. It is also important to identify correct dissection planes and accurately define tumor extension, thus to achieve higher rates of R0 resections [67].

3. Surgical treatment

Surgical resection is the first-line treatment in non-cirrhotic and compensated cirrhotic livers [5]. The aim of surgery is to achieve R0 resection while preserving enough future remnant liver, in order to avoid postoperative liver failure [68]. Therefore, the most appropriate surgical technique is chosen according to principles of oncological radicality, safety and the least invasiveness [69], considering that HCC tends to be a recurrent disease (recurrence rate 40–70%), and so re-resection or noninvasive treatments are often needed [70].

Large nodules, major intrahepatic vessels invasion, portal branches and hepatic vein thrombosis do not contraindicate to surgery as soon as R0 resection can be achieved [71], keeping in mind that a well-preserved liver function is necessary to perform radical hepatic resections [72]. Surgery can be even performed in case of HCV and HBV hepatitis as long as there is metabolic syndrome-related hepatopathy or cirrhosis is compensated. (Child-Pugh $\leq$ 8; MELD $\leq$ 9) [73].

Patient performance status is also a factor that has to be considered while planning a surgical resection of the liver. Advanced age is not a contraindication, as long as these patients are carefully selected, according to their general condition, performance status, life expectancy and treatment tolerability [56].

In some cases, surgery may be a *bridging* treatment to liver transplant in patients with advanced cirrhosis and HCC, when waiting time exceeds 6–8 months [74].

Impaired liver function, insufficient future remnant liver, advanced tumor stage and poor performance status are absolute contraindications to surgical resection [73]. Liver resection could not be performed in the case of Child-Pugh > 8, MELD $\geq$ 9, bilirubin $\geq$ 3 mg/dl associated with INR $\geq$ 1.7 or PT < 50%, platelet count < 50,000/μl, indocyanine green retention at 15 minutes >22% and portal vein pressure gradient >10 mmHg without possible TIPS [72, 73]. Extended portal or vena caval thrombosis and extrahepatic disease reveal an advanced HCC stage and contraindicate surgical resection [73]. Patients not eligible for surgery are those with ECOG performance status 4, ASA index > 3, Charlson's index > 3–4 and older than 70 years with comprehensive geriatric assessment (CGA) = 3 or systemic diseases with severe prognosis (life expectancy < 12 months) [56].

Intrahepatic recurrence after surgical treatment is often linked to portal venous invasion, both macroscopic (MPVI) and microscopic (mPVI). MPVI can be preoperatively detected by CT, MRI and US, whereas mPVI is very difficult to diagnose preoperatively. In order to reduce recurrence rates due to mPVI, in young and fit patients, anatomic liver resection (ALR) should be preferred to nonanatomic liver resection (NALR) [75]. ALR should be taken into account especially in patients who have solitary PVI (in a single portal vein branch) or a higher risk of mPVI linked to α-fetoprotein ≥ 20 ng/ml, PIVKA-II ≥ 100 mAU/ml, tumor size ≥ 5 cm and a confluent lesion morphology [76, 77]. Some authors suggest that during anatomic resection, it is better to avoid excessive rotation of the liver, perform an early extrahepatic ligation of the portal pedicle of the resected segment(s) before parenchymal transection and obtain an adequate surgical margin to decrease the risk of recurrences [71].

On the other hand, NALR allows *parenchyma-sparing* surgery that, though associated to higher recurrence rates, is indicated in elderly and cirrhotic patients suffering from early HCC, where an anatomic resection would sacrifice an excessive amount of the parenchyma (**Figure 4**) [75].

Surgery is proved to be superior to RF in terms of local recurrences for nodules >2 cm [19, 78], but in the case of multinodular HCC, in selected patients, they can be combined together to achieve a better outcome, compared to TACE or TARE, whose role remains palliative (**Figure 5**) [35, 64, 78].

3.1 Major hepatectomies

All liver resections involving three or more liver segments of Couinaud are considered major hepatectomies. Most commonly performed resections are right hepatectomy, left hepatectomy, right-extended hepatectomy, left-extended hepatectomy and median hepatectomy [69]. Major hepatectomy is frequently required to achieve a complete tumor removal (**Figure 6**) [79].

Healthy livers may be resected as much as 70% without major complications; cirrhotic or hepatopathic patients shall be cautiously submitted to resection after precise FRL analysis in terms of future remnant liver function (FRLF) and volume [54]. Liver resections for HCC related to NAFLD and metabolic syndrome are encumbered by important rates of complications (13–20%) and mortality (2%); procedure risk profile in this condition is closer to that burdening cirrhotic livers rather than non-cirrhotic ones [5].

Age is not a contraindication to major hepatectomy, because elderly patients' liver, when healthy, have comparable regeneration rates to younger ones, while patients' performance status and liver residual function are more important [80].

Major hepatectomies can be performed safely in either open or mini-invasive approaches [81].

Open approach is more invasive, but it offers great advantages in a better view on the operative field, allowing a complete administration in organ mobilization and a prompt control of bleeding (**Figure 7**). Open approach is indicated in the case of upper abdominal adhesions, respiratory impairment and advanced liver fibrosis. In severe respiratory disease, pneumoperitoneum worsens gas exchange; therefore, laparoscopic- and robot-assisted resection are contraindicated [82]. In the case of upper abdominal adhesions, it is hard to induce an adequate pneumoperitoneum to insert trocars and instrument safely, and open approach is the one indicated [83]. Advanced liver fibrosis makes the organ stiffer and difficult to mobilize with laparoscopic graspers [84]. The *liver hanging manoeuver* (*LHM*), which is a technique of passing a tape along the retrohepatic avascular space and suspending the liver during parenchymal transection, facilitates anterior approach of major hepatectomy and minimizes bleeding by elevation of the liver along its deeper parenchymal plane [85, 86].

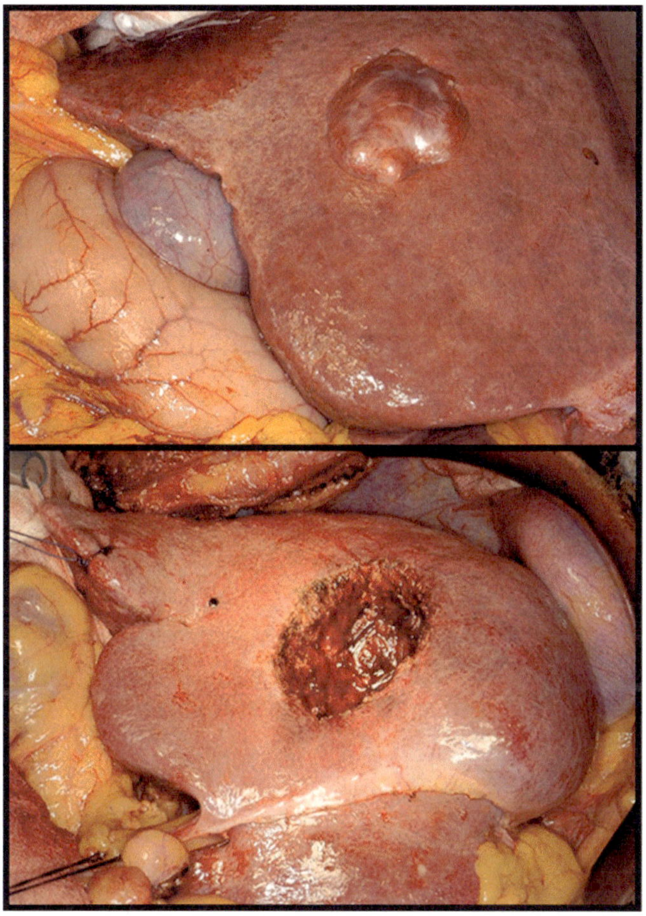

Figure 4.
Wedge resection (NALR) in the NAFLD liver. HHC located in V/VIII segment.

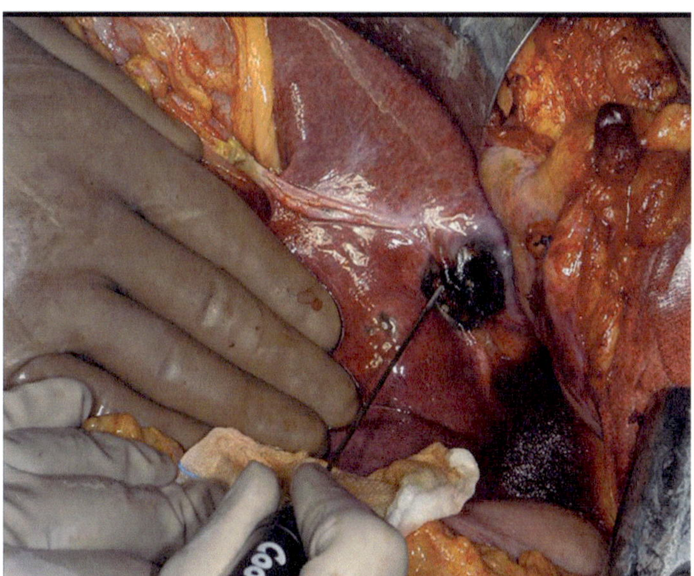

Figure 5.
Intraoperative RF in HCC nodule of II segment.

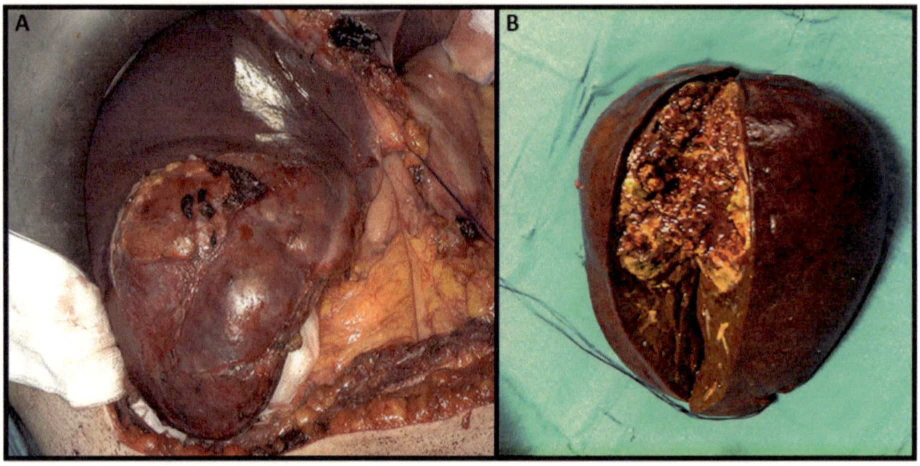

Figure 6.
(A) Large HCC In non-cirrhotic live requiring right hepatectomy. (B) Extended right hepatectomy in NAFLD, surgical sample showing a 11-cm HCC.

Minimally invasive liver surgery has strongly progressed during the last 20 years [87].

Laparoscopic approach is proven as being safe and presents good outcomes in terms of hospitalization and morbidity. However, the main disadvantage of this approach is the lack of control when a huge bleeding occurs, but the LHM reducing bleeding risk makes the procedure safer.

Robotic-assisted resection is the newest technology in hepatobiliary surgery. Compared to laparoscopy, robotic instruments allow wide-angle rotation; therefore, it is easier and faster to perform sutures and ligatures. Four-arm *da Vinci Si* enables the surgeon to perform safer resections, reduced bleeding and major dexterity, particularly in hilar time and in vena cava detachment time. One of the major disadvantages of the robot is its cost [88, 89].

HCC is a fast-spreading tumor, particularly in the vascular system; therefore, major resections in large or multinodular tumors allow the most radical removal; however, consistent volume of the functioning liver is also resected, increasing risks of liver impairment in cirrhotic and hepatopathic patients [90].

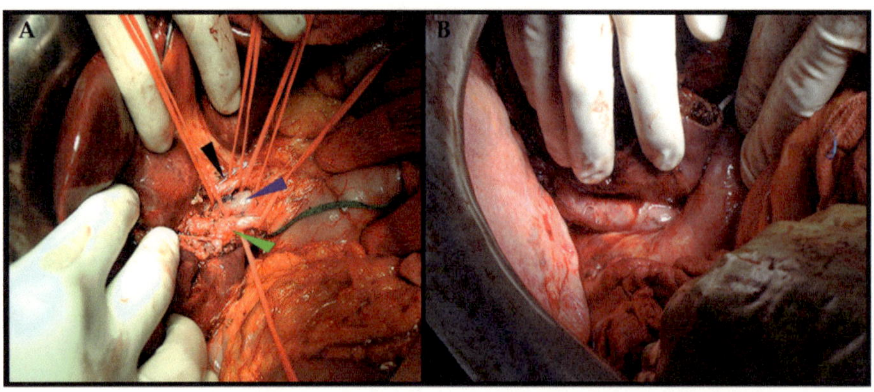

Figure 7.
(A) Dissection of liver hilum. Elements are indicated by arrows: choledocus (green), portal vein (blue), hepatic artery (black). (B) Caval detachment in bisegmentectomy (VI–VII).

3.2 Limited hepatectomies

Limited hepatectomy means resection of two or less segments of Couinaud, like left lobectomy, involving segments II and III, and bisegmentectomy of VI–VII and VI–V, that are the most common (**Figure 8**). Limited hepatectomies are indicated in the case of single or multiple HCC nodules located in one or two adjacent liver segments [69], especially when early diagnosed. Otherwise non-followed up patients are often diagnosed with advanced or multinodular HCC, which are eligible to more extended hepatectomies only.

Limited hepatectomies tend to preserve liver function, so analysis of FRLF and FRLV is often unnecessary in healthy patients, while it is mandatory in compensated cirrhosis due to higher resection risk and distorted liver anatomy [73].

Limited resection is often performed with mini-invasive surgical technique, such as laparoscopic- or robot-assisted surgery. Although expert surgeons are able to resect safely even posterior and subdiaphragmatic lesions, these techniques have some limits. Laparoscopy, in fact, has prolonged surgical times for liver mobilization due to difficulties in parenchyma manipulation, arduous bleeding control and necessity of a major experience of the surgeon.

Robotic liver resection (RLR) allows to go beyond laparoscopic disadvantages, thanks to superior flexibility of its arms. For this reason, RLRs are considered safe, even in deep parenchyma or posterior segment [89]. It is comparable to open approach considering the oncological radicality, but it presents the same advantages of laparoscopy in terms of length of hospital stay and postoperative complications. Conversion rate from robotic to open approach ranges from 0 to 8.8% [87].

Open surgery shall be chosen in the case of contraindications to other approaches such as respiratory impairment that is worsened by pneumoperitoneum or excessive difficulties in liver manipulation; the surgeon's experience remains an important variable in surgical indications, and safety of intervention shall always drive the choice [82, 84].

Nonanatomic liver resection, or wedge resection, is reserved for early HCC (BCLC 0 or A), particularly in the elderly, suffering from advanced cirrhosis or exophytic lesions in hypertrophic segments, where anatomic resection would determine too extensive healthy parenchyma loss [75].

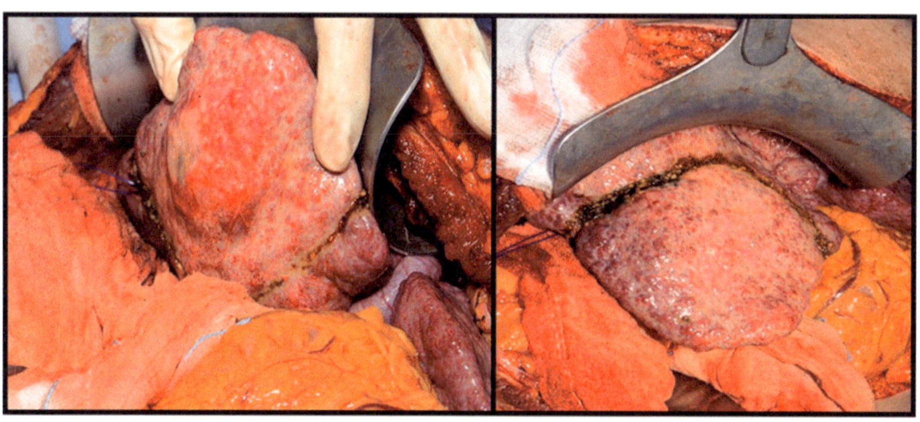

Figure 8.
Anatomic resection of segment VI in cirrhotic live. HCC diameter 2.5 cm.

3.3 Staged hepatectomies

Staged hepatectomies in HCC treatment are the most recent innovation, first introduced to treat multiple colorectal metastases, now under evaluation for extended hepatectomies in advanced HCC patients [91]. The main issue related to this technique is that most HCC patients are cirrhotic or hepatopathics, and cirrhosis limits parenchyma regeneration in a significant way [91, 92].

Extended resection is feasible when the future remnant liver is ≥40% for cirrhotic patients, ≥30% in patients with severe steatosis or fibrosis without cirrhosis and ≥20% in those with normal liver function [93].

Several strategies can be carried out in order to increase future remnant liver volume (FRLV), improve resectability and reduce postoperative risk of liver failure (PLF) in patients with inadequate FRLV. These techniques include preoperative portal vein embolization (PVE) or ligation (PVL), sequential transarterial chemoembolization and PVE, two-stage hepatectomy (TSH), preoperative Yttrium-90 (^{90}Y) radioembolization (RE) and associated liver partition and portal vein ligation for staged hepatectomy (ALPPS) [93]. Parenchyma hypertrophy shall be assessed using CT volumetry before performing second-stage hepatectomy [94].

ALPPS is indicated in non-cirrhotic patients with insufficient remnant liver or in the case of PVE failure [93, 95, 96]. This procedure allows higher and faster hypertrophy rates compared to other strategies, due to parenchyma transection and collateral portal branches ligation, especially in hepatopathics; such advantages have been seen also in cirrhotic patients [92]. Moreover, it reduces risk of HCC progression thanks to the shorter time interval between operations. On the other hand, it is associated with high risk of PLF (27%) probably due to portal hyperperfusion, major perioperative complications and mortality [97]. Some authors suggest that the use of anterior approach combined with hanging manoeuver allows higher control and safety during ALPPS procedure [92]. Only few case series have been published about staged hepatectomy for HCC, more perspective research is still necessary, even if this technique is proofing effective and beneficial in selected patients [98].

3.4 Complication

Postoperative complications have higher incidence and severity in cirrhotic patients [99].

Postoperative live failure (PLF) is the most life-threatening complication following hepatic resection, especially in cirrhotics [93]. It is defined as the decrease in liver synthetic, excretory and/or detoxifying functions after resection [100]. It can be associated with insufficient future liver volume, prolonged operative time, prolonged ischemia, massive intra- and postoperative bleeding, hemodynamic instability, bile duct obstruction, drug-induced injury, viral reactivation and sepsis [90]. It occurs after the fifth day in 4–19% of cases, and it is characterized by various symptoms and signs, such as ascites, pleural effusion, prolonged cholestasis, coagulation disorders, elevated serum lactate levels, hyperbilirubinemia, hypoalbuminemia, hypoglycaemia and hepatic encephalopathy [90, 93].

Bile leakage is another severe postoperative complication. It occurs in 4–17% of cases with comparable incidences in laparoscopic and open approaches [101]. It can induce further complications, such as extrahepatic abscess, requiring reoperation; otherwise it is usually managed with interventional radiology [100].

Postoperative ascites is common, and it may be caused by portal flow resistance increase and serum albumin loss. It can be treated with diuretics, sodium restriction or albumin infusion [100]. Persistent ascites is associated to higher risks of spontaneous bacterial peritonitis (SBP) and mortality.

Clotting disorders are frequent after extended hepatectomies and in cirrhotic patients, who may already have preoperative low platelet count. They can manifest as PT and aPTT prolongation, increase in levels of fibrinogen degradation products and platelet levels reduction [100].

Surgical site infection may occurs within 30 days after resection [100].

Postoperative pneumonia and respiratory disturbs (acute lung injury, acute respiratory distress syndrome) rarely occur after liver resection, especially in the elderly [100].

Resected patients shall be rapidly mobilized postoperatively; feeding shall start early, together with intravenous liquid restriction. Nonadequately selected patients may also suffer from postoperative acute renal failure or hepatorenal syndrome [100].

Mini-invasive surgical approaches allow lower postoperative complications, such as ascites, pleural effusion and hospital-acquired infections [87, 99, 102].

4. Follow-up

HCC recurrence within 5 years after hepatic resection occurs in 40–70% of patients [70, 103, 104]. Several recurrence risk factors should be carefully considered while planning postoperative surveillance (**Table 4**) [70].

Intrahepatic recurrent HCC can develop from an intrahepatic metastasis (IM type) or arise from de novo multicentric carcinogenesis (MO type) due to the underlying chronic liver disease. These two HCC types can be distinguished according to their clinic-pathological characteristics and recurrence-free interval [70].

Early recurrence occurs within 2 years from primary resection, and they seem associated with intrahepatic metastasis, whereas late recurrences can show up more than 2 years after surgery, and they are linked to multicentric occurrence [105].

Differentiating them is important because MO, compared to IM, is associated with higher survival rate after repeated resection and better prognosis [106].

RHCCs have the same imaging features of primary HCC, so they shall be detected and diagnosed using the same methods of primary HCC diagnosis.

US, CT or MRI and AFP determination should be performed after surgical resection.

Surgical factors	Non-anatomical resection Positive histologic margin (R1 or R2) Necessity of transfusion due to significant bleeding Iatrogenic tumor escape or rupture
Clinicopathological factors	Low tumor differentiation Advanced tumor stage Tumor rupture, damaged capsule Tumor diameter > 5 cm Tumor number ≥ 3 Vascular tumor thrombus Lymph node invasion Adjacent organ invasion satellite lesion High level of AFP before operation Increased AFP level 2 months after operation
Patient's factor	Underlying chronic liver disease: active hepatitis infection or cirrhosis

Wen et al. [70].

Table 4.
Risk factors of postoperative recurrence.

US should be performed every 6 months within the first 5 years after surgical treatment; a second level imaging study is requested at the first year and repeated after 12–18 months according to the underlying liver status [5]. Resected patients for HCC, who received direct-acting antiviral (DAA) therapy for HCV negativization, are commonly kept in a less intensive follow-up with US every 12–18 months, for a persistent recurrence risk is maintained [107].

Once detected, RHCC shall be carefully assessed in order to plan the best therapy. Re-resection is the treatment of choice if nodule is resectable and patient is eligible for surgery; so, disease-free time, performance status, future remnant liver volume and function, cirrhosis, portal hypertension and other aspects should be evaluated again before repeating operation. Only about 20% of patients with recurrent HCC receive surgical treatment [105]. Multiple resections could be performed after major or limited primary hepatectomy [70, 108].

Both open and laparoscopic resections can be carried out, but laparotomy is generally preferred, since intra-abdominal adhesions limit laparoscopic approach [109]. Five-year survival rate higher than 70% can be achieved in well-selected patients, despite repeated treatments [103, 104].

Prognosis after repeated resections is linked to clinic-pathological characteristics of primary HCC and recurrence interval. Particularly a disease-free period longer than 1 year after primary resection, single primary HCC and negative portal invasion are positive prognostic factors after second resection [105, 108].

Other possible locoregional therapies for recurrent illness are RFA, MWA and TACE. Liver transplantation could be taken into account in selected patients with worsened liver function and falling within transplant criteria [70, 103].

Incidence of extrahepatic metastases (EHM) after hepatectomy is low (range 5–20%) [108, 110]. High-serum alpha-fetoprotein levels, after liver resection or transplant, is suspicious for extrahepatic recurrence; thus serial cross-sectional total body imaging is mandatory to identify them, and palliative R0 resection may be performed in fit patients with quality of life and survival benefits [27].

5. Conclusion

HCC is a deadly malignancy either in cirrhotic and non-cirrhotic patients. A well-timed follow-up and detection of patients at risk are fundamental, since diagnosis at early stage allows more aggressive and effective treatments. HCC in non-cirrhotic liver will be more often diagnosed, particularly in the case of NASH and NAFLD, because they are followed up more strictly.

In recent years, indications to surgery have not changed substantially, while a lot has been introduced in terms of imaging, which is nowadays an essential support in preoperative planning, intraoperative guide and postoperative follow-up. Staged hepatectomy techniques have shown interesting results and will become part of clinical practice in the future, especially in treatment of non-cirrhotic patients. Surgery remains the most effective treatment against HCC, since complete resections allow important survival benefits at 3, 5 and 10 years.

Author details

Stefania Brozzetti[1*], Simone Bini[1], Chiara D'Alterio[1], Chiara De Lucia[1], Leonardo Luca Chiarella[1], Katia Fazzi[1] and Michele Di Martino[2]

1 Department of Surgery "Pietro Valdoni", Policlinico Umberto I, University of Rome La Sapienza, Rome, Italy

2 Deparment of Radiological Sciences, Policlinico Umberto I, University of Rome La Sapienza, Rome, Italy

*Address all correspondence to: stefania.brozzetti@uniroma1.it

IntechOpen

© 2019 The Author(s). Licensee IntechOpen. This chapter is distributed under the terms of the Creative Commons Attribution License (http://creativecommons.org/licenses/by/3.0), which permits unrestricted use, distribution, and reproduction in any medium, provided the original work is properly cited.

References

[1] Bray F, Ferlay J, Soerjomataram I, Siegel RL, Torre LA, Jemal A. Global cancer statistics 2018: GLOBOCAN estimates of incidence and mortality worldwide for 36 cancers in 185 countries. CA: A Cancer Journal for Clinicians. 2018;**68**(6):394-424. DOI: 10.3322/caac.21492

[2] Forner A, Reig M, Bruix J. Hepatocellular carcinoma. Lancet. 2018;**391**(10127):1301-1314. DOI: 10.1016/S0140-6736(18)30010-2

[3] Desai A, Sandhu S, Lai J-P, Sandhu DS. Hepatocellular carcinoma in non-cirrhotic liver: A comprehensive review. World Journal of Hepatology. 2019;**11**(1):1-18. DOI: 10.4254/wjh.v11.i1.1

[4] Brozzetti S, Bini S, Luca Chiarella L, Fazzi K, Di Martino M, Bezzi M. HCC in elderly patients. Curative intraoperative strategies and management in recurrences. Liver Cancer. InTechOpen; 2018. DOI: 10.5772/intechopen.79748

[5] Galle PR, Forner A, Llovet JM, et al. EASL clinical practice guidelines: Management of hepatocellular carcinoma. Journal of Hepatology. 2018;**69**(1):182-236. DOI: 10.1016/j.jhep.2018.03.019

[6] Hackl C, Schlitt HJ, Kirchner GI, Knoppke B, Loss M. Liver transplantation for malignancy: Current treatment strategies and future perspectives. World Journal of Gastroenterology. 2014;**20**(18):5331-5344. DOI: 10.3748/wjg.v20.i18.5331

[7] Durand F, Levitsky J, Cauchy F, Gilgenkrantz H, Soubrane O, Francoz C. Age and liver transplantation. Journal of Hepatology. 2019;**70**(4):745-758. DOI: 10.1016/j.jhep.2018.12.009

[8] Mazzaferro V, Regalia E, Doci R, et al. Carcinomas in patients with cirrhosis. The New England Journal of Medicine. 1996;**334**(11):693-699. DOI: 10.1056/NEJM199603143341104

[9] Sposito C, Mazzaferro V, Bhoori S, et al. Milan criteria in liver transplantation for hepatocellular carcinoma: An evidence-based analysis of 15 years of experience. Liver Transplantation. 2011;**17**(S2):S44-S57. DOI: 10.1002/lt.22365

[10] Mazzaferro V, Llovet JM, Miceli R, et al. Predicting survival after liver transplantation in patients with hepatocellular carcinoma beyond the Milan criteria: A retrospective, exploratory analysis. The Lancet Oncology. 2009;**10**(1):35-43. DOI: 10.1016/S1470-2045(08)70284-5

[11] Lei JY, Wang WT, Yan LN. Up-to-seven criteria for hepatocellular carcinoma liver transplantation: A single center analysis. World Journal of Gastroenterology. 2013;**19**(36):6077-6083. DOI: 10.3748/wjg.v19.i36.6077

[12] Belghiti J, Durand F. Criteria for liver transplantation for hepatocellular carcinoma: What is an acceptable outcome? Liver International. 2011;**31**(Suppl. 1):161-163. DOI: 10.1111/j.1478-3231.2010.02413.x

[13] Peng Y, Qi XGX. Child-Pugh versus MELD score for the assessment of prognosis in liver cirrhosis. Medicine. 2016;**95**(8):1-29. DOI: 10.1097/MD.0000000000002877

[14] Marroni CP, de Mello Brandão AB, Hennigen AW, et al. MELD scores with incorporation of serum sodium and death prediction in cirrhotic patients on the waiting list for liver transplantation: A single center experience in southern Brazil. Clinical Transplantation. 2012;**26**(4):E395-E401. DOI: 10.1111/j.1399-0012.2012.01688.x

[15] Valapour M, Skeans MA, Smith JM, et al. OPTN/SRTR 2015 annual data report: Lung. American Journal of Transplantation. 2017;**17**:357-424. DOI: 10.1111/ajt.14129

[16] Changyong E, Wang D, Yu Y, Liu H, Ren HJT. Efficacy comparison of radiofrequency ablation and hepatic resection for hepatocellular carcinoma: A meta-analysis. Journal of Cancer Research and Therapeutics. 2017;**13**(4):625-630. DOI: 10.4103/jcrt.JCRT_406_17

[17] Vogl TJ, Nour-Eldin NEA, Hammerstingl RM, Panahi B, Naguib NNN. Microwave ablation (MWA): Basics, technique and results in primary and metastatic liver neoplasms—Review article. RöFo - Fortschritte auf dem Gebiet der Röntgenstrahlen und der bildgebenden Verfahren. 2017;**189**(11):1055-1066. DOI: 10.1055/s-0043-117410

[18] Jiang Y-Q, Wang Z-X, Deng Y-N, Yang Y, Wang G-Y, Chen G-H. Efficacy of hepatic resection vs. radiofrequency ablation for patients with very-early-stage or early-stage hepatocellular carcinoma: A population-based study with stratification by age and tumor size. Frontiers in Oncology. 2019;**9**(February):1-10. DOI: 10.3389/fonc.2019.00113

[19] Cucchetti A, Piscaglia F, Cescon M, Ercolani G, Pinna AD. Systematic review of surgical resection vs radiofrequency ablation for hepatocellular carcinoma. World Journal of Gastroenterology. 2013;**19**(26):4106-4118. DOI: 10.3748/wjg.v19.i26.4106

[20] Tan W, Deng Q, Lin S, Wang Y, Xu G. Comparison of microwave ablation and radiofrequency ablation for hepatocellular carcinoma: A systematic review and meta-analysis. International Journal of Hyperthermia. 2019;**36**(1):264-272. DOI: 10.1080/02656736.2018.1562571

[21] Wu B, Zhou J, Ling G, Zhu D, Long Q. CalliSpheres drug-eluting beads versus lipiodol transarterial chemoembolization in the treatment of hepatocellular carcinoma: A short-term efficacy and safety study. World Journal of Surgical Oncology. 2018;**16**(1):1-8. DOI: 10.1186/s12957-018-1368-8

[22] Hyun D, Cho SK, Shin SW, et al. Early stage hepatocellular carcinomas not feasible for ultrasound-guided radiofrequency ablation: Comparison of transarterial chemoembolization alone and combined therapy with transarterial chemoembolization and radiofrequency ablation. Cardiovascular and Interventional Radiology. 2016;**39**(3):417-425. DOI: 10.1007/s00270-015-1194-0

[23] Qian J, Feng GS, Vogl T. Combined interventional therapies of hepatocellular carcinoma. World Journal of Gastroenterology. 2003;**9**(9):1885-1891. DOI: 10.3748/wjg.v9.i9.1885

[24] Vilana R, Bruix J, Bru C, Ayuso C, Solé MRJ. Tumor size determines the efficacy of percutaneous ethanol injection for the treatment of small hepatocellular carcinoma. Hepatology. 1992;**16**(2):353-357

[25] Facciorusso A, Serviddio G, Muscatiello N. Local ablative treatments for hepatocellular carcinoma: An updated review. World Journal of Gastrointestinal Pharmacology and Therapeutics. 2016;**7**(4):477-489. DOI: 10.4292/wjgpt.v7.i4.477

[26] Gough-palmer AL, Michal W, Gedroyc W, Gough-palmer AL, Witold WM. Laser ablation of hepatocellular carcinoma—A review. World Journal of Gastroenterology. 2008;**14**(47):7170-7174. DOI: 10.3748/wjg.14.7170

[27] Brozzetti S, Bini S, Fazzi K, et al. Case-report: Metastases in a low-stage middle-graded HCC in cleared HCV

infection, non-cirrhotic liver: Surgical therapy. Case Report—Open Access. International Journal of Surgery Case Reports. 2018;**47**:19-21. DOI: 10.1016/j.ijscr.2018.04.013

[28] Siddique O, Yoo ER, Perumpail RB, et al. The importance of a multidisciplinary approach to hepatocellular carcinoma. Journal of Multidisciplinary Healthcare. 2017;**10**:95-100. DOI: 10.2147/JMDH.S128629

[29] Subramanian KKK, Tandon M, Pandey CK, Jain P. Patients with cirrhosis of liver operated for non-transplant surgery: A retrospective analysis. Journal of Clinical and Translational Hepatology. 2019;7(X): 1-6. DOI: 10.14218/jcth.2018.00043

[30] Maithel SK, Kneuertz PJ, Kooby DA, Scoggins CR, Weber SM, Martin RCG, et al. Importance of low preoperative platelet count in selecting patients for resection of hepatocellular carcinoma: A multi-institutional analysis. Journal of the American College of Surgeons. 2011;**212**(4):638-648. DOI: 10.1016/j.jamcollsurg.2011.01.004

[31] Maida M, Orlando E, Cammà CCG. Staging systems of hepatocellular carcinoma: A review of literature. World Journal of Gastroenterology. 2014;**20**(15):4141-4150. DOI: 10.3748/wjg.v20.i15.4141

[32] Barone C, Koeberle D, Metselaar H, Parisi G, Sansonno D, Spinzi G. Multidisciplinary approach for HCC patients: Hepatology for the oncologists. Annals of Oncology. 2013;**24**(Supplement 2):ii15-ii23. DOI: 10.1093/annonc/mdt053

[33] Chawla A, Ferrone C. Hepatocellular carcinoma surgical therapy: Perspectives on the current limits to resection. Chinese Clinical Oncology. 2018;**7**(5):48-48. DOI: 10.21037/cco.2018.08.12

[34] Guglielmi A, Ruzzenente A, Conci S, et al. Hepatocellular carcinoma: Surgical perspectives beyond the Barcelona clinic liver cancer recommendations. World Journal of Gastroenterology. 2014;**20**(24):7525-7533. DOI: 10.3748/wjg.v20.i24.7525

[35] Torzilli G, Belghiti J, Kokudo N, Takayama T, Capussotti L, Nuzzo G, et al. A snapshot of the effective indications and results of surgery for hepatocellular carcinoma in tertiary referral centers. Annals of Surgery. 2013;**257**(5):929-937. DOI: 10.1097/sla.0b013e31828329b8

[36] Vitale A, Saracino E, Boccagni P, et al. Validation of the BCLC prognostic system in surgical hepatocellular cancer patients. Transplantation Proceedings. 2009;**41**(4):1260-1263. DOI: 10.1016/j.transproceed.2009.03.054

[37] Bolondi L, Burroughs A, Dufour JF, Galle PR, Mazzaferro V, Piscaglia F, et al. Heterogeneity of patients with intermediate (BCLC B) hepatocellular carcinoma: Proposal for a subclassification to facilitate treatment decisions. Seminars in Liver Disease. 2012;**1**(212):348-359. DOI: 10.1055/s-0032-1329906

[38] Yang X, Pan L, Wang L, et al. Systematic review of single large and/or multinodular hepatocellular carcinoma: Surgical resection improves survival. Asian Pacific Journal of Cancer Prevention. 2015;**16**(13):5541-5547. DOI: 10.7314/APJCP.2015.16.13.5541

[39] Cheung TT, Ng KK, Chok KS, et al. Combined resection and radiofrequency ablation for multifocal hepatocellular carcinoma: Prognosis and outcomes. World Journal of Gastroenterology. 2010;**16**(24):3056-3062. DOI: 10.3748/wjg.v16.i24.3056

[40] Simon CJ, Dupuy DE, Iannitti DA, et al. Intraoperative triple antenna hepatic microwave ablation.

American Journal of Roentgenology. 2006;**187**(4):333-340. DOI: 10.2214/AJR.05.0804

[41] Aghoram R, Cai P, Dickinson JA. Alpha-foetoprotein and/or liver ultrasonography for screening of hepatocellular carcinoma in patients with chronic hepatitis B. Cochrane Database of Systematic Reviews. 2012;**9**:1-24. DOI: 10.1002/14651858.CD002799.pub2

[42] Singal A, Volk ML, Waljee A, et al. Meta-analysis: Surveillance with ultrasound for early-stage hepatocellular carcinoma in patients with cirrhosis. Alimentary Pharmacology & Therapeutics. 2009;**30**(1):37-47. DOI: 10.1111/j.1365-2036.2009.04014.x

[43] Bolondi L. Screening for hepatocellular carcinoma in cirrhosis. Journal of Hepatology. 2003;**39**(6):1076-1084. DOI: 10.1016/s0168-8278(03)00349-0

[44] Kee KM, Lu SN. Diagnostic efficacy of ultrasound in hepatocellular carcinoma diagnosis. Expert Review of Gastroenterology & Hepatology. 2017;**11**(4):277-279. DOI: 10.1080/17474124.2017.1292126

[45] Hennedige T, Kundapur S. Imaging of hepatocellular carcinoma: Diagnosis, staging and treatment monitoring. Cancer Immaging. 2012;**12**:530-547. DOI: 10.1102/1470-7330.2012.0044

[46] Ayuso C, Rimola J, García-Criado Á. Imaging of HCC. Abdominal Imaging. 2012;**37**(2):215-230. DOI: 10.1007/s00261-011-9794-x

[47] Zhang BYB. Combined alpha fetoprotein testing and ultrasonography as a screening test for primary liver cancer. Journal of Medical Screening. 1999;**6**:108-110. DOI: 10.1136/jms.6.2.108

[48] Saitta C, Raffa G, Alibrandi A, et al. PIVKA-II is a useful tool for diagnostic characterization of ultrasound-detected liver nodules in cirrhotic patients. Medicine (United States). 2017;**96**(26):1-5. DOI: 10.1097/MD.0000000000007266

[49] Kim TK, Jang H. Contrast-enhanced ultrasound in the diagnosis of nodules in liver cirrhosis. World Journal of Gastroenterology. 2014;**20**(13):3590-3596. DOI: 10.3748/wjg.v20.i13.3590

[50] Cantisani V, David E, Meloni FM, et al. Recall strategies for patients found to have a nodule in cirrhosis: Is there still a role for CEUS?. Medical Ultrasonography. 2015;**17**(4):515-520. DOI: 10.11152/mu.2013.2066.174.rsp

[51] Russo FP, Imondi A, Lynch EN, Farinati F. When and how should we perform a biopsy for HCC in patients with liver cirrhosis in 2018? A review. Digestive and Liver Disease. 2018;**50**(7):640-646. DOI: 10.1016/j.dld.2018.03.014

[52] Zhang Y, Fowler K, Hamilton G, et al. Liver fat imaging—A clinical overview of ultrasound, CT, and MR imaging. The British Journal of Radiology. 2018;**91**(March):1-12. DOI: 10.1259/bjr.20170959

[53] Bolog N, Andreisek G, Oancea IMA. CT and MR imaging of hepatocellular carcinoma. Journal of Gastrointestinal and Liver Diseases. 2011;**20**(2):181-189

[54] Guglielmi A, Ruzzenente A, Conci S, Valdegamberi A, Iacono C. How much remnant is enough in liver resection? Digestive Surgery. 2012;**29**(1):6-17. DOI: 10.1159/000335713

[55] Wile G, Gorden L, Caserta MP, Sakala M, Shen P. Presurgical planning for hepatobiliary malignancies. Magnetic Resonance Imaging Clinics of North America. 2014;**22**(3):447-465. DOI: 10.1016/j.mric.2014.04.003

[56] Brozzetti S, Bezzi M, de Sanctis GM, et al. Elderly and very elderly patients with hepatocellular carcinoma: Strategy for a first line treatment. Annali Italiani di Chirurgia. 2014;**85**(2):120-128

[57] Christ B, Dahmen U, Herrmann KH, et al. Computational modeling in liver surgery. Frontiers in Physiology. 2017;**8**(Nov). DOI: 10.3389/fphys.2017.00906

[58] Willatt JM, Hussain HK, Adusumilli S, Marrero JA. MR imaging of hepatocellular carcinoma in the cirrhotic liver: Challenges and controversies. Radiology. 2008;**247**(2):311-330. DOI: 10.1148/radiol.2472061331

[59] Yang X, Qiu Z, Ran R, et al. Prognostic importance of bile duct invasion in surgical resection with curative intent for hepatocellular carcinoma using PSM analysis. Oncology Letters. 2018;**16**(3):3593-3602. DOI: 10.3892/ol.2018.9108

[60] Park DH, Lee KS, Lee D, et al. Clinical features and outcomes of patients with hepatocellular carcinoma complicated with bile duct invasion. Clinical and Molecular Hepatology. 2017;**23**(2):160-169. DOI: 10.3350/cmh.2016.0088

[61] Orimo T, Kamiyama T, Yokoo H, et al. Hepatectomy for hepatocellular carcinoma with bile duct tumor thrombus, including cases with obstructive jaundice. Annals of Surgical Oncology. 2016;**23**(8):2627-2634. DOI: 10.1245/s10434-016-5174-7

[62] Qiao W, Yu F, Wu L, Li B, Zhou Y. Surgical outcomes of hepatocellular carcinoma with biliary tumor thrombus: A systematic review. BMC Gastroenterology. 2016;**16**(1):4-10. DOI: 10.1186/s12876-016-0427-2

[63] Yeh CN, Jan YY, Lee WC, Chen MF. Hepatic resection for hepatocellular carcinoma with obstructive jaundice due to biliary tumor thrombi. World Journal of Surgery. 2004;**28**(5):471-474. DOI: 10.1007/s00268-004-7185-y

[64] Heimbach JK, Kulik LM, Finn RS, et al. AASLD guidelines for the treatment of hepatocellular carcinoma. Hepatology. 2018;**67**(1):358-380. DOI: 10.1002/hep.29086

[65] Sigrist RMS, Liau J, El Kaffas A, Chammas MC, Willmann JK. Ultrasound elastography: Review of techniques and clinical applications. Theranostics. 2017;7(5):1303-1329. DOI: 10.7150/thno.18650

[66] Gong N-M. Intraoperative US and contrast-enhanced intraoperative US during hepatic resection for patients with hepatocellular carcinoma in liver cirrhosis1. Clinical Hemorheology and Microcirculation. 2018:1-16. DOI: 10.3233/ch-180431

[67] Fan MH, Chang AE. Resection of liver tumors: Technical aspects. Surgical Oncology. 2002;**10**(4):139-152. DOI: 10.1016/S0960-7404(02)00002-6

[68] Pulitano C, Crawford M, Joseph D, Aldrighetti L, Sandroussi C. Preoperative assessment of postoperative liver function: The importance of residual liver volume. Journal of Surgical Oncology. 2014;**110**(4):445-450. DOI: 10.1002/jso.23671

[69] Pang YY, Strasberg SM. The Brisbane 2000 terminology of liver anatomy and resections (HPB 2000;**2**:333-339). HPB Journal. 2002;**4**(2):99. author reply 99-100. DOI: 10.1080/136518202760378489

[70] Wen T, Jin C, Facciorusso A, et al. Multidisciplinary management of recurrent and metastatic hepatocellular carcinoma after resection: An international expert consensus. HepatoBiliary Surgery and Nutrition.

2018;**7**(5):353-371. DOI: 10.21037/hbsn.2018.08.01

[71] Tsai TJ, Chau GY, Lui WY, et al. Clinical significance of microscopic tumor venous invasion in patients with resectable hepatocellular carcinoma. Surgery. 2000;**127**(6):603-608. DOI: 10.1067/msy.2000.105498

[72] Hackl C, Schlitt HJ, Renner P, Lang SA. Liver surgery in cirrhosis and portal hypertension. World Journal of Gastroenterology. 2016;**22**(9):2725-2735. DOI: 10.3748/wjg.v22.i9.2725

[73] Zamora-Valdes D, Taner TND. Surgical treatment of hepatocellular carcinoma. Cancer Control. 2017;**24**(3): 1-15. DOI: 10.1177/1073274817729258

[74] Belghiti J, Cortes A, Abdalla EK, et al. Resection prior to liver transplantation for hepatocellular carcinoma. Annals of Surgery. 2003;**238**(6):885-893. DOI: 10.1097/01.sla.0000098621.74851.65

[75] Zhou Y, Xu D, Wu L, Li B. Meta-analysis of anatomic resection versus non-anatomic resection for hepatocellular carcinoma. Langenbeck's Archives of Surgery. 2011;**396**(7):1109-1117. DOI: 10.1007/s00423-011-0784-9

[76] Shimada S, Kamiyama T, Yokoo H, et al. Clinicopathological characteristics of hepatocellular carcinoma with microscopic portal venous invasion and the role of anatomical liver resection in these cases. World Journal of Surgery. 2017;**41**(8):2087-2094. DOI: 10.1007/s00268-017-3964-0

[77] Kajiyama K, Maehara Y, Shirabe K, et al. Prognosis of hepatocellular carcinoma accompanied by microscopic portal vein invasion. World Journal of Gastroenterology. 2009;**15**(21):2632. DOI: 10.3748/wjg.15.2632

[78] Tsang Y-M, Huang G-T, Lee P-H, et al. Liver resection improves the survival of patients with multiple hepatocellular carcinomas. Annals of Surgical Oncology. 2009;**16**(4):848-855. DOI: 10.1245/s10434-008-0282-7

[79] Strasberg SM, Belghiti J, Clavien P-A, et al. The Brisbane 2000 terminology of liver anatomy and resections. HPB Journal. 2000;**2**(3):333-339. DOI: 10.1016/S1365-182X(17)30755-4

[80] Yasuda S, Nomi T, Hokuto D, Yoshikawa T, Matsuo Y, Sho M. Liver regeneration after major liver resection for hepatocellular carcinoma in the elderly. Journal of Investigative Surgery. 2018:1-7. DOI: 10.1080/08941939.2018.1517839. [E-pub ahead of print]

[81] Fruscione M, Pickens R, Baker EH, et al. Robotic-assisted versus laparoscopic major liver resection: analysis of outcomes from a single center. HPB Journal. 2019. DOI: 10.1016/j.hpb.2018.11.011. [E-pub ahead of print]

[82] Cavalcante AN, Gurrieri C, Sprung J, Schroeder DR, Weingarten TN. Isoflurane and postoperative respiratory depression following laparoscopic surgery: A retrospective propensity-matched analysis. Bosnian Journal of Basic Medical Sciences. 2018;**18**(1):95-100. DOI: 10.17305/bjbms.2017.2478

[83] Leoni S, Piscaglia F, Serio I, et al. Adherence to AASLD guidelines for the treatment of hepatocellular carcinoma in clinical practice: Experience of the bologna liver oncology group. Digestive and Liver Disease. 2014;**46**(6):549-555. DOI: 10.1016/j.dld.2014.02.012

[84] Giovanardi F, Lai Q, Bertacco A, Vitale A. Resection for hepatocellular cancer: overpassing old barriers. Translational Gastroenterology and Hepatology. 2018;**3**(1):64-64. DOI: 10.21037/tgh.2018.09.13

[85] Ogata S, Belghiti J, Varma D, et al. Two hundred liver hanging maneuvers for major hepatectomy. Annals of Surgery. 2007;**245**(1):31-35. DOI: 10.1097/01.sla.0000224725.40979.0a

[86] J. B. Editorial perspective: Resection of large hepatocellular carcinoma using the combination of liver hanging maneuver and anterior approach. World Journal of Surgery. 2010;**34**:1879-1880. DOI: 10.1007/s00268-010-0593-2

[87] Machairas N, Papaconstantinou D, Tsilimigras DI, et al. Comparison between robotic and open liver resection: A systematic review and meta-analysis of short-term outcomes. Updates in Surgery. 2019;**71**(1):39-48. DOI: 10.1007/s13304-019-00629-0

[88] Liu R, Wakabayashi G, Kim H-J, et al. International consensus statement on robotic hepatectomy surgery in 2018. World Journal of Gastroenterology. 2019;**25**(12):1432-1444. DOI: 10.3748/wjg.v25.i12.1432

[89] Fahrner R, Rauchfuß F, Bauschke A, Kissler H, Settmacher U, Zanow J. Robotic hepatic surgery in malignancy: Review of the current literature. Journal of Robotic Surgery. 2019. DOI: 10.1007/s11701-019-00939-w. [E-pub ahead of print]

[90] Khan AS, Garcia-Aroz S, Ansari MA, et al. Assessment and optimization of liver volume before major hepatic resection: Current guidelines and a narrative review. International Journal of Surgery. 2018;**52**:74-81. DOI: 10.1016/j.ijsu.2018.01.042

[91] Cai X, Tong Y, Yu H, et al. The ALPPS in the Treatment of Hepatitis B – Related Hepatocellular Carcinoma With Cirrhosis : A Single-Center Study and Literature Review. Surgical Innovation. 2017:1-7. DOI: 10.1177/1553350617697187

[92] Vennarecci G, Levi Sandri GBEG. Performing the ALPPS procedure by anterior approach and liver hanging maneuver. Annals of Surgery. 2016;**263**(1):e11. DOI: 10.1097/SLA.0000000000001007

[93] Tustumi F, Ernani L, Coelho FF, et al. Preoperative strategies to improve respectability for hepatocellular carcinoma: A systematic review and meta-analysis. HPB Journal. 2018;**20**(12):1109-1118. DOI: 10.1016/j.hpb.2018.06.1798

[94] Sparrelid E, Jonas E, Tzortzakakis A, et al. Dynamic Evaluation of Liver Volume and Function in Associating Liver Partition and Portal Vein Ligation for Staged Hepatectomy. Journal of Gastrointestinal Surgery. 2017:967-974. DOI: 10.1007/s11605-017-3389-y

[95] De Santibañes E, Alvarez FA, Ardiles V. How to avoid postoperative liver failure: A novel method. World Journal of Surgery. 2012;**36**(1):125-128. DOI: 10.1007/s00268-011-1331-0

[96] Schnitzbauer AA, Lang SA, Goessmann H, et al. Right portal vein ligation combined with in situ splitting induces rapid left lateral liver lobe hypertrophy enabling 2-staged extended right hepatic resection in small-for-size settings. Annals of Surgery. 2012;**255**(3):405-414. DOI: 10.1097/SLA.0b013e31824856f5

[97] Zhou Z, Xu M, Lin N, et al. Associating liver partition and portal vein ligation for staged hepatectomy versus conventional two-stage hepatectomy: A systematic review and meta-analysis. World Journal of Surgical Oncology. 2017;**15**(1):1-10. DOI: 10.1186/s12957-017-1295-0

[98] Vennarecci G, Ferraro D, Tudisco A, et al. The ALPPS procedure: Hepatocellular carcinoma as a main indication. An Italian single-center experience. Updates in Surgery. 2018;**71**(1):67-75. DOI: 10.1007/s13304-018-0596-3

[99] Chen K, Pan Y, Zhang B, Liu X, Maher H, Zheng X. Laparoscopic versus open surgery for hepatocellular carcinoma: A meta-analysis of high-quality case-matched studies. Canadian Journal of Gastroenterology and Hepatology. 2018;**2018**:1-15. DOI: 10.1155/2018/1746895

[100] Ishii M, Mizuguchi T, Harada K, et al. Comprehensive review of post-liver resection surgical complications and a new universal classification and grading system. World Journal of Hepatology. 2014;**6**(10):745-751. DOI: 10.4254/wjh.v6.i10.745

[101] Xiong JJ, Altaf K, Javed MA, Huang W, Mukherjee R, Mai G, et al. Meta-analysis of laparoscopic vs open liver resection for hepatocellular carcinoma. Hepatology Research. 2012;**18**(45):6657-6668. DOI: 10.3748/wjg.v18.i45.6657

[102] Swaid F, Geller DA. Minimally invasive primary liver cancer surgery. Surgical Oncology Clinics of North America. 2019;**28**(2):215-227. DOI: 10.1016/j.soc.2018.11.002

[103] Faber W, Seehofer D, Neuhaus P, et al. Repeated liver resection for recurrent hepatocellular carcinoma. Journal of Gastroenterology and Hepatology. 2011;**26**(7):1189-1194. DOI: 10.1111/j.1440-1746.2011.06721.x

[104] Joliat GR, Allemann P, Labgaa I, Demartines N, Halkic N. Treatment and outcomes of recurrent hepatocellular carcinomas. Langenbeck's Archives of Surgery. 2017;**402**(5):737-744. DOI: 10.1007/s00423-017-1582-9

[105] Lacaze L, Scotté M, Nicolle C. Surgical treatment of intra hepatic recurrence of hepatocellular carcinoma. World Journal of Hepatology. 2015;7(13):1755-1760. DOI: 10.4254/wjh.v7.i13.1755

[106] Yang SL, Luo YY, Chen M, et al. A systematic review and meta-analysis comparing the prognosis of multicentric occurrence and vs. intrahepatic metastasis in patients with recurrent hepatocellular carcinoma after hepatectomy. HPB Journal. 2017;**19**(10):835-842. DOI: 10.1016/j.hpb.2017.06.002

[107] Schietroma I, Scheri GC, Pinacchio C, Statzu M, Pascale FG. Hepatitis C Virus and Hepatocellular Carcinoma-Pathogenetic Mechanisms and Impact of Direct-Acting Antivirals. Open Virology Journal. 2018;(12):16-25. DOI: 10.2174/1874357901812010016

[108] Minagawa M, Makuuchi M, Takayama T, Kokudo N. Selection criteria for repeat hepatectomy in patients with recurrent hepatocellular carcinoma. Annals of Surgery. 2003;**238**(5):703-710. DOI: 10.1097/01.sla.0000094549.11754.e6

[109] Song KD, Lim HK, Rhim H, et al. Repeated hepatic resection versus radiofrequency ablation for recurrent hepatocellular carcinoma after hepatic resection: A propensity score matching study. Radiology. 2015;**275**(2):599-608. DOI: 10.1148/radiol.14141568

[110] Hatzaras I, Bischof DA, Fahy B, Cosgrove D, Pawlik TM. Treatment options and surveillance strategies after therapy for hepatocellular carcinoma. Annals of Surgical Oncology. 2014;**21**(3):758-766. DOI: 10.1245/s10434-013-3254-5

Section 2

Role of Surgery in the Management of Hepatic Diseases

Chapter 6

Ischemic Preconditioning Directly or Remotely Applied on the Liver to Reduce Ischemia-Reperfusion Injury in Resections and Transplantation

Maria Eugenia Cornide-Petronio, Mónica B. Jiménez-Castro, Jordi Gracia-Sancho and Carmen Peralta

Abstract

Ischemia-reperfusion (I/R) injury is an important cause of liver damage occurring during surgical procedures. In liver resection, I/R causes post-operative transaminasemia and liver function failure. In liver transplantation, I/R causes graft dysfunction, ranging from biochemical abnormalities to primary non-function of the transplanted organ. Ischemic preconditioning is a surgical strategy to reduce the severity of I/R and improve post-operative outcomes by prior exposure to a brief period of vascular occlusion directly to the target organ or remotely to a distant vascular bed. This chapter aims to discuss the different ischemic preconditioning strategies in both liver resection surgery and liver transplantation. In addition, we will describe the differences of such surgical strategies in both steatotic and non-steatotic livers in both preclinical experiments and clinical practice. Such information may be useful to guide the design of the effective ischemic preconditioning methods in the surgery of hepatic resections and liver transplantation.

Keywords: ischemia-reperfusion injury, liver resections, liver transplantation, ischemic preconditioning, remote ischemic preconditioning

1. Introduction

Ischemia-reperfusion (I/R) injury is a phenomenon in which cellular damage in a hypoxic organ is accentuated following the oxygen restoration [1–3], being a major pathophysiological event and cause of morbidity and mortality in liver resections and transplantation [4]. Despite the attempts to solve this problem, hepatic I/R is an unresolved problem. In addition, hepatic steatosis is a major risk factor for liver surgery, as it is associated with an increased complication index and postoperative mortality after major liver resection and transplantation, since steatotic livers show impaired regenerative response and reduced tolerance to I/R injury compared with non-steatotic ones. Of note, the prevalence of steatosis ranges from 24 to 45%

 IntechOpen

of the population and consequently a further increase in the number of steatotic livers submitted to surgery is to be expected [5]. These observations highlight the need to develop protective strategies in liver surgical conditions.

The mechanisms involved in liver I/R injury are complicated, mainly including microcirculation failure and oxidative stress [4]. A wide range of strategies has been attempted in order to mitigate I/R injury, mainly pharmacological treatments focused on gene therapy, improvement of preservation solutions, among others. However, an effective treatment is still lacking [4] since is difficult to achieve by targeting individual mechanism. Surgical strategies such as the ischemic preconditioning (IPC) technique noted for its effectiveness, as it activates several protective pathways against I/R injury in experimental models should be considered. IPC can be either applied directly to the target organ [6] or remotely (RIPC) to a distant vascular bed [7]. The benefits of the IPC and RIPC observed in experimental models of hepatic warm and cold ischemia [8, 9] prompted human trials of ischemic preconditioning. However, controversial results have been showed in the clinical practice. Therefore, the present chapter aims to describe the current knowledge of the IPC and RIPC in liver resections and liver transplantation of both steatotic and non-steatotic livers. In addition, the scientific controversies regarding the possible beneficial effects of these techniques, in experimental, translational and clinical studies in the setting of liver surgery will be discussed.

2. Ischemic preconditioning

Preconditioning the liver with ischemia involves a brief period of portal triad clamping usually between 5 and 15 min followed by a brief period of reperfusion (10–20 min) before a prolonged period of ischemia [10] (**Figure 1**). The exact mode of action of the IPC in the prevention of post-operative hepatic complication has not yet been fully comprehended. The molecular basis for IPC consists of a sequence of events in which in response to the triggers of IPC, a signal must be generated and transduced into an intracellular message leading to the effector mechanism

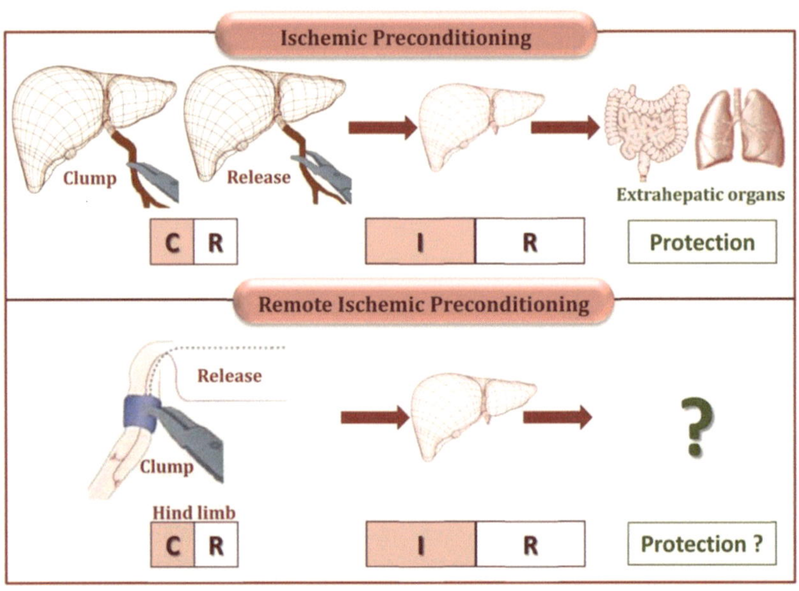

Figure 1.
Schematic illustration of ischemic preconditioning and remote ischemic preconditioning.

of protection [11, 12]. As in the pathophysiology of hepatic I/R, in the modulation of hepatic injury induced by IPC, there is a complex interaction between different mechanisms and cell types [13].

2.1 IPC in experimental models

Over the years, studies with experimental animal models have reported numerous positive effects of IPC on the alleviation of hepatic I/R injury and improvements of post-operative liver functioning. Various combinations of ischemia and reperfusion periods have been tested showing similar beneficial effects: lower aminotransferase levels, reduced hepatocellular injury, and higher survival rates [14]. IPC protected against mitochondrial ROS and thus reduce the oxidative stress-mediated damage in liver I/R injury [15–18]. However, Rüdiger et al. showed that IPC is beneficial in liver submitted to an ischemic period of up to 75 min, but not for more prolonged ischemia [19].

2.1.1 IPC in warm ischemia without liver resection

IPC modulates several molecular pathways involving in I/R. When long periods of liver ischemia occur in hepatectomy or transplantation, the lack of oxygenation induces the rapid ATP consume to generate energy for cellular metabolism, resulting in adenosine production. The accumulation of adenosine provokes its transformation to hypoxanthine and xanthine leading to ROS production. IPC (5 min of ischemia/10 min reperfusion) modulates oxidative stress since reduces the accumulation of xanthine and the conversion of xanthine dehydrogenase (XDH) to xanthine oxidase (XO). IPC (5 min of ischemia/10 min reperfusion) inhibits this ROS generating system, xanthine/XOD [11–13]. The activation of adenosine receptor A2 induced by IPC stimulates the activity of various intracellular kinases, like protein kinase C (PKC)-specifically PKC-δ- and p38 mitogen-activated protein kinase (p38MAPK) [20]. The activation of p38 and c-Jun N-terminal kinase (JNK-1) induced by IPC (10 min of ischemia/10 min reperfusion) is associated with increased cyclin D1 expression and entry into the cell cycle [21]. In addition to this, activation of p38 by different pharmacological strategies mimicking IPC effects, including agonists of the adenosine A2 receptor, carbon monoxide (CO), NO, and atrial natriuretic peptide (ANP) has been considered to be a crucial mechanism of hepatoprotection in the setting of liver surgery [22]. Moreover, autophagic flux is enhanced by liver IPC (10 min of ischemia/10 min reperfusion), since endothelial nitric oxide synthase (eNOS)-derived NO activates autophagy via phosphorylation of p38 MAPK [23]. On the other hand, the mechanism involved in the benefits of IPC might be different dependently of the type of the liver [1]. Indeed, in the presence of steatosis, IPC (5 min of ischemia/10 min reperfusion) reduces MAPK activation (JNK and p38), and this is associated with protection against hepatic I/R injury [24, 25]. The involvement of sirtuin-1 (SIRT1) induction in the benefits of IPC (5 min of ischemia/10 min reperfusion) on normothermic hepatic conditions has been reported [26]. Thus, SIRT1 inhibition decreased the expression of extracellular signal-regulated protein kinases (ERK) and augmented p38 protein levels [26]. ERK activation during IPC (5 min of ischemia/10 min reperfusion) protects against I/R injury in steatotic livers, by inhibiting apoptosis [27], whereas treatment with a p38 activator abolished the benefits of IPC on hepatic damage [24]. In addition, inactivation of GSK-3β by IPC (10 min of ischemia/10–15 min reperfusion) induces β-catenin signaling and subsequently up-regulates anti-apoptotic factors, such as Bcl-2 and survivin, leading to a significant amelioration of liver I/R injury [28, 29]. **Figure 2** shows some of the protective mechanisms of IPC in the hepatic I/R injury.

2.1.2 IPC in liver resections under warm ischemia

The beneficial effects of IPC (10 min of ischemia/5 min reperfusion) in liver partial hepatectomy (PH) have been shown to be linked to better ATP recovery, NO production, antioxidant activities, and regulation of endoplasmic reticulum stress. All of this limited mitochondrial damage and apoptosis. In addition, the ERK1/2 and p38 MAPK activation induced by IPC in PH favors liver regeneration [30]. Furthermore, IPC (10 min of ischemia/10 min of reperfusion) can initiate hepatocyte proliferation action by a signaling mechanism involving TNF-α/IL-6 signal pathway [31]. In contrast, Qian et al. found that IPC impaired residual liver regeneration after major PH without portal blood bypass in rats. In this case, IPC was of 5 min ischemia/10 min reperfusion [32]. Another study testing regenerative capacity of the liver after IPC (10 min ischemia/10 min reperfusion) and PH showed that, despite IPC decreased hepatic injury, it did not influence the regeneration up to 48 h [33].

2.1.3 IPC in reduced-size orthotopic liver transplantation

In a reduced-size orthotopic liver transplantation (ROLT) rat model, IPC (10 min ischemia/10 min reperfusion) has been suggested that potentiates hepatocyte proliferation via TNF-α/IL-6-dependent pathway [34]. In addition, authors described that IPC inhibits IL-1 through NO, increases HGF, and reduces TGF-β to finally promote regeneration [34]. In addition, by another pathway independent

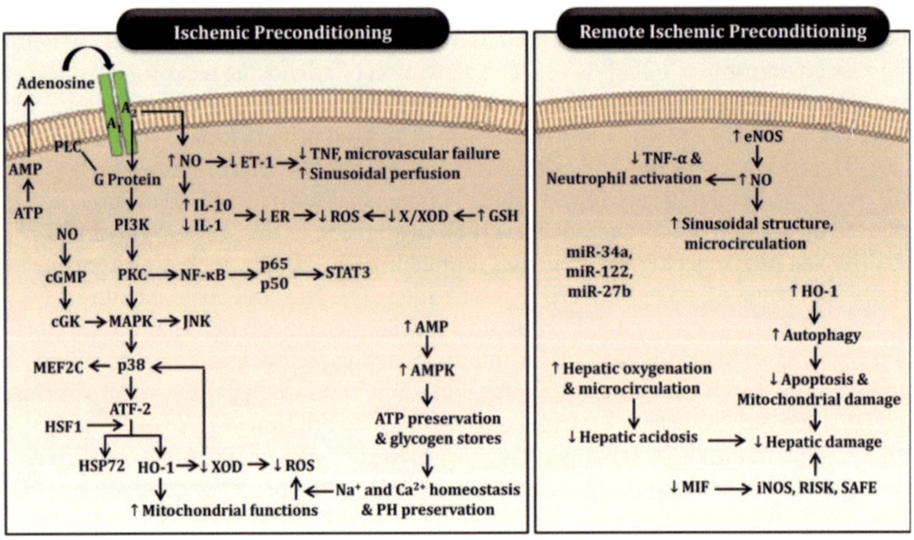

Figure 2.

Protective mechanisms propose of ischemic preconditioning and remote ischemic preconditioning in the hepatic ischemia-reperfusion injury. A2-R: adenosine 2 receptor; AMP: adenosine monophosphate; AMPK: AMP-activated protein kinase; ATF-2: activating transcription factor-2; ATP: adenosine triphosphate; cGMP: guanosine 3′,5′-cyclic monophosphate; eNOS: endothelial nitric oxide synthase; ER: endoplasmic reticulum; ET-1: endothelin-1; GSH: glutathione; HO-1: heme oxygenase-1; HSF-1: heat shock transcription factor-1; HSP72: heat-shock protein 72; IL: interleukin; iNOS: inducible nitric oxide synthase; JNK: jun N-terminal kinase; MAPK: mitogen-activated protein kinase; MEF2c: myocyte enhancer factor-2; MIF: macrophage migration inhibitory factor; NF-κB: factor nuclear factor-kappa B; NO: nitric oxide; PI3K: phosphatidylinositol 3-kinase; PKC: protein kinase C; PLC: phospholipase C; ROS: reactive oxygen species; STAT3: signal transducer and activator of transcription-3; TNF: tumor necrosis factor; X/XOD: xanthine/ xanthine oxidase.

of NO, IPC induced over-expression of heat shock protein 70 (HSP70) and heme-oxigenase-1 (HO-1) [35]. HO-1 protects against I/R injury, whereas the benefits resulting from HSP70 are mainly related to hepatocyte proliferation [35]. In addition, when steatotic grafts from living donors were transplanted applying IPC, the incidence of necrosis was reduced and the expression of both pro-autophagic beclin-1 and LC3 was increased [36]. On the other hand, in a rat model of ROLT with 70 or 90% hepatectomy, IPC (10 min ischemia/15 min reperfusion) impaired hepatic proliferative response by decreasing IL-6 and blunting cell cycle progression through a mechanism at least partially independent of STAT3 [37].

2.1.4 IPC in orthotopic liver transplantation

IPC (5 min ischemia/10 min reperfusion) has protected liver grafts in an experimental model of orthotopic liver transplantation (OLT) by modulation of xanthine/XOD system [38]. IPC reduced cAMP generation, thus ameliorating hepatic injury and survival of recipients with steatotic grafts [39]. In addition, AMPK activation by IPC (5 min ischemia/10 min reperfusion) increased the accumulation of adiponectin in steatotic liver grafts. This increased resistin and activated PI3K/Akt pathway, thus protecting steatotic livers against damage that follows transplantation [40]. However, it should be noted that in experimental liver transplantation from cadaveric donors, brain death abrogates the benefits of IPC (5 min ischemia/10 min reperfusion) in both steatotic and non-steatotic liver transplantation [41, 42]. Indeed, in the setting of liver transplantation, the inflammatory response induced by brain dead, present in the liver before the induction of IPC, would interact with various mechanistic aspects of IPC and block the eventual IPC response. Thus, Jimenez-Castro et al. have demonstrated that the treatment with acetylcholine protected liver grafts from the deleterious effects induced by brain death [41]. Under these conditions, the application of IPC was useful to improve the post-operative outcomes after transplantation.

In addition to the liver, the benefits of IPC in experimental models of warm ischemia and liver transplantation have been observed in extrahepatic organs. Thus, IPC protects against lung damage associated with liver transplantation. The application of IPC in liver before I/R can prevent the release of both TNF and xanthine/XOD from the liver to the circulation. This regulated the P-selectin up-regulation and the neutrophil accumulation in remote organs such as lung and splanchnic organs [43].

2.2 IPC in clinical trials

The benefits of IPC observed in experimental models of hepatic resections and liver transplantation [8, 9] prompted human trials of IPC. The benefits of this surgical strategy have been evidenced in patients submitted to liver resections, protecting both steatotic and non-steatotic livers [44]. However, different results have been reported on the effects of IPC in the clinical practice of liver transplantation [45, 46].

2.2.1 IPC in liver resections

The first clinical trial testing IPC in patients undergoing major PH was reported by Clavien et al. [47]. Authors conclude that IPC (10 min ischemia/10 min reperfusion) is a protective strategy against hepatic ischemia in humans, particularly in young patients requiring a prolonged period of inflow occlusion and in the presence of steatosis [44, 47]. Other clinical trials also suggest that IPC (10 min ischemia/10 min reperfusion) provides both better intraoperative hemodynamic stability and anti-ischemic effects compared with intermittent clamping [48, 49]. Regarding the molecular basis of IPC (10 min ischemia/10 min reperfusion) in clinical PH, its beneficial effects have been shown to be linked to the down-regulation of potentially cytotoxic functions of PMNLs elicited by the Pringle Maneuver [50]. In addition, IPC (10 min ischemia/15 min reperfusion) increased the generation of adenosine and attenuated the degradation of purines in patients undergoing PH. Moreover, IPC appeared to attenuate apoptotic response of the liver remnant after resection [51]. Other clinical trial revealed that IPC (10 min ischemia/10 min reperfusion) stimulated the expression of the IL-1-RA, inducible nitric oxide synthase (iNOS), and Bcl-2 which decreased the inflammatory response and abrogated liver I/R injury [52]. Interestingly, since the ischemic period and pathophysiology are similar in partial hepatectomy and living donor liver transplantation, IPC could reduce damage and improve liver regeneration failure, a relevant risk factor in living donor liver transplantation [34]. Moreover, IPC could be implemented as an appropriate surgical strategy for the use of suboptimal livers, such as steatotic ones, in the clinical practice. Different results indicate that in patients with liver cirrhosis, IPC (5 min ischemia/5 min reperfusion) has been a suitable method to decrease liver I/R injury [53, 54]. Recently, the protective mechanism of IPC in patients with liver cirrhosis subjected to PH has been associated with changes in MAPK pathways [54]. In contrast, IPC applied for 15 min followed by 5 min reperfusion did not improve liver tolerance to I/R injury after PH in patients with liver cirrhosis [55]. In fact, RIPC did not induce changes in the postoperative levels of transaminases, bilirubin, and albumin nor reduced the morbidity and mortality rates and the duration of hospitalization [55].

2.2.2 IPC in orthotopic liver transplantation

Clinical trials in liver transplantation report different results on the effects of IPC against hepatic I/R injury. An IPC of 10 min ischemia/10 min reperfusion before liver transplantation reduced inflammatory response, improved ischemia tolerance, and decreased early graft function [56]. However, although the application of IPC (10 min ischemia/15 min reperfusion) reduced hepatocellular necrosis, it showed no clinical benefits [57]. In the largest prospective randomized trial of 10 min period IPC in liver transplantation from cadaveric donors, I/R injury was greater when IPC was applied [45], and it was called the "IPC paradox." This was in accordance with the results obtained in experimental model of liver transplantation from cadaveric donors indicating that brain death abrogates the benefits of IP on post-operative outcomes [41, 42]. In fact, a microarray analysis in a randomized trial of 10 min IPC in deceased donor liver transplantation identified alteration of the expression of different antioxidant, immunological, lipid biosynthesis, cell development and growth transcripts, which are associated with hepatic damage [58].

3. Remote ischemic preconditioning

RIPC is a surgical technique by which preconditioning of one organ or vascular bed provides protection to distant organs or vascular beds during a sustained period of ischaemia (**Figure 1**). Few experimental and clinical studies, most of them from the last years, have addressed the effects of RIPC in livers submitted to I/R.

3.1 RIPC in experimental models

3.1.1 RIPC in warm ischemia without liver resection

When RIPC is applied in the hind limb, it reduced hepatic warm I/R injury of mice, rats, and rabbits. RIPC (5–10 min ischemia/5–10 min reperfusion) has been shown to improve hepatic oxygenation and microcirculation and to reduce hepatic acidosis and damage [59, 60]. RIPC (4 min ischemia/4 min reperfusion) induced eNOS activation, leading to NO production to preserve sinusoidal structure and blood flow [61]. In addition, RIPC (5 min ischemia/5 min reperfusion) regulated the expressions of iNOS and eNOS and the expressions of miR-34a, miR-122, and miR-27b injury related miRs in fatty livers, thus attenuating I/R injury [62, 63]. RIPC (10 min ischemia/10 min reperfusion) also induced the up-regulation of HO-1, induced autophagy, and then reduced the damaged mitochondria to inhibit apoptosis and eventually protect hepatic cells from I/R injury [64, 65]. Moreover, RIPC (5 min ischemia/5 min reperfusion) reduced neutrophil activation and adhesion and TNF-α [66]. Controversial results have been described in a rat model in which RIPC protocol included 3 cycles of 10 min ischemia interspersed with 10 min of reperfusion periods [67]. Regarding the hemodynamic and microcirculatory alterations, RIPC protocol had beneficial effect; however, the histopathological findings were paradox [67, 68]. In addition to RIPC in the hind limb, when RIPC (5 min ischemia/5 min reperfusion) is applied in kidney, it has also been shown to protect liver against I/R injury, improving blood flow, histology, and redox-state [69]. **Figure 2** shows some of the protective mechanisms of RIPC in the hepatic I/R injury.

3.1.2 RIPC in liver resections

A recent study in mice showed that RIPC (3 cycles of 5 min of ischemia each followed by 5 min of reperfusion) applied in the right femoral vascular bundle did not affect regeneration after 70%-PH [70]. However, of clinical interest, the same protocol of RIPC improved liver weight gain and hepatocyte mitoses after 90%-PH [70].

3.1.3 RIPC in orthotopic liver transplantation

In an experimental model of OLT, RIPC based on 4 cycles of 5 min of ischemia and 5 min of reperfusion was applied on the infrarenal aorta. The results suggested that RIPC might confer potent protection against the detrimental effects of I/R injury including apoptosis and inflammation [71]. In addition, authors suggest that HO-1 overexpression could play an orchestrating role in RIPC (5 min ischemia/5 min reperfusion)-mediated organ protection [71]. In addition, a recent study showed that the same protocol of RIPC also exhibits protective effects, as indicated by increased portal venous flow and microcirculation, as well as decreased AST and ALT levels and a reduced Suzuki score in a model of OLT [72]. Authors suggest that the RIPC inhibited the macrophage migration inhibitory factor (MIF), which resulted in the modulation of further downstream pro-survival mechanisms (iNOS, RISK-, SAFE-pathways), protecting graft injury [72].

3.2 RIPC in clinical trials

Only three studies dated in 2017 and 2018 have addressed the effects of RIPC in the clinical liver surgery.

3.2.1 RIPC in liver resections

In major HP, RIPC was shown to reduce liver I/R injury as indicated by a reduction in post-operative transaminases and increased ICG clearance [73]. To induce RIPC, a tourniquet was inflated to induce 10 min of ischemia and then deflated for 10 min to reperfuse the leg. This was repeated twice prior to commencing the operation. RIPC has potential to reduce liver injury following PH [73]. In addition, other clinical trial where RIPC was induced by three cycles of 5 min of ischemia of right upper limb followed by 5 min of reperfusion showed hepatic cytoprotective effects assessed by cholinesterase and bilirubin levels during liver resection [74]. Authors suggest that a shorter protocol of RIPC is safe and of equal effect, although the mechanisms of this effect must be investigated in future studies [74].

3.2.2 RIPC in orthotopic liver transplantation

The first trial to investigate the feasibility of RIPC in liver transplant recipients was addressing by Robertson et al. [75]. The trial involved randomization of adult recipients undergoing deceased donor liver transplantation. To induce RIPC, a tourniquet was inflated for 5 min and then deflated for 5 min to reperfuse the leg. This was repeated twice and completed prior to the transplant procedure. Authors demonstrated that RIPC is feasible, acceptable to patients and safe in this group of patients but clinical benefits within the first 3 months post transplantation were not detected [75]. Authors suggest that 5 min cycles are insufficient to create localized ischemia in the limb [75].

4. Conclusion

Surgical strategies such as the induction of IPC or RIPC could be of clinical interest in human liver resections and liver transplantation in both steatotic and non-steatotic livers. Both IPC and RIPC are easy to apply, inexpensive and does not require the use of drugs with potential side effects, but it requires a period of pre-ischemic manipulation for organ protection. These preconditioning techniques have been demonstrated to be promising tools for the reduction of hepatic I/R injury in different warm and cold ischemia models. Therefore, the potential applications of IPC and RIPC in human liver surgery are numerous. The benefits of IPC and RIPC have been evidenced in patients submitted to partial hepatectomy in both steatotic and non-steatotic livers. In our view, IPC and RIPC could resolve, at least partially, the lack of liver grafts available for transplant, since it can improve the post-operative outcome of liver grafts from extended criteria donors. However, controversial results on the effects of IPC and RIPC have been reported in the clinical practice of liver transplantation. It should be considered that the underlying mechanisms of both IPC and RIPC and their relevance in liver surgery remain poorly understood. Indeed, as stated along this chapter, most of the experimental studies have been focused on the molecular changes occurring during IPC and RIPC in non-brain-dead donors. Moreover, most of the experimental studies of IPC and RIPC have been performed only in I/R injury models, without hepatic resections or liver transplantation. The tolerance to I/R injury induced by either IPC or RIPC is dependently of the number of cycles of I/R and their duration as well as the surgical procedures. The clinical application of strategies designed at benchside will depend on the use of experimental models of IPC and RIPC that resemble as much as possible the clinical conditions. Multidisciplinary research groups should devote additional efforts to better understand the molecular mechanisms of IPC and RIPC during the different clinical liver surgery setting to ultimately develop useful surgical strategies aimed at reducing I/R damage.

Acknowledgements

This research was supported by the Ministerio de Economía y Competitividad (project grant SAF-2015-64857-R) Madrid, Spain; the European Union (FondosFeder, "una manera de hacer Europa"); by CERCA Program/Generalitat de Catalunya; by the Secretaria d'Universitats i Recerca (Grant 2017SGR-551) Barcelona, Spain. J Gracia-Sancho received continuous funding from the Instituto de Salud Carlos III (currently FIS PI17/00012) and the CIBEREHD, from Ministerio de Ciencia, Innovación y Universidades.

Conflict of interest

The authors declare that they have no conflict of interest.

Author details

Maria Eugenia Cornide-Petronio[1†], Mónica B. Jiménez-Castro[2†], Jordi Gracia-Sancho[3] and Carmen Peralta[1,4,5*]

1 Institut d'Investigacions Biomèdiques August Pi i Sunyer (IDIBAPS), Barcelona, Spain

2 Transplant Biomedicals, S.L., Barcelona, Spain

3 Barcelona Hepatic Hemodynamic Laboratory, Institut d'Investigacions Biomèdiques August Pi i Sunyer (IDIBAPS), Hospital Clínic de Barcelona, Centro de Investigaciones Biomédicas en Red en Enfermedades Hepáticas y Digestivas (CIBEREHD), Barcelona, Spain

4 Centro de Investigación Biomédica en Red de Enfermedades Hepáticas y Digestivas (CIBEREHD), Barcelona, Spain

5 Facultad de Medicina, Universidad International de Cataluña, Barcelona, Spain

*Address all correspondence to: cperalta@clinic.ub.es

† Both authors contributed equally to this work.

IntechOpen

© 2019 The Author(s). Licensee IntechOpen. This chapter is distributed under the terms of the Creative Commons Attribution License (http://creativecommons.org/licenses/by/3.0), which permits unrestricted use, distribution, and reproduction in any medium, provided the original work is properly cited. CC BY

References

[1] Serafin A, Rosello-Catafau J, Prats N, Xaus C, Gelpi E, Peralta C. Ischemic preconditioning increases the tolerance of fatty liver to hepatic ischemia-reperfusion injury in the rat. The American Journal of Pathology. 2002;**161**:587-601. DOI: 10.1016/S0002-9440(10)64214-9

[2] Clavien P, Harvey P, Strasberg S. Preservation and reperfusion injuries in liver allografts. An overview and synthesis of current studies. Transplantation. 1992;**53**:957-978

[3] Huguet C, Gavelli A, Chieco P, Bona S, Harb J, Joseph J, et al. Liver ischemia for hepatic resection: where is the limit? Surgery. 1992;**111**:251-259

[4] Fu P, Li W. Nitric oxide in liver ischemia-reperfusion injury. In: Muriel P, editor. Liver Pathophysiology. London: Elsevier INC; 2017. pp. 125-127

[5] Safwan M, Collins KM, Abouljoud MS, Salgia R. Outcome of liver transplantation in patients with prior bariatric surgery. Liver Transplantation. 2017;**23**:1415-1421. DOI: 10.1002/lt.24832

[6] Murry CE, Jennings RB, Reimer KA. Preconditioning with ischemia: A delay of lethal cell injury in ischemic myocardium. Circulation. 1986;**74**:1124-1136

[7] Przyklenk K, Bauer B, Ovize M, Kloner RA, Whittaker P. Regional ischemic 'preconditioning' protects remote virgin myocardium from subsequent sustained coronary occlusion. Circulation. 1993;**87**:893-899

[8] Desai KK, Dikdan GS, Shareef A, Koneru B. Ischemic preconditioning of the liver: a few perspectives from the bench to bedside translation. Liver Transplantation. 2008;**14**:1569-1577. DOI: 10.1002/lt.21630

[9] Bahde R, Spiegel HU. Hepatic ischaemia-reperfusion injury from bench to bedside. The British Journal of Surgery. 2010;**97**:1461-1475. DOI: 10.1002/bjs.7176

[10] Suyavaran A, Thirunavukkarasu C. Preconditioning methods in the management of hepatic ischemia reperfusion-induced injury: Update on molecular and future perspectives. Hepatology Research. 2017;**47**:31-48. DOI: 10.1111/hepr.12706

[11] Serafín A, Fernández-Zabalegui L, Prats N, Wu ZY, Roselló-Catafau J, Peralta C. Ischemic preconditioning: tolerance to hepatic ischemia-reperfusion injury. Histology and Histopathology. 2004;**19**:281-289. DOI: 10.14670/HH-19.281

[12] Cutrin JC, Perrelli MG, Cavalieri B, Peralta C, Rosell Catafau J, Poli G. Microvascular dysfunction induced by reperfusion injury and protective effect of ischemic preconditioning. Free Radical Biology & Medicine. 2002;**33**:1200-1208. DOI: 10.1016/S0891-5849(02)01017-1

[13] Massip-Salcedo M, Roselló-Catafau J, Prieto J, Avíla MA, Peralta C. The response of the hepatocyte to ischemia. Liver International. 2007;**27**:6-16. DOI: 10.1111/j.1478-3231.2006.01390.x

[14] Theodoraki K, Tympa A, Karmaniolou I, Tsaroucha A, Arkadopoulos N, Smyrniotis V. Ischemia/reperfusion injury in liver resection: a review of preconditioning methods. Surgery Today. 2011;**41**:620-629. DOI: 10.1007/s00595-010-4444-4

[15] Quarrie R, Cramer BM, Lee DS, Steinbaugh GE, Erdahl W, Pfeiffer DR, et al. Ischemic preconditioning decreases mitochondrial proton leak and reactive oxygen species production in the postischemic heart. The Journal

of Surgical Research. 2010;**165**:5-14. DOI: 10.1016/j.jss.2010.09.018

[16] Jaeschke H, Woolbright BL. Current strategies to minimize hepatic ischemia–reperfusion injury by targeting reactive oxygen species. Transplantation Reviews (Orlando, Fla.). 2012;**26**:103-114. DOI: 10.1016/j.trre.2011.10.006

[17] Osman AS, Osman AH, Kamel MM. Study of the protective effect of ischemic and pharmacological preconditioning on hepatic ischemic reperfusion injury induced in rats. JGH Open. 2017;**1**:105-111. DOI: 10.1002/jgh3.12018

[18] Gabiatti G, Grezzana-Filho TJM, Cerski CTS, Bofill C, Valle S, Corso CO. Topical hepatic hypothermia associated with ischemic preconditioning. Histopathological and biochemical analysis of ischemia reperfusion damage in a 24 hour model 1. Acta Cirúrgica Brasileira. 2018;**33**:924-934. DOI: 10.1590/s0102-865020180100000007

[19] Rüdiger HA, Kang KJ, Sindram D, Riehle HM, Clavien PA. Comparison of ischemic preconditioning and intermittent and continuous inflow occlusion in the murine liver. Annals of Surgery. 2002;**235**:400-407

[20] Yun N, Lee SM. Activation of protein kinase C delta reduces hepatocellular damage in ischemic preconditioned rat liver. The Journal of Surgical Research. 2013;**185**:869-876. DOI: 10.1016/j.jss.2013.07.005

[21] Teoh N, Leclercq I, Pena AD, Farrell G. Low-dose TNF-alpha protects against hepatic ischemia-reperfusion injury in mice: implications for preconditioning. Hepatology. 2003;**37**:118-128. DOI: 10.1053/jhep.2003.50009

[22] Alchera E, Dal Ponte C, Imarisio C, Albano E, Carini R. Molecular mechanisms of liver preconditioning. World Journal of Gastroenterology. 2010;**16**:6058-6067. DOI: 10.3748/wjg.v16.i48.6058

[23] Shin JK, Kang JW, Lee SM. Enhanced nitric oxide-mediated autophagy contributes to the hepatoprotective effects of ischemic preconditioning during ischemia and reperfusion. Nitric Oxide. 2016;**58**:10-19. DOI: 10.1016/j.niox.2016.05.007

[24] Massip-Salcedo M, Casillas-Ramirez A, Franco-Gou R, Bartrons R, Ben Mosbah I, Serafin A, et al. Heat shock proteins and mitogen-activated protein kinases in steatotic livers undergoing ischemia-reperfusion: some answers. The American Journal of Pathology. 2006;**168**:1474-1485. DOI: 10.2353/ajpath.2006.050645

[25] Massip-Salcedo M, Zaouali MA, Padrissa-Altés S, Casillas-Ramirez A, Rodés J, Roselló-Catafau J, et al. Activation of peroxisome proliferator-activated receptor-alpha inhibits the injurious effects of adiponectin in rat steatotic liver undergoing ischemia-reperfusion. Hepatology. 2008;**47**:461-472. DOI: 10.1002/hep.21935

[26] Pantazi E, Zaouali MA, Bejaoui M, Serafin A, Folch-Puy E, Petegnief V, et al. Silent information regulator 1 protects the liver against ischemia-reperfusion injury: implications in steatotic liver ischemic preconditioning. Transplant International. 2014;**27**:493-503. DOI: 10.1111/tri.12276

[27] Terada K, Kaziro Y, Satoh T. Analysis of Ras-dependent signals that prevent caspase-3 activation and apoptosis induced by cytokine deprivation in hematopoietic cells. Biochemical and Biophysical Research Communications. 2000;**267**:449-455. DOI: 10.1006/bbrc.1999.1955

[28] Ko JS, Gwak MS, Kim GS, Shin YH, Ryu S, Kim JS, et al. The protective effect of ischemic preconditioning

against hepatic ischemic-reperfusion injury under isoflurane anesthesia in rats. Transplantation Proceedings. 2013;**45**:1704-1707. DOI: 10.1016/j.transproceed.2012.08.026

[29] Yan Y, Li G, Tian X, Ye Y, Gao Z, Yao J, et al. Ischemic preconditioning increases GSK-3β/β-catenin levels and ameliorates liver ischemia/reperfusion injury in rats. International Journal of Molecular Medicine. 2015;**35**:1625-1632. DOI: 10.3892/ijmm.2015.2153

[30] Ben Mosbah I, Duval H, Mbatchi SF, Ribault C, Grandadam S, Pajaud J, et al. Intermittent selective clamping improves rat liver regeneration by attenuating oxidative and endoplasmic reticulum stress. Cell Death & Disease. 2014;**5**:e1107. DOI: 10.1038/cddis.2014.65

[31] Jin LM, Jin SF, Liu YX, Zhou L, Xie HY, Yan S, et al. Ischemic preconditioning enhances hepatocyte proliferation in the early phase after ischemia under hemi-hepatectomy in rats. Hepatobiliary & Pancreatic Diseases International. 2012;**11**:521-526. DOI: 10.1016/S1499-3872(12)60217-3

[32] Qian Y, Liu Z, Geng X. Lack of protection of ischaemic preconditioning in the rat model of major hepatectomy with ischaemia reperfusion injury. Asian Journal of Surgery. 2008;**31**:140-147. DOI: 10.1016/S1015-9584(08)60075-5

[33] Gomez D, Homer-Vanniasinkam S, Graham AM, Prasad KR. Role of ischaemic preconditioning in liver regeneration following major liver resection and transplantation. World Journal of Gastroenterology. 2007;**13**: 657-670. DOI: 10.3748/wjg.v13.i5.657

[34] Franco-Gou R, Peralta C, Massip-Salcedo M, Xaus C, Serafín A, Roselló-Catafau J. Protection of reduced-size liver for transplantation. American Journal of Transplantation. 2004;**4**:1408-1420. DOI: 10.1111/j.1600-6143.2004.00532.x

[35] Franco-Gou R, Roselló-Catafau J, Casillas-Ramirez A, Massip-Salcedo M, Rimola A, Calvo N, et al. How ischaemic preconditioning protects small liver grafts. The Journal of Pathology. 2006;**208**:62-73. DOI: 10.1002/path.1859

[36] Esposti DD, Domart MC, Sebagh M, Harper F, Pierron G, Brenner C, et al. Autophagy is induced by ischemic preconditioning in human livers formerly treated by chemotherapy to limit necrosis. Autophagy. 2010;**6**:172-174

[37] Yao A, Li X, Pu L, Zhong J, Liu X, Yu Y, et al. Impaired hepatic regeneration by ischemic preconditioning in a rat model of small-for-size liver transplantation. Transplant Immunology. 2007;**18**:37-43. DOI: 10.1016/j.trim.2007.02.002

[38] Fernández L, Carrasco-Chaumel E, Serafín A, Xaus C, Grande L, Rimola A, et al. Is ischemic preconditioning a useful strategy in steatotic liver transplantation? American Journal of Transplantation. 2004;**4**:888-899. DOI: 10.1111/j.1600-6143.2004.00447.x

[39] Jiménez-Castro MB, Casillas-Ramirez A, Massip-Salcedo M, Elias-Miro M, Serafin A, Rimola A, et al. Cyclic adenosine 3′,5′-monophosphate in rat steatotic liver transplantation. Liver Transplantation. 2011;**17**:1099-1110. DOI: 10.1002/lt.22359

[40] Jiménez-Castro MB, Casillas-Ramírez A, Mendes-Braz M, Massip-Salcedo M, Gracia-Sancho J, Elias-Miró M, et al. Adiponectin and resistin protect steatotic livers undergoing transplantation. Journal of Hepatology. 2013;**59**:1208-1214. DOI: 10.1016/j.jhep.2013.07.015

[41] Jiménez-Castro MB, Meroño N, Mendes-Braz M, Gracia-Sancho J, Martínez-Carreres L, Cornide-Petronio ME, et al. The effect of brain death in rat steatotic and non-steatotic liver

transplantation with previous ischemic preconditioning. Journal of Hepatology. 2015;**62**:83-91. DOI: 10.1016/j.jhep.2014.07.031

[42] Cornide-Petronio ME, Negrete-Sánchez E, Mendes-Braz M, Casillas-Ramírez A, Bujaldon E, Meroño N, et al. The effect of high-mobility group box 1 in rat steatotic and nonsteatotic liver transplantation from donors after brain death. American Journal of Transplantation. 2016;**16**:1148-1159. DOI: 10.1111/ajt.13560

[43] Peralta C, Fernández L, Panés J, Prats N, Sans M, Piqué JM, et al. Preconditioning protects against systemic disorders associated with hepatic ischemia-reperfusion through blockade of tumor necrosis factor-induced P-selectin up-regulation in the rat. Hepatology. 2001;**33**:100-113. DOI: 10.1053/jhep.2001.20529

[44] Clavien PA, Selzner M, Rüdiger HA, Graf R, Kadry Z, Rousson V, et al. A prospective randomized study in 100 consecutive patients undergoing major liver resection with versus without ischemic preconditioning. Annals of Surgery. 2003;**238**:843-850. DOI: 10.1097/01.sla.0000098620.27623.7d

[45] Koneru B, Shareef A, Dikdan G, Desai K, Klein KM, Peng B, et al. The ischemic preconditioning paradox in deceased donor liver transplantation-evidence from a prospective randomized single blind clinical trial. American Journal of Transplantation. 2007;7:2788-2796. DOI: 10.1111/j.1600-6143.2007.02009.x

[46] Robertson FP, Magill LJ, Wright GP, Fuller B, Davidson BR. A systematic review and meta-analysis of donor ischaemic preconditioning in liver transplantation. Transplant International. 2016;**29**:1147-1154. DOI: 10.1111/tri.12849

[47] Clavien PA, Yadav S, Sindram D, Bentley RC. Protective effects of ischemic preconditioning for liver resection performed under inflow occlusion in humans. Annals of Surgery. 2000;**232**:155-162. DOI: 10.1097/00000658-200008000-00001

[48] Nuzzo G, Giuliante F, Vellone M, De Cosmo G, Ardito F, Murazio M, et al. Pedicle clamping with ischemic preconditioning in liver resection. Liver Transplantation. 2004;**10**:S53-S57. DOI: 10.1002/lt.20045

[49] Choukèr A, Schachtner T, Schauer R, Dugas M, Löhe F, Martignoni A, et al. Effects of Pringle manoeuvre and ischaemic preconditioning on haemodynamic stability in patients undergoing elective hepatectomy: a randomized trial. British Journal of Anaesthesia. 2004;**93**:204-211. DOI: 10.1093/bja/aeh195

[50] Choukèr A, Martignoni A, Schauer R, Dugas M, Rau HG, Jauch KW, et al. Beneficial effects of ischemic preconditioning in patients undergoing hepatectomy: the role of neutrophils. Archives of Surgery. 2005;**140**:129-136. DOI: 10.1001/archsurg.140.2.129

[51] Arkadopoulos N, Kostopanagiotou G, Theodoraki K, Farantos C, Theodosopoulos T, Stafyla V, et al. Ischemic preconditioning confers antiapoptotic protection during major hepatectomies performed under combined inflow and outflow exclusion of the liver. A randomized clinical trial. World Journal of Surgery. 2009;**33**:1909-1915. DOI: 10.1007/s00268-009-0117-0

[52] Barrier A, Olaya N, Chiappini F, Roser F, Scatton O, Artus C, et al. Ischemic preconditioning modulates the expression of several genes, leading to the overproduction of IL-1Ra, iNOS, and Bcl-2 in a human model of liver ischemia-reperfusion. The FASEB Journal. 2005;**19**:1617-1626. DOI: 10.1096/fj.04-3445com

[53] Li SQ, Liang LJ, Huang JF, Li Z. Ischemic preconditioning protects liver from hepatectomy under hepatic inflow occlusion for hepatocellular carcinoma patients with cirrhosis. World Journal of Gastroenterology. 2004;**10**:2580-2584. DOI: 10.3748/wjg.v10.i17.2580

[54] Wang L, Feng L, Rong W, Liu M, Wu F, Yu W, et al. Regional ischemic preconditioning has clinical value in cirrhotic HCC through MAPK pathways. Journal of Gastrointestinal Surgery. 2018. DOI: 10.1007/s11605-018-3960-1

[55] Ye B, Zhao H, Hou H, Wang G, Liu F, Zhao Y, et al. Ischemic preconditioning provides no additive clinical value in liver resection of cirrhotic and non-cirrhotic patients under portal triad clamping: A prospective randomized controlled trial. Clinics and Research in Hepatology and Gastroenterology. 2014;**38**:467-474. DOI: 10.1016/j.clinre.2014.03.013

[56] Azoulay D, Del Gaudio M, Andreani P, Ichai P, Sebag M, Adam R, et al. Effects of 10 minutes of ischemic preconditioning of the cadaveric liver on the graft's preservation and function: the ying and the yang. Annals of Surgery. 2005;**242**:133-139. DOI: 10.1097/01.sla.0000167848.96692.ad

[57] Cescon M, Grazi GL, Grassi A, Ravaioli M, Vetrone G, Ercolani G, et al. Effect of ischemic preconditioning in whole liver transplantation from deceased donors. A pilot study. Liver Transplantation. 2006;**12**:628-635. DOI: 10.1002/lt.20640

[58] Raza A, Dikdan G, Desai KK, Shareef A, Fernandes H, Aris V, et al. Global gene expression profiles of ischemic preconditioning in deceased donor liver transplantation. Liver Transplantation. 2010;**16**:588-599. DOI: 10.1002/lt.22049

[59] Tapuria N, Junnarkar SP, Dutt N, Abu-Amara M, Fuller B, Seifalian AM, et al. Effect of remote ischemic preconditioning on hepatic microcirculation and function in a rat model of hepatic ischemia reperfusion injury. HPB: The Official Journal of the International Hepato Pancreato Biliary Association. 2009;**11**:108-117. DOI: 10.1111/j.1477-2574.2009.00006.x

[60] Kanoria S, Glantzounis G, Quaglia A, Dinesh S, Fusai G, Davidson BR, et al. Remote preconditioning improves hepatic oxygenation after ischaemia reperfusion injury. Transplant International. 2012;**25**:783-791. DOI: 10.1111/j.1432-2277.2012.01481.x

[61] Abu-Amara M, Yang SY, Quaglia A, Rowley P, de Mel A, Tapuria N, et al. Nitric oxide is an essential mediator of the protective effects of remote ischaemic preconditioning in a mouse model of liver ischaemia/reperfusion injury. Clinical Science (London, England). 2011;**121**:257-266. DOI: 10.1042/CS20100598

[62] Duan YF, Sun DL, Chen J, Zhu F, An Y. MicroRNA-29a/b/c targets iNOS and is involved in protective remote ischemic preconditioning in an ischemia-reperfusion rat model of non-alcoholic fatty liver disease. Oncology Letters. 2017;**13**:1775-1782. DOI: 10.3892/ol.2017.5623

[63] Duan YF, An Y, Zhu F, Jiang Y. Remote ischemic preconditioning protects liver ischemia-reperfusion injury by regulating eNOS-NO pathway and liver microRNA expressions in fatty liver rats. Hepatobiliary & Pancreatic Diseases International. 2017;**16**:387-394. DOI: 10.1016/S1499-3872(17)60006-7

[64] Lai IR, Chang KJ, Chen CF, Tsai HW. Transient limb ischemia induces remote preconditioning in liver among rats: the protective role of heme oxygenase-1. Transplantation. 2006;**81**:1311-1137. DOI: 10.1097/01.tp.0000203555.14546.63

[65] Wang Y, Shen J, Xiong X, Xu Y, Zhang H, Huang C, et al. Remote ischemic preconditioning protects against liver ischemia-reperfusion injury via heme oxygenase-1-induced autophagy. PLoS One. 2014;**9**:e98834. DOI: 10.1371/journal.pone.0098834

[66] Tapuria N, Junnarkar S, Abu-Amara M, Fuller B, Seifalian AM, Davidson BR. Modulation of microcirculatory changes in the late phase of hepatic ischaemia-reperfusion injury by remote ischaemic preconditioning. HPB: The Official Journal of the International Hepato Pancreato Biliary Association. 2012;**14**:87-97. DOI: 10.1111/j.1477-2574.2011.00407.x

[67] Magyar Z, Varga G, Mester A, Ghanem S, Somogyi V, Tanczos B, et al. Is the early or delayed remote ischemic preconditioning the more effective from a microcirculatory and histological point of view in a rat model of partial liver ischemia-reperfusion? Acta Cirúrgica Brasileira. 2018;**33**:597-608. DOI: 10.1590/s0102-865020180070000005

[68] Magyar Z, Mester A, Nadubinszky G, Varga G, Ghanem S, Somogyi V, et al. Beneficial effects of remote organ ischemic preconditioning on micro-rheological parameters during liver ischemia-reperfusion in the rat. Clinical Hemorheology and Microcirculation. 2018;**70**:181-190. DOI: 10.3233/CH-170351

[69] Czigány Z, Turóczi Z, Ónody P, Harsányi L, Lotz G, Hegedüs V, et al. Remote ischemic perconditioning protects the liver from ischemia-reperfusion injury. The Journal of Surgical Research. 2013;**185**:605-613. DOI: 10.1016/j.jss.2013.07.018

[70] Kambakamba P, Linecker M, Schneider M, Kron P, Limani P, Tschuor C, et al. Novel benefits of remote ischemic preconditioning through VEGF-dependent protection from resection-induced liver failure in the mouse. Annals of Surgery. 2018;**268**:885-893. DOI: 10.1097/SLA.0000000000002891

[71] Czigany Z, Bleilevens C, Beckers C, Stoppe C, Möhring M, Fülöp A, et al. Limb remote ischemic conditioning of the recipient protects the liver in a rat model of arterialized orthotopic liver transplantation. PLoS One. 2018;**13**:e0195507. DOI: 10.1371/journal.pone.0195507

[72] Emontzpohl C, Stoppe C, Theißen A, Beckers C, Neumann UP, Lurje G, et al. The role of macrophage migration inhibitory factor in remote ischemic conditioning induced hepatoprotection in a rodent model of liver transplantation. Shock. 2018. DOI: 10.1097/SHK.0000000000001307

[73] Kanoria S, Robertson FP, Mehta NN, Fusai G, Sharma D, Davidson BR. Effect of remote ischaemic preconditioning on liver injury in patients undergoing major hepatectomy for colorectal liver metastasis: a pilot randomised controlled feasibility trial. World Journal of Surgery. 2017;**41**:1322-1330. DOI: 10.1007/s00268-016-3823-4

[74] Rakić M, Patrlj L, Amić F, Aralica G, Grgurević I. Comparison of hepatoprotective effect from ischemia-reperfusion injury of remote ischemic preconditioning of the liver vs local ischemic preconditioning of the liver during human liver resections. International Journal of Surgery. 2018;**54**:248-253. DOI: 10.1016/j.ijsu.2018.05.001

[75] Robertson FP, Goswami R, Wright GP, Imber C, Sharma D, Malago M, et al. Remote ischaemic preconditioning in orthotopic liver transplantation (RIPCOLT trial): a pilot randomized controlled feasibility study. HPB: The Official Journal of the International Hepato Pancreato Biliary Association. 2017;**19**:757-767. DOI: 10.1016/j.hpb.2017.05.005

Chapter 7

Challenging Issues in Hepatic Adenoma

Mirela Patricia Sîrbu Boeți, Beatrice Tivadar, Ioana G. Lupescu, Vlad Herlea, Mirela Boroș, Dana Tomescu and Vladislav Brașoveanu

Abstract

Hepatic adenoma is known as a benign lesion encountered mainly in female patients and classically linked to the administration of oral contraceptives. In the last decade, the risk factors for its occurrence have changed and so did the sex ratio. The histopathological classification of hepatic adenomas was found to be related with certain genetic mutations that determine the risk for malignancy. The diagnosis of hepatic tumor is correlated with clinical and imaging data in an effort not only to rule out other tumors but also to distinguish the subtype of adenoma, which is very important for the management of the patient. The ultimate diagnosis is established by pathologists by routine histopathological and specific immunohistochemical staining. There are two major issues that pathologists need to recognize: the presence of β-catenin gene mutation and/or malignant degeneration. The best imaging examination is considered to be MRI. However, along with MRI, ultrasound and computer tomography have proved themselves to be effective not only in evaluating the number, size, localization, and complications of hepatic adenomas, but also in identifying their subtype. A detailed presentation of characteristics of all groups of hepatic adenoma is provided. The means of management of hepatic adenomas are documented and decisional algorithm is explained, based on certain criteria.

Keywords: hepatic adenoma, hepatocellular adenoma, liver adenoma, adenomatosis, hepatectomy, laparoscopic hepatectomy, liver transplantation, liver imaging

1. Introduction

Hepatic adenoma (HA) is a rare, benign tumor of epithelial origin (2% of all liver tumors [1]) that develops usually in healthy liver [2] and is known to occur mainly in young female patients, having been linked to the prolonged use of oral contraceptives [3]. In Europe and North America, it has an incidence of 3/100,000/year [4]. Even though multiple hepatic adenomas have been described in the literature, this is a rare occurrence, most of the adenomas being solitary (70–80%), and thus, often asymptomatic unless they become complicated (voluminous adenomas causing upper quadrant pain and/or rupture of the tumor with hemoperitoneum and malignant transformation) [5]. Hepatocellular adenoma is a term sometimes used instead of hepatic adenoma, being correct in contradiction to liver adenoma

 IntechOpen

or liver cell adenoma, which are less desirable because these two can also include the bile duct adenoma [6]. Even though the prognosis of this type of tumor is not well established, it is important to differentiate it from other hepatic tumors since the hepatic adenoma has a particular therapeutic management. Differential diagnosis however can be challenging, but can be achieved preoperatively by imaging techniques. Positive diagnosis is a histopathological one and is often obtained postoperatively [7].

2. Epidemiology

The incidence of HA has increased in recent years, but at the same time, imaging techniques have improved, and therefore, this higher incidence might be explained by the better diagnostic techniques nowadays available. Also, in recent years, it seems to be a change in epidemiology, as more cases of HA in male patients are described, particularly in Europe and Asia. This may be caused by an increased incidence of obesity, another recognized risk factor of HA. Moreover, in recent years, more and more cases of malignant transformation of HA have been reported, and this also might be a result of improved histopathological diagnosis.

Although the link between HA and use or oral contraceptive in women of childbearing age is maintained, recent studies have shown other emerging important risk factors such as metabolic syndrome [8].

3. Risk factors

The most important risk factor seems to be the use of oral contraceptives. Hepatic adenoma used to be exceptionally rare before the age of oral contraceptives, but after these became popular as a contraceptive solution, more and more cases of HA were reported. In women who were long-time users of oral contraceptives, the incidence was 1 in 30–40,000, whereas in women who have never used oral contraceptives, the incidence was 1 in 1 million, which proves a strong link between these two. Hepatic adenomas in women with prolonged use of oral contraceptives tend to be more numerous, more voluminous, and with a higher risk of spontaneous rupture and bleeding [9–12].

Another important risk factor that became even more important than other known risk factors, such as glycogen storage diseases and diabetes mellitus type 2 alone, is the metabolic syndrome. Obesity is more and more prevalent in the general population, and thus, it became a more important risk factor in this pathology. Weight loss should be considered as the first therapeutic option in the management of HA in obese patients [13]. A recent study has proved that bariatric-induced weight loss results in significant regression of HA in severely obese women, which emphasizes the role of overweight in HA pathophysiology [14]. Even more so, patients with metabolic syndrome and hepatic adenomas seem to be associated with a higher rate of malignization [8]. The association between oral contraceptive use and metabolic syndrome on one hand and HA on the other tends to prove an important hormonal sensitivity of the tumor (obesity is associated with higher estrogen levels), and this is supported by the fact that adenomas may stop their evolution or even regress as a result of oral contraceptive cessation [15]. In spite of this, immunohistological studies failed to prove the direct effect of these hormones via steroid receptors in normal and adenomatous hepatic tissue, and so the mechanism by which high estrogen levels may cause an adenomatous transformation is still incompletely understood [16]. As a hyperestrogenic state, pregnancy has also been incriminated as a risk factor, and there have been many reports of ruptured HAs in pregnant patients with a very high mortality for both mother and child [16–19].

Apart from estrogen, use of anabolic androgens has also been linked to a higher incidence in HAs, which is being proved not only in body builders but also in patients treated with steroids for Fanconi syndrome, aplastic anemia, etc. Cessation of steroid use has also been linked to regression in size of HAs [15].

Hepatic adenoma has also been linked to glycogen storage disease and hepatocyte nuclear factor 1A maturity onset diabetes of the young (HNF1A MODY). The incidence is 51% in patients with type I glycogen storage disease and 25% in those with type III glycogen storage disease (GSD) [8]. Hepatic adenoma in GSD occurs before the age of 20 years, is more common in males, and is typically multiple. Dietary therapy and correction of insulin, glucose, and glucagon levels have been proved to lead to regression of adenomas [15]. The mechanism by which GSD is involved in the development of HA is also unknown.

Finally, there seems to be a genetic predisposition, and nowadays, HAs are believed to result from specific genetic mutations involving TCF1 (transcription factor 1 gene), IL6ST (interleukin 6 signal transducer gene), and CTNNB1 (β catenin-1 gene) [20].

4. Pathology

HAs present as solitary lesions in most cases (70–80%), although multiple adenomas can exist of variable sizes. HAs usually occur in the right hepatic lobe. Macroscopically, HAs present as a smooth, tan-colored lesion, well demarcated from the normal hepatic tissue in spite of not having a capsule, often with areas of hemorrhage and necrosis (**Figure 1**). Large blood vessels that surround it are the source of hemorrhage in a complicated adenoma. The lack of a fibrous capsule means that the bleeding can extend into the liver parenchyma unrestricted.

Microscopically, adenomas are made of adenoma cells, which are typically larger than normal hepatocytes and contain glycogen and lipid inclusions (**Figures 2** and **3**). The nuclei are small and regular and mitoses are infrequent. The normal architecture of hepatic tissue is severely disrupted, with no portal tracts of bile ducts, while adenoma cells are disposed in trabeculae interspersed with arteries and thin-walled blood vessels and sinusoids. The absence of bile ducts is a notable feature that helps in the differential diagnosis of HA with non-neoplastic liver tissue and focal nodular hyperplasia. Kupffer cells may only rarely be present in HA.

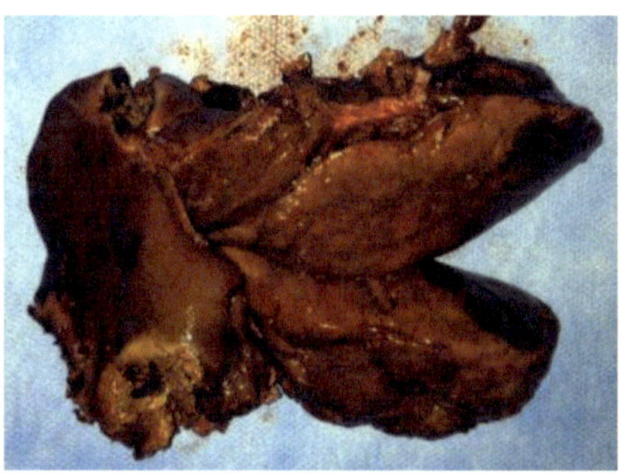

Figure 1.
Resected specimen after mesohepatectomy for a large IHA.

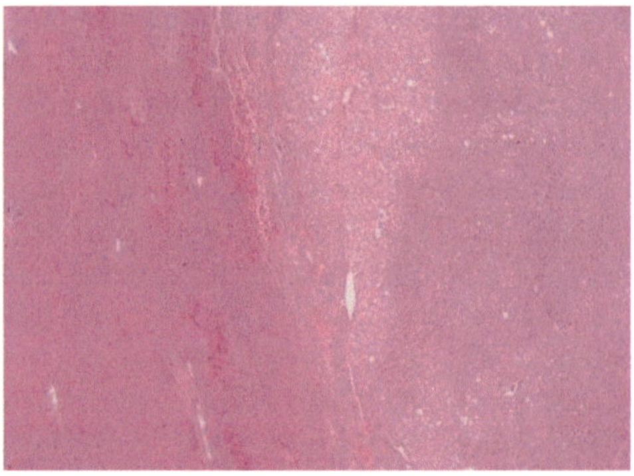

Figure 2.
Normal liver (left) and hepatocellular adenoma (right), HE ×40.

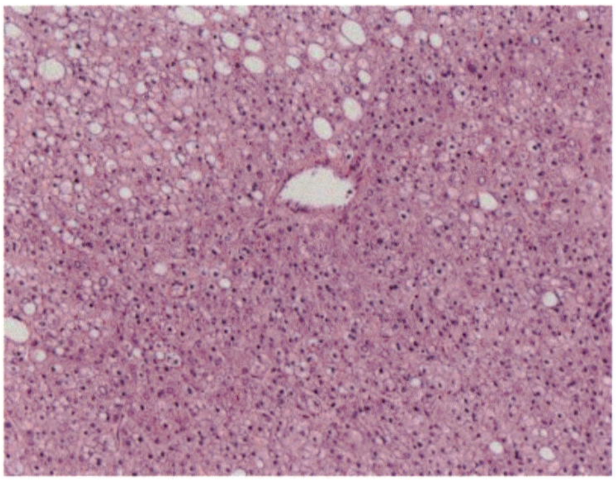

Figure 3.
Hepatocellular adenoma—benign hepatocytes (large, clear, and pale due to accumulation of glycogen) arranged in plates, cords, and sheets, HE ×200.

Similarities with a well differentiated hepatocellular carcinoma (Edmonson I) makes the differential diagnosis a challenging one.

Based on an extensively characterized clinical, morphological, phenotypical, and genotypical profile, four distinct subtypes of HA have been identified [3, 21]:

1. Hepatocyte nuclear factor-1 (HNF-1)—mutated HAs (H-HA)

2. β-Catenin-mutated hepatic adenomas (β-HA)

3. Inflammatory hepatic adenomas (which harbor mutations involving the interleukin-6 signal transducer) (IHA)

4. Unclassified hepatic adenomas (U-HA).

Inflammatory and HNF1-mutated hepatic adenomas are the most frequent subtypes (80%).

The first group (H-HA) comprises 35–40% of all patients and almost exclusively includes women. It is related to the presence of transcription factor 1 gene mutations that inactivate hepatocyte nuclear factor 1α (HNF-1α). The nonfunctioning HNF-1α protein promotes lipogenesis and hepatocellular proliferation. Moreover, abnormal HNF-1α protein determines silencing of liver fatty acid-binding protein FABP1. FABP1 is a gene positively regulated by HNF-1α and expressed in normal liver tissue, but in H-HA its downregulation results in impaired fatty acid trafficking in hepatocytes, which causes intracellular fat deposition [22]. H-HA is sometimes associated with maturity-onset diabetes of the young (MODY), type 3, and familial hepatic adenomatosis. Half of these patients have multiple HAs. More than 90% have a history of oral contraceptive use. The tumors are characterized by marked steatosis (**Figures 4**–**7**), a very low risk of complications, and a low risk of malignant transformation. On immunohistochemistry staining, H-HA is LFABP (liver fatty acid binding protein) negative, which is in contrast with normal expression in the surrounding nontumoral liver [21]. The sharp contrast between tumor and adjacent parenchyma in terms of steatosis and LFABP expression enables delineation of tumor borders which are often irregular and lobulated with often small HA foci in vicinity.

The second group comprises 10–15% of all patients, includes mainly men, and is characterized by the presence of mutations that activate β-catenin and cellular abnormalities. β-Catenin is encoded by catenin β 1 gene (CTNNB1) on chromosome 3p21 and represents an important downstream effector of the Wnt/β-catenin pathway. This pathway is important in liver embryogenesis, cell adhesion, growth, zonation, and regeneration [22]. An activating β-catenin mutation is also associated with specific conditions such as glycogen storage disorders or androgen administration. The phenotype is represented by cellular atypia with high nuclear-cytoplasmic ratio, nuclear atypia, and pseudoglandular growth pattern. It is identified by immunohistochemistry due to a strong expression of glutamine synthetase with or without aberrant cytoplasmic and nuclear expression of β-catenin. β-HA has the highest risk of malignant transformation than other HA subtypes, and it is very difficult to be distinguished from the well-differentiated hepatocellular carcinoma (HCC). Some risk factors are related to β-HA, such as male hormone administration, glycogenosis, and familial polyposis.

The third group (IHA) includes 50% of all patients and is most common in overweight women who suffer from metabolic syndrome or have had prolonged estrogen exposure. Patients with IHA demonstrate both serum and lesional indicators of an active inflammatory response. IHA is characterized histological by inflammation, marked sinusoidal dilatation or congestion, numerous thick-walled arteries, and ductular reaction (**Figures 8** and **9**). This subgroup was previously named 'telangiectatic focal nodular hyperplasia.' The extent of congestion, peliosis, and hemorrhage is different from case to case. Steatosis may be present in IHA but is not as extensive as in H-HA. In case of multiple tumors, the amount of steatosis

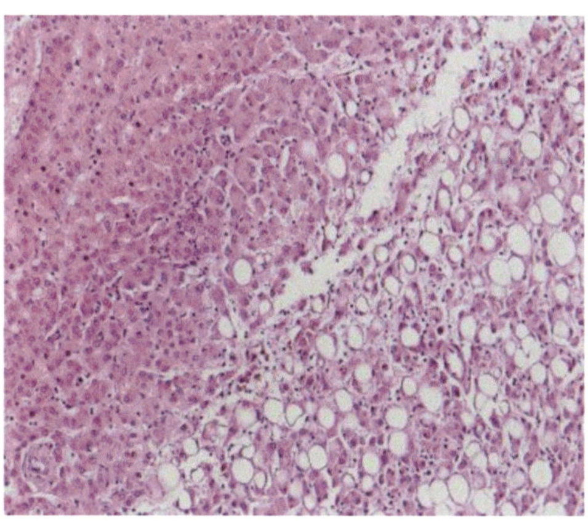

Figure 4.
Hepatocellular adenoma—HNF1 alpha mutated subtype—steatosis within the tumor, HE ×200.

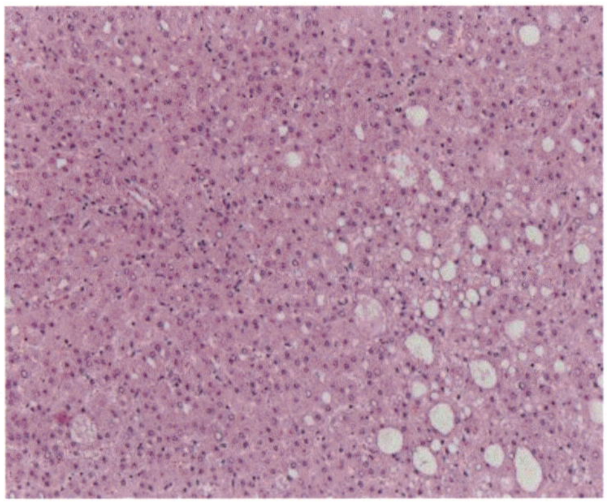

Figure 5.
Hepatocellular adenoma—HNF1 alpha mutated subtype—steatosis and pseudoglandular formations, HE ×200.

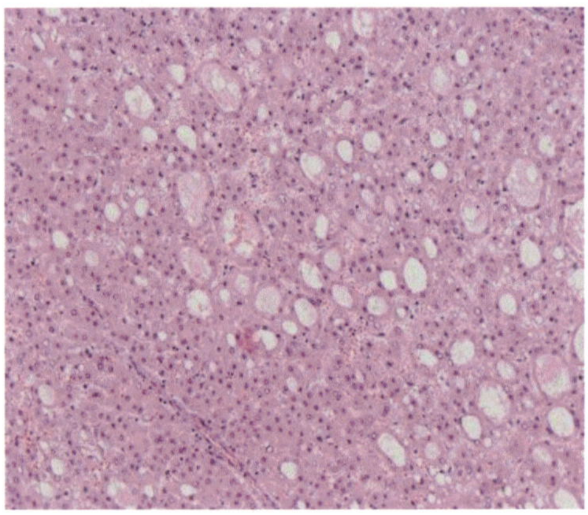

Figure 6.
Hepatocellular adenoma—HNF1 alpha mutated subtype—pseudoglandular formations and steatosis within the tumor, HE ×200.

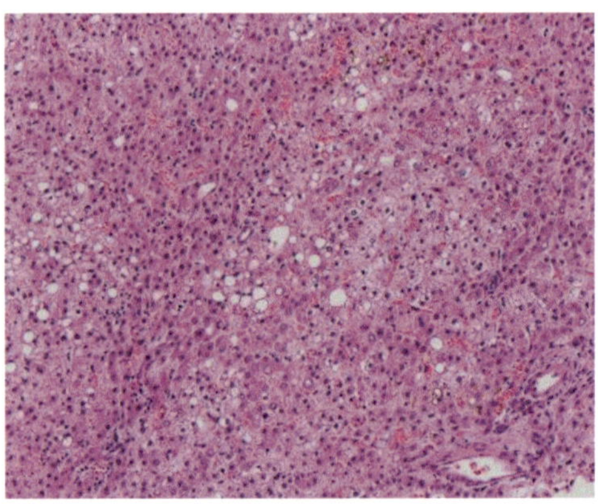

Figure 7.
Hepatocellular adenoma—steatosis within the tumor, HE ×200.

varies among the tumors in the same patient. Immunohistochemically, it is distinctive by a strong expression of inflammation-associated proteins such as serum amyloid A and C-reactive protein at mRNA and protein levels. The genetics of this

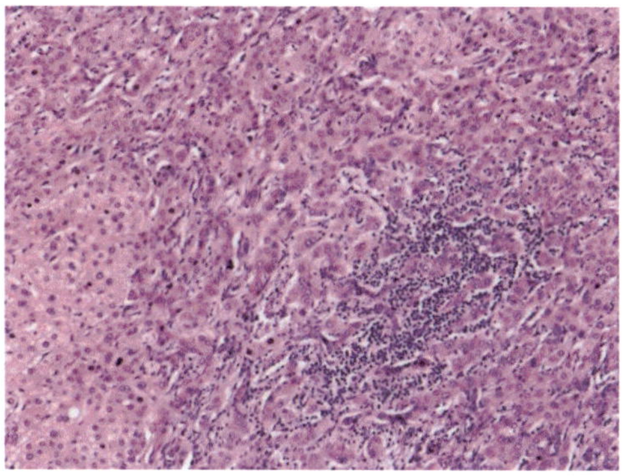

Figure 8.
Hepatocellular adenoma—inflammatory subtype, HE ×200.

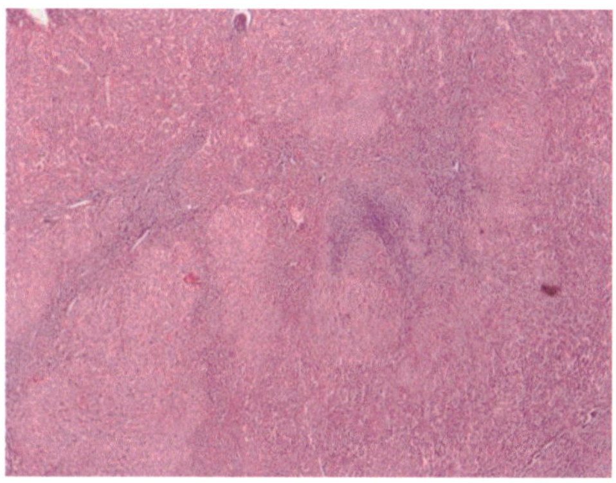

Figure 9.
Hepatocellular adenoma—inflammatory subtype, HE ×40, with sinusoidal dilatation and hemorrhage within the tumor.

group is related to activation of the JAK/STAT pathway underlined by mutations in different genes. In 60%, there are somatic gain-of-function mutations of the interleukin-6 signal transducer gene (IL6ST), which is located at chromosome 5q11 and encodes for glycoprotein 130. Gain-of-function mutations in glycoprotein 130 activate JAK–STAT-3 without interleukin-6 binding. The other 40% show overexpression of wild-type glycoprotein 130, which activates STAT-3 through an unidentified mechanism. Marked peliosis is probably caused by suppression of albumin gene, insulin-like growth factor gene IGF1, and/or transthyretin gene. Mutations of β-catenin may coexist in 10% of IHA (β-IHA). These patients may have signs and symptoms of systemic inflammatory syndrome, manifested as fever, leukocytosis, and elevated serum levels of CRP. Abnormal results of liver function tests may occur, with elevation of alkaline phosphatase and γ-glutamyl transferase. Systemic AA amyloidosis is a rare complication of HA which causes nephrotic syndrome with deteriorating renal function. Resection of the tumor is followed by improvement in renal function and a marked decrease of the serum concentrations of acute phase proteins [23].

The last group that is unclassified (UHA) accounts for 5–10% of adenomas. For this group, the genotype is unknown and the phenotype and immunohistochemistry—unspecific. In this group is also included HA that cannot be classified due to near-total necrosis or hemorrhage [21].

The first important thing for the pathologist is to correctly identify the β-catenin-activated HA and to decide when immunostaining is needed. Morphology and additional immunohistochemical markers can discriminate between different types of HA in more than 90% of cases [24]. Identification of beta-catenin positive adenomas has important implications in the decision for surveillance and treatment of these patients. Even if very specific, nuclear β-catenin immunostaining is of low sensitivity in accurate detection of β-HA and β-IHA due to uneven staining distribution or focal nuclear staining. Therefore, additional molecular biology is required. It is recommended to perform glutamine synthetase (GS) staining on every single HA, because GS is one of the target genes in case of β-catenin activation, and it is usually diffusely and strongly expressed in β-catenin-activated HA. GS staining can also be patchy or diffuse but less intense and still be an indication of β-catenin-activating mutations, but in this case, a molecular analysis must be performed to confirm it.

The second important thing for the pathologist is to correctly recognize foci of HCC inside HA. The problem is to avoid overdiagnosis in case of mild or focal cellular atypia. Some HAs may look worrisome due to the presence of architectural distortion, thicker liver cell plates, extensive pseudogland formation, and decreased reticulin framework together with increased CD34 staining (**Figure 10**). These are called "atypical HA," "borderline lesions," and, recently, "well-differentiated hepatocellular neoplasms of uncertain malignant potential." Reticulin staining (**Figure 11**) is the most powerful tool to identify foci of definite malignant transformation, especially in association with architectural distortion, cellular atypia, and increased CD34 staining. Glypican 3 is also very useful when it is positive (**Figure 12**), but its negativity does not rule out malignancy [25]. In most cases of HA and occasionally in HCC, the CD34 staining intensity is variable in different areas and virtually all HCCs have homogenous CD34-positive staining intensity and density [26]. Total loss of reticulin network and diffuse increased CD34 expression, possible presence of glypican 3, and increased MIB1 staining are indications for HCC foci. HSP70 can be also useful. There is no specific phenotype of HCC developed from HA, but some observed that these HCC are often pigmented or cholestatic.

The pathologist needs enough samples, some of them at the junction with the nontumoral liver. For immunohistochemical results, it is mandatory to have a biopsy of the nontumoral liver for comparison.

Interestingly, certain magnetic resonance imaging (MRI) features seem to correlate with the histologic subtypes, suggesting that it may be possible to classify them by MRI [7]. HNF1-inactivated HA and inflammatory HA can particularly be diagnosed by radiologists with considerable accuracy.

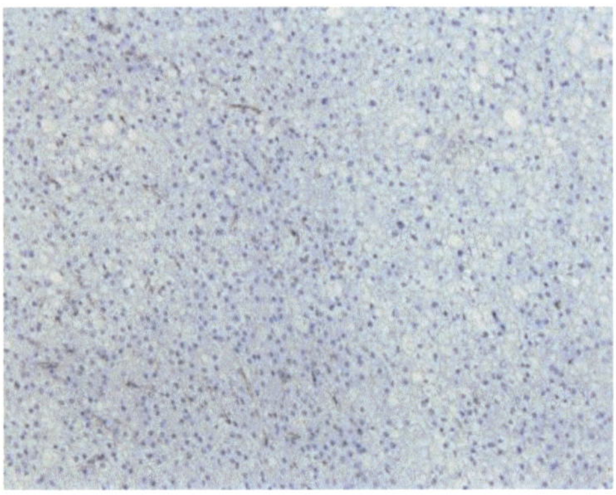

Figure 10.
Hepatocellular adenoma—CD34 immunohistochemical stain for endothelial cells, few sinusoids are seen in the tumor, ×200.

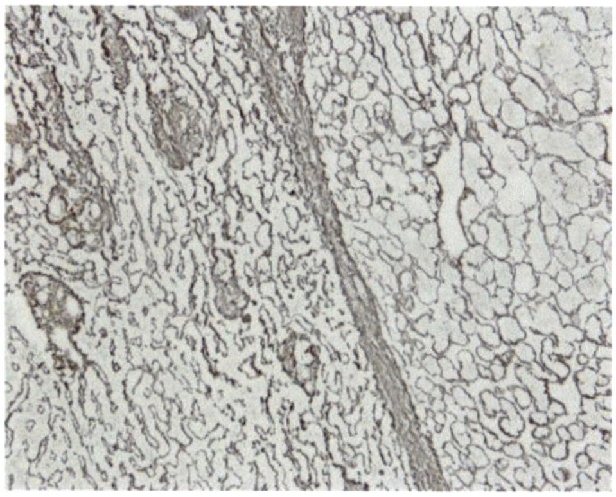

Figure 11.
Hepatocellular adenoma—reticulin stain—left normal liver and right hepatocellular adenoma—there is no loss of reticulin network, Gomori ×200.

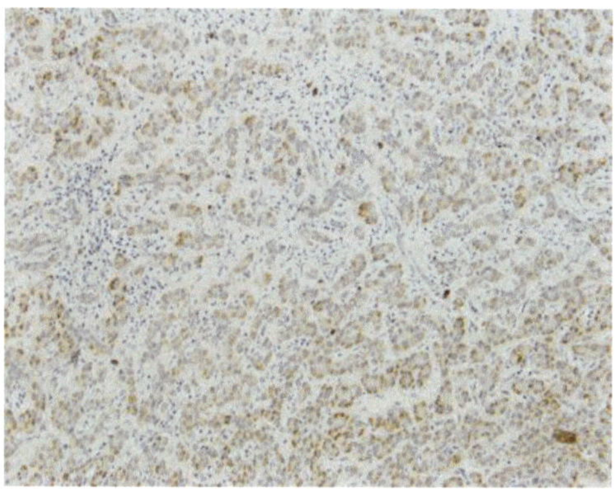

Figure 12.
Hepatocellular adenoma—HNF1 alpha mutated subtype—mild lipofuscin deposits revealed by glypican 3 immunohistochemical stain, ×200.

4.1 Adenomatosis

Adenomatosis is a distinct clinical entity and was first described in 1985 [27] and since then has been defined by the presence of more than 10 adenomas, involving both hepatic lobes, in the absence of glycogen storage diseases, prolonged use of steroids, or resolution with steroid cessation [28]. It is estimated that adenomatosis affects both men and women, and, unlike HA, is correlated with a higher risk of impaired liver function, manifested as an increase in serum alkaline phosphatase and GGT levels [27] and also with a higher risk of bleeding. Instead, the malignant degeneration does not correlate with the number of lesions. There are two different patterns of adenomatosis: (1) the massive pattern, which is defined by the existence of larger lesions, up to 10 cm, that often result in gross hepatomegaly with deformed contour of the liver and (2) the multifocal pattern, which is characterized by smaller lesions, with diameter less than 4 cm, that rarely deform the liver, but has a tendency to progress fast and become symptomatic [29]. The etiology of hepatic adenomatosis is suspected to be linked to congenital or acquired abnormalities of hepatic vasculature. In a study of 15 patients with adenomatosis, 5 had abnormalities in hepatic vasculature: congenital absence of portal vein, portal venous thrombosis with cavernous modification, and intrahepatic portosystemic shunts [1, 30].

The conditions that predispose to adenomatosis and evolution of the disease are poorly understood, since the medical literature reports only information in regard to individual cases or small case series, but some similarities with the HA are evident: the tendency toward hemorrhage (especially in adenomas larger than 4 cm) and the risk of malignant transformation. Adenomas in hepatic adenomatosis may be of inflammatory, hepatocyte nuclear factor 1 alpha mutated, or beta-catenin mutated subtype.

5. Signs and symptoms

Most commonly, HA goes unnoticed due to its lack of signs and symptoms, but when it does become symptomatic, it is either due to its increase in volume, tumor necrosis, or complications such as life-threatening intra-abdominal bleeding due to spontaneous rupture of the highly vascularized tumor. Sudden, severe pain with hypotension in a patient with HA indicates rupture into the peritoneum, an event associated with a mortality of up to 20 percent if not identified and/or treated accordingly [9, 31, 32]. The risk of bleeding is difficult to estimate overall, but it is quite high in patients with symptomatic HAs (25–64%). Tumor size that exceeds 35 mm has been associated with an increased risk of bleeding [33]. The risk of bleeding depends on the localization of the tumor. Exophytic lesions (protruding from liver) had the highest risk of bleeding (67%), followed by subcapsular ones (19%) and at last intrahepatic HA (11%). Lesions in segments II and III had more bleeds than those in the right liver (34% versus 19%). The visualization on imaging of peripheral or central arteries represents a risk of bleeding comparative with no visible vascularization in the lesion [33]. Also a long history of contraceptive use and recent hormonal use are risk factors for bleeding from HA. Young age seems to be associated with an increased incidence of HA rupture, independent of hormonal treatment duration, suggesting a need for careful surveillance or prophylactic treatment in this population [34]. Bleeding is graded as intratumoral (grade I), intrahepatic (grade II), or extrahepatic (grade III) and represents a potentially life-threatening complication in patients with HAs.

Hepatic adenomas are diagnosed when they cause epigastric or upper quadrant pain or during an imaging study done for unrelated ailments, and less commonly when an abdominal mass is palpated on clinical examination. When HA is sufficiently large and compresses bile ducts, jaundice may become another sign.

6. Diagnosis and differential diagnosis

There are no specific serologic markers or laboratory findings for HA, but certain findings can lead the diagnosis away from an adenoma and toward a liver cell carcinoma in case of an increased serum alpha-fetoprotein, or toward a metastasis in the case of increased serum tumor markers for digestive tract tumors [35].

The definite diagnosis in this pathology is naturally a histological one; however, obtaining it preoperatively means making a biopsy from a fragile and highly vascular tissue, with significant risk of bleeding. Having to deal with a benign lesion, and given the fact that the amount of tissue obtained is rarely enough or suitable for a diagnosis, this risk is not justified. Thus, the diagnosis of this tumor is based on analyzing a combination of epidemiologic and clinical data and imaging studies, but often the confirmation of the diagnosis is done by the pathologist, after the hepatic resection.

Usually a HA is suspected in a young adult with a singular and asymptomatic hepatic lesion, but a thorough differential diagnosis should be made and often this proves to be difficult. The differential diagnosis between adenomas and focal nodular hyperplasia is usually challenging, but can be done, most of the times, based on imaging characteristics.

6.1 Imaging in liver adenomas

Imaging in adenomas includes mostly ultrasound, contrast-enhanced ultrasound (CEUS), multislice computer tomography (MSCT), and magnetic resonance imaging (MRI) (**Figure 13**).

6.1.1 Ultrasound

The most accessible, cost-friendly, and probably responsible for most discoveries of asymptomatic HA is the ultrasound, even though it cannot distinguish it from other liver tumors. On gray scale ultrasound, HA is seen as a well-defined solid, echogenic mass, but sometimes as complex hyper/hypoechoic, heterogeneous mass with anechoic areas due to fat, hemorrhage, necrosis, and calcifications; a capsule may also be seen [36]. Color Doppler US can aid in the distinction from FNH in the absence of a central arterial signal, FNH having characteristic intratumoral and peritumoral vessels [37, 38]. Contrast-enhanced ultrasound with sulfur hexafluoride microbubbles (SonoVue or Lumason) greatly improves diagnosis as compared to US without contrast.

6.1.2 Computer tomography

One of the most accurate imaging tools in diagnosing a HA is contrast enhanced computed tomography (CECT), on which it appears as a well demarcated tumor, with characteristic peripheral enhancement during the early phase with subsequent centripetal flow during the portal venous phase. A heterogeneous consistency is usually a sign of necrosis, hemorrhage, or fibrosis [5].

Multiphasic computed tomography (CT) has a detection rate of 100% for adenomas, which is however different per type of examination: nonenhanced 86%, hepatic arterial-dominant phase (HAP) 100%, portal venous-dominant phase (PVP) 82%, and delayed 88%. Tumor margins are well defined by a low-attenuation pseudocapsule in 86% of adenomas and the surface appears smooth, without lobulated contour, in 95%. Tumor fat and calcifications are uncommon (7%, respectively 5%). Other than areas of fat, hemorrhage, or necrosis, the adenomas show homogenous enhancement, especially on PVP and delayed-phase scans [39].

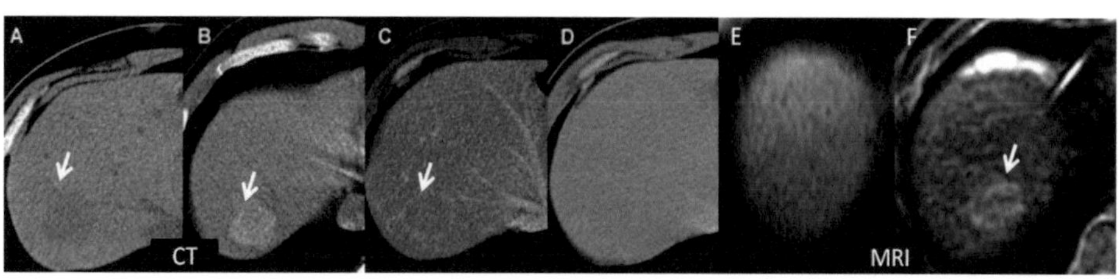

Figure 13.
HA located in segment VII as shown by imaging on NECT (A), CECT—arterial phase (B), portal venous phase (C), parenchymal phase (D), MRI T1w (E), and T2w (F). Atoll sign characterized by a hyper intense band in the periphery and isodensity in the center of the lesion with respect of the surrounding liver is relevant on CT in portal venous phase (C). A hyperintense rim in T2 wi is described in inflammatory adenoma (arrow in F).

MSCT technique: nonenhanced CT and enhanced triphasic CT: in arterial (30–35 s after the bolus tracker detection), portal venous (60–80 s after contrast medium injection), and equilibrium/late phases (after 3–5 min). 1.5 ml/kg of nonionic iodinated contrast material is injected into an antecubital vein with a rate of 3 ml/s using a power injector.

CT findings are depending on HA subtype. On nonenhanced CT (NECT), hemorrhage within tumor is seen on as hyperdense foci, intratumoral lipid as hypodense foci (negative density), and focal coarse calcifications are rarely seen (**Figure 14**). On contrast-enhanced (CECT), encapsulation is present in ~20% of HAs, best seen on the late phase (**Figure 14**). Hypervascularity is most intense and persistent in inflammatory subtype of HA (**Figure 15**).

CT is most useful in distinguishing a HA from other liver tumors or lesions: (1) focal nodular hyperplasia which has a characteristic central star-shaped hypodense scar, (2) hemangiomas with their peripheral enhancement on arterial phase and progressive centripetal fill-in pattern, (3) liver cell carcinoma which has a particular wash-in, wash-out pattern, and (4) singular liver metastases with no fat or hemorrhage.

6.1.3 Magnetic resonance imaging (MRI)

6.1.3.1 MRI technique

Unenhanced conventional sequences: T2w is useful in detection of focal liver lesions. T2* is important in the evaluation of iron content and chemical shift artifact sequences; T1 in/out of phase is important to delineate steatosis or intralesional lipomatous content; ssFSE short TE/long TE makes differentiation between cysts and solid mass; and diffusion is the most sensitive sequence for liver lesion detection.

Contrast enhanced T1: multiphase dynamic 3D acquisitions without and with intravenous injection of 0.1 ml/kgbw of extracellular or liver-specific contrast paramagnetic agents (Gd-EOB-DTPA) in arterial phase (AP): detection of hypervascular lesions, portal venous phase (PVP), late phase (LP), and hepatobiliary phase (HBP).

Imaging key features in HAs are: hypervascularity, fat content, hemorrhage, and encapsulation. MRI shows some elements better than CT (lipid and hemorrhage). HA shows no substantial uptake or retention in contrast enhanced MRI with Gadoxetate (Primovist). MRI features for adenomas are distinct from FNH. T1WI: mass with heterogeneous signal intensity; increased signal intensity (due to fat or recent hemorrhage); decreased signal intensity (necrosis, calcification, old hemorrhage) T1 + C: heterogeneous, hypervascular liver mass with foci of fat or hemorrhage in a young woman.

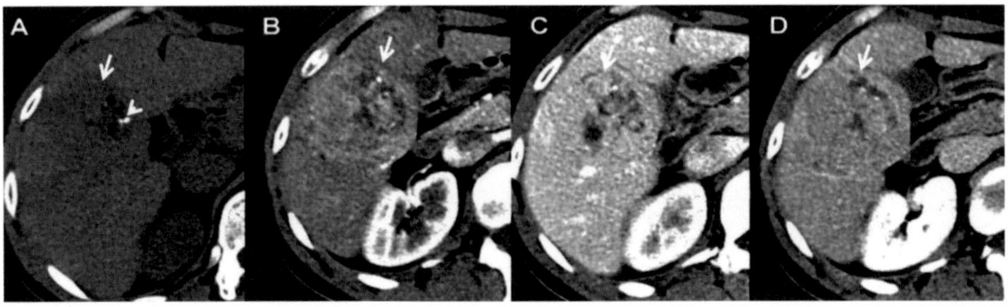

Figure 14.
NECT with large liver mass with central calcifications, small lipomatous inclusions, solid components and necrosis (A), CECT—arterial phase (B), portal venous phase (C), and parenchymal phase (D).

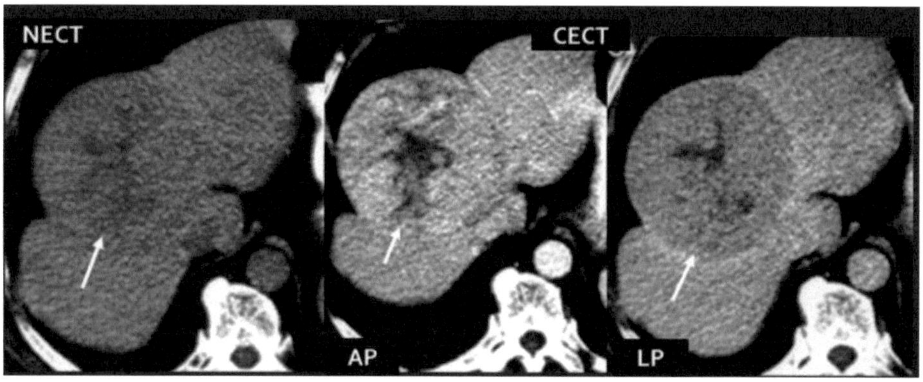

Figure 15.
CT evaluation: liver adenoma with central necrotic area and encapsulation (arrow).

6.1.3.2 MRI evaluation

Some MRI findings of HAs are similar to CT findings, but MRI is usually more sensitive in detecting fat from hemorrhage. The appearance of HAs on MRI is highly variable, especially in T1, but if contrast medium is used, then it may be better characterized, showing early arterial enhancement and becoming nearly isointense to liver on delayed images.

On T1-weighted images (T1wi), HA appears as a heterogeneous signal intensity mass. The increased signal of HA is due to fat and recent hemorrhage, and the decreased signal intensity is due to necrosis, calcification, or old hemorrhage. A fibrous pseudocapsule may be seen in HA as a hypointense rim. In T2wi, the mass appears heterogeneous; increased signal intensity corresponds to old hemorrhage or necrosis, and the decreased signal intensity is due to the fat or recent hemorrhage. The peripheral rim (fibrous pseudocapsule) in HA appears hypointense in liver parenchyma (**Figure 16**). After contrast injection (T1wi + C) in arterial phase, adenomas are heterogeneous hypervascular masses (inflammatory HA+++) and in delay phase a pseudocapsule, which is hyperintense comparative to the normal liver, can be seen. After Gadoxetate-enhanced MR (Gd-EOB-DTPA), in HA there is no substantial contrast uptake or retention on hepatobiliary phase [40].

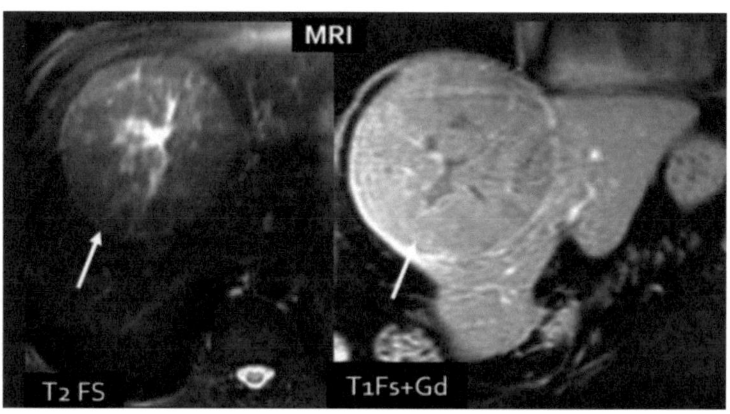

Figure 16.
MRI evaluation: liver adenoma with central necrotic area and pseudocapsule hyperintense to the surrounding liver (arrow).

MRI with hepatobiliary agents is an important tool not only in differential subtype definition but even in surveillance with early identification of complications and discovery of some signs of HA malignant degeneration [41]. Lesion enlargement and heterogeneity of signal intensity and of contrast enhancement are signs of malignant transformation [42].

Imaging recommendations: the best imaging tool is represented by Gadoxetate-enhanced MRI including multiphase and hepato-biliary phase acquisition [43]. The best sequence to evaluate fat into HA is T1wi with in and opposed TE.

6.1.3.3 Classification of HAs based on imaging examinations

MRI is the imaging modality of choice for characterization of HA subtypes [22]. Inflammation, abnormal rich vascularization, peliotic areas, and abundant fatty infiltration are pathologic findings differently present in the HA subtypes at multiparametric MRI [41].

HNF1A-mutated adenoma (H-HA): on MRI, the diffuse and homogenous fat deposition within HA-H determines a specific imaging pattern: on T1-weighted Gradient-Echo MR, it is hyper- or isointense, with diffuse signal drop-off with the use of chemical shift sequence (**Figure 17**). On T2-weight MR, images appears isointense to slightly hyperintense. Gadolinium-enhanced T1-weighted MR images show moderate enhancement in the arterial phase, with no persistent enhancement in the portal venous and delayed phases. Generally, its size is less than 5 cm, and there are minimal risks of bleeding and malignant transformation [22]. At multidetector CT, macroscopic fat deposits can be identified and establish the diagnosis of H-HA. On CEUS, it has iso- to moderately increased vascularity, mixed filling in the arterial phase after contrast and isoechoic appearance in the portal venous and delayed phases.

β-catenin-mutated hepatic adenoma (β-HA): there are no distinctive patterns established on MRI, multidetector CT, or CEUS, but they usually are hypervascular with evidence of hemorrhage or necrosis within tumor. Besides the fact that has the highest risk of malignant transformation (> 10%), it may mimic hepatocellular carcinoma with strong enhancement during arterial phase and with portal venous wash-out.

Inflammatory hepatic adenoma (IHA): includes those previously called "telangiectatic HA." It has specific patterns on MRI due to less fat content, sinusoidal dilation, peliotic areas, and abnormal vessels. On T1-weighted Gradient-Echo MR images, it is depicted as isointense or mildly hyperintense, without signal drop-off with the use of chemical sequence, and on T2-weighted MR images, it becomes bright (diffusely hyperintense). On Gadolinium-enhanced T1-weighted MR images, it shows intense enhancement during arterial phase that persists in

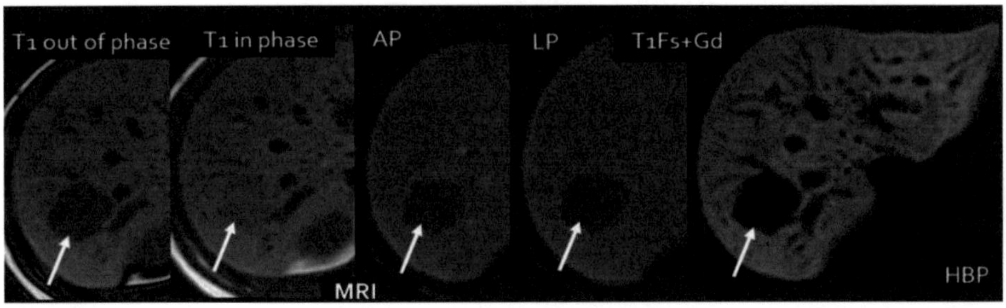

Figure 17.
HNF1A-mutated HA: diffuse lipid deposition within HA best seen using T1 with TE in and out of phase (arrow).

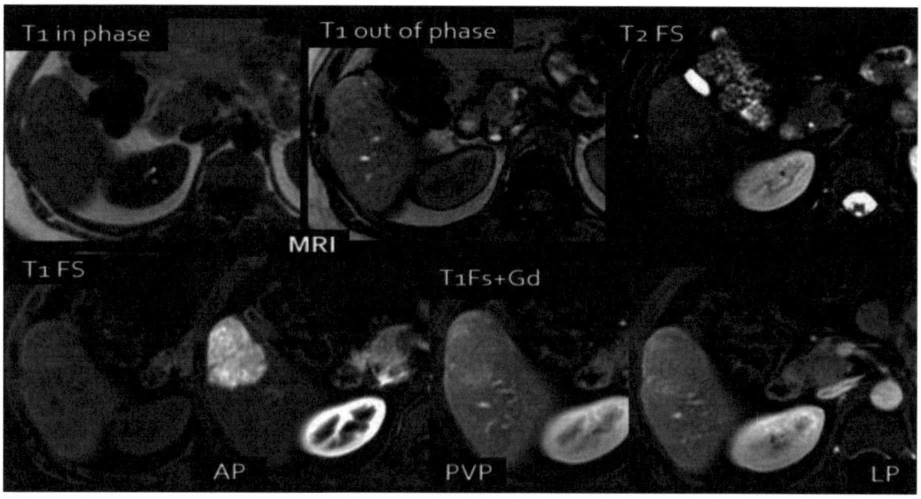

Figure 18.
Inflammatory liver adenoma: hyperintensity T2 wi and hypervascularity of the liver mass through the late AP, and discreetly hyperintense in portal and late phase.

the portal venous and delayed phases (**Figure 18**). The atoll sign is specific for IHA and may be due to sinusoidal dilatation. In up to 30% of cases, there is evidence of hemorrhage, and a 10% likelihood of malignant degeneration is estimated. At multidetector CT, IHA is depicted as heterogeneously hyperattenuating mass in NECT and in CECT shows enhancement features similar to those at MRI. At CEUS, it has arterial vascularity with centripetal filling, a sustained enhanced rim and central wash-out in the late venous phase.

Unclassified hepatic adenoma (U-HA) does not fit other profiles of HA subtypes.

6.1.3.4 Differential imaging diagnostic of adenomas

Hepatocellular carcinoma (HCC) may be hard to distinguish on imaging or pathology. Biliary, vascular, nodal invasion and metastases of HCC typically occur in older, cirrhotic men [42, 45]. Adenoma occurs in young, healthy women.

Fibrolamellar HCC is shown as a large, lobulated mass with scar and septa inside. Vascular, biliary invasion and metastases are common.

Focal nodular hyperplasia (FNH) is depicted on MRI + C in arterial phase as a homogeneously enhancing mass and in all other phases as an isodense mass comparative to normal liver. In T2WI, a scar is typically seen as hyperintense. On delayed phase MR, FNH uniformly retains Gadoxetate [44, 45]. Gadoxetic acid-enhanced MRI can differentiate between HA and FNH with a high sensitivity and specificity [46].

Hypervascular metastases are usually multiple. The primary tumor (i.e., thyroid, breast, kidney, or endocrine) must be searched for. CT + C or MRI + C in arterial phase shows heterogeneous enhancement. In portal and delayed phases, hypervascular metastases may appear isodense, hypodense, or hypointense.

6.2 Nuclear medicine studies

Most HAs have a decreased uptake of Gallium and colloid, early and retained uptake of hepatobiliary agents, and no uptake on PET scanning.

If radiological studies cannot distinguish HA from HCC and FNH, a combination of radionuclide imaging, including technetium (99mTc)-sulfur colloid sulfur-colloid,

Ga, and technetium-99 pyridoxyl-5-methyltryptophan (PMT) uptake may help establish the correct diagnosis [47]. Most adenomas do not take up technetium Tc-99m sulfur colloid so they appear as a "cold" spot in the parenchyma of the liver. This examination is not particularly good in diagnosing an adenoma but in distinguishing one from a FNH, which shows equal or greater uptake of the radiolabeled agent compared with surrounding liver [48]. 99mTc-labeled DISIDA (dimethyliminoacetic acid) liver scintigraphy has also been used by some authors for diagnosis of HA [47].

Positron emission tomography (PET) scanning with fluorine-18-fluorodeoxyglucose (^{18}FDG) is useful in differentiating HAs from malignant tumors, because malignant tumors show uptake of ^{18}FDG but not benign tumors, with some exceptions like inflammation and abscess.

Although CEUS, CT, MRI, and nuclear studies help in characterization of hepatic lesions as adenomas, the findings sometimes are nonspecific, and biopsy and/or resection may still be necessary.

6.3 Detection of malignant transformation

The pathogenesis of malignant transformation of hepatocellular adenoma is still poorly understood. Some light was recently shed on the mechanisms of hepatocarcinogenesis, which suggest the importance of telomerase reverse transcriptase (TERT) promoter mutations beside the early event of β-catenin mutation. Apparently, only the β-catenin mutations that occur on exon 3 and not those on exon 7–8 are involved in malignant transformation of HA [49]. It still remains unclear if hepatocellular carcinoma emerges from hepatocellular adenoma or if the lesions are coincident. Malignant transformation of hepatocellular adenoma has been reported in 4% of women and 47% of men with HA [50]. The risk of malignancy is very high for β-HA, which is most frequently associated with glycogenosis type 1, androgenic hormone intake (many of these tumors expressing androgen receptors in men), and familial polyposis. It is important to remind that no HA subtype is devoid of risk of malignant transformation. Men are predisposed to hepatocellular carcinoma regardless of etiology, and for this reason, surgical treatment is strongly recommended for male patients diagnosed with HA. For women, an older age (50 years or older) or a younger age (15 years or less) is a risk factor for malignant degeneration that must be taken into account to refer these patients to surgeon for resection or at least to a hepatologist for very close and careful surveillance.

At present, no clinical assessment can distinguish between HA and degenerated HA, and no rules for surveillance of HA in both sexes are clearly defined according to subtypes. The methods and the periodicity of following these patients are variable. Radiological assessments could include CEUS, multidetector raw CT, and dynamic MRI. CEUS allows more sensitive recognition and specific exclusion of malignancy compared with CT and dynamic MRI and has the advantage that can be repeatedly performed without the risk associated with allergic reactions or radiation exposure. Moreover, MRI has the disadvantage that cannot be performed everywhere in the world because the technical skills and expertise are very much geographically dependent. Two main features must be taken into consideration at reassessment of these patients with HA: the size of the tumor and, more important, the hemodynamic changes that precede the tumor growth [50]. Malignant degenerations are considered when the tumor was first iso-attenuated when compared with normal liver during the nonenhanced and delayed phases and appeared homogenous in the early phase but, at a later examination, it becomes enhanced in the early phase and hypo-attenuated in the delayed phase. Also, the presence of a nodule within a nodule during the arterial phase is known as a sign of malignancy. β-HA often has cytological atypia and pseudoglandular pattern, and it is sometimes almost impossible to identify HCC.

7. Management and current guidelines

The surgeons must be convinced that HA subtypes are important for the management of the patients. From now on, a diagnosis of HA cannot be conceived without group classification. The number and location of HA play a great role in management, but various clinical conditions such as age, sex, etiology, background liver, or comorbidities must be taken into consideration. Other aspects also play a role in decision making, like where the patient lives, the degree of his/her anxiety, and cost of surveillance. The management of patients with HA must be planned by a complex team formed by surgeons, hepatologists, pathologists, radiologists, gastroenterologist, molecular biologists, and geneticists.

There are no clear guidelines for the management of HA, because the treatment depends on many factors such as HA size, number, localization, gender, age, presence of symptoms, and complications.

In young women treated with contraceptive pills, asymptomatic lesions under 5 cm in diameter should be kept under close observation with CT/CEUS repeated every 6 months [51] and repeated alpha-feto-protein, all the while ceasing to use contraceptive pills [52]. Any modification in imaging suggesting a malignant transformation or an increase in the serum tumor marker should lead to liver resection. There are some authors who advocate resection of adenomas of any size given their risk of malignization and bleeding, if the resection can be performed with acceptable risk. The facts that surgical excision guarantees a definitive diagnosis and long-term cure favor the universal indication of surgery for HA [53].

7.1 Surgical resection

The indications for surgery in nonemergent cases are: HA > 5 cm, female patients taking oral contraceptives with HA > 3 cm [47], HA with growing size, HA with HCC or dysplastic foci, β-catenin-activated HA, imaging features of malignant transformation, increased serum alpha fetoprotein, HA in males regardless of the tumor size, HA in GSD, symptomatic patients, or when malignancy cannot be excluded [54]. The type of resection depends mainly on number, size, histological type, and localization of HA. The resection techniques vary from simple enucleation to liver transplantation [55]. Liver resection for HA can be anatomic or nonanatomic. Anatomic resections reported in the literature for HA refer to minor hepatectomies that imply the removal of the tumor with one or two segments of the liver [56], but also major hepatectomies like left and right hemihepatectomy, mesohepatectomy [57], and left or right extended hepatectomy [26, 58]. Nonanatomical resections are wedge resections [59]. Enucleation seems to be a choice for such benign tumor, but is not advisable due to the risk of remnant tumor that can cause tumor recurrence or, worse, malignant degeneration, especially for β-catenin HA. It was speculated that the classical 1 cm oncological safety margin could be lowered to 0.5 cm for HA. The safety margin at the edge of resection is mandatory, if any suspicion of HCC exists.

Surgery in elective cases is less than 1% and most tumors can be operated laparoscopically, with significant advantages [59–61]. A better cosmetic result, a shorter hospitalization (4 days) with early return to normal life, and a lower incisional rate are the main advantages that laparoscopy has comparative with open approach. However, laparoscopy should be performed only in specialized centers with extensive experience in both hepatic and laparoscopic surgery.
The first non-anatomical laparoscopic liver resection for HA reported by Ferzli et al. [62] in 1995 was followed one year later by the first anatomic laparoscopic resection for HA performed by Azagra et al. [63]. Pure laparoscopic procedure can be performed for HA with no mortality and reduced morbidity even in

hemodynamic stable patients with ruptured HA [61]. Moreover, some surgeons consider laparoscopic surgery the standard of care for the treatment of HA [59]. Hand-assisted or "hybrid" techniques are also optional approaches [64] and the parietal incision is later used for specimen retrieval. In pure laparoscopic surgery, the specimen is retrieved through a Pfannenstiel incision even when the tumor is as large as 180 mm [61].

Pringle maneuver can be of great use to minimize the intraoperative blood loss and it is used by surgeons both in laparotomy and laparoscopy. Some authors consider it unnecessary for laparoscopic left lateral sectionectomy [60]. Instead, others perform the maneuver for both atypical and anatomical resections. Laparoscopy is restricted by the localization of HA involving segments VII and VIII. The half-Pringle maneuver was associated for right posterior sectionectomy and resulted in less bleeding [65].

Total vascular exclusion of the liver is routinely recommended in high dorsal resections for HA [66].

Intraoperative blood transfusion is rarely needed and generally is performed in case of ruptured bleeding adenoma. Conversion of laparoscopy to laparotomy should be considered just in case of too much bleeding and difficulties for the anesthesiologist to stabilize the patient.

The high rates of mortality and morbidity previously reported after liver resection for bleeding HA are recently denied by new evidences [30]. Emergency resection of ruptured HA has a mortality rate of 5–10%, whereas elective surgery has a mortality rate of less than 1% [67]. These results are explained nowadays by the availability of improved hemostatic techniques, excellent anesthesia support, and postoperative intensive care. In the past, in the presence of signs of hemorrhagic shock, the mortality was as high as 20% for resection [68]. At present, the mortality for such patients trends toward zero. Nonsurgical strategies such as arterial embolization or gauze packing have been recommended in order to stabilize the patient and delay resection to an elective setting. There are situations when intraperitoneal bleeding from a ruptured adenoma is self-limited and a laparotomy is done just for biopsy. A recent bleeding adenoma does not necessarily need resection. After this acute bleeding, some of these tumors regress, others are stationary, and few rebleed. Transarterial embolization (TAE) can not only stabilize the patient but also obtain complete avoidance of surgical intervention. Sometimes, repeated embolization is needed to achieve hemostasis. However, liver resection remains the best means to achieve hemostasis and also to obtain a thorough histology.

7.2 Liver transplantation

Liver transplantation is an extraordinary choice in a few selected patients, with multiple HAs, giant HAs [69], or recurrent adenomas that are not technically resectable [70]. Those HAs considered unresectable are either in close proximity to major vascular structures or the liver hilum or less than 20% of viable hepatic parenchyma remains after resection. Liver transplantation for recurrent HA is a more technically demanding procedure if compared to the cases with chronic liver disease due to the presence of postoperative adhesions that must be divided before reaching the liver and also due to difficulties in liver implantation when at least a major hepatic vein and hepatic pedicle are absent after major hepatectomy [70]. Transplanted liver is generally harvested from a cadaveric donor but living liver transplantation has also been reported [71]. Due to an expanding armamentarium and experience in angiographically controlling bleeding from a ruptured HA, liver transplantation as an ultimate life-rescue therapy remains exceptionally rare, being reported for spontaneous intra-partum rupture of hepatocellular adenoma [72] (**Algorithm 1**).

Algorithm 1. Management in hepatic adenoma.

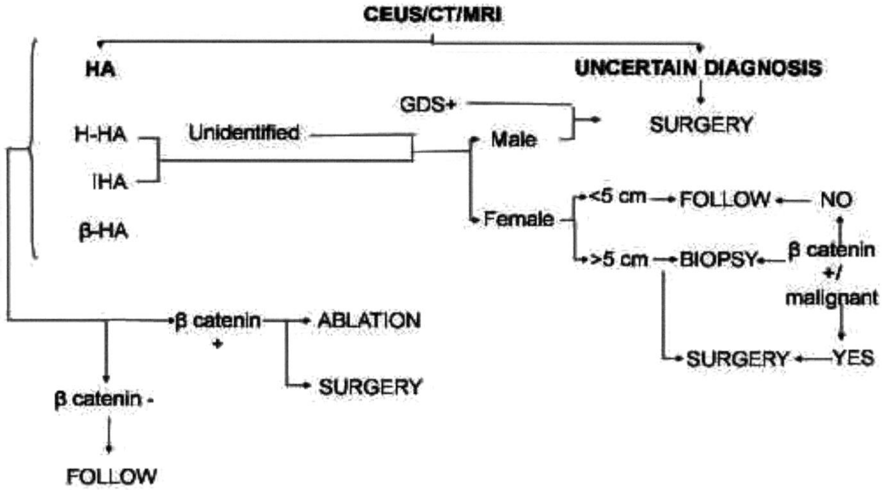

7.3 Management of liver adenomatosis

The management of cases with liver adenomatosis is cumbersome. All women with adenomatosis must discontinue exogenous hormone therapy and should avoid pregnancies. In the massive pattern of adenomatosis, if larger lesions comprise a single lobe, a hemihepatectomy or more limited hepatic resection (**Figure 19**) could be a wise choice. Laparoscopic left lateral sectionectomy can be a good approach for those patients expecting a future liver transplantation [73] (**Algorithm 2**).

Algorithm 2. Management in liver adenomatosis.

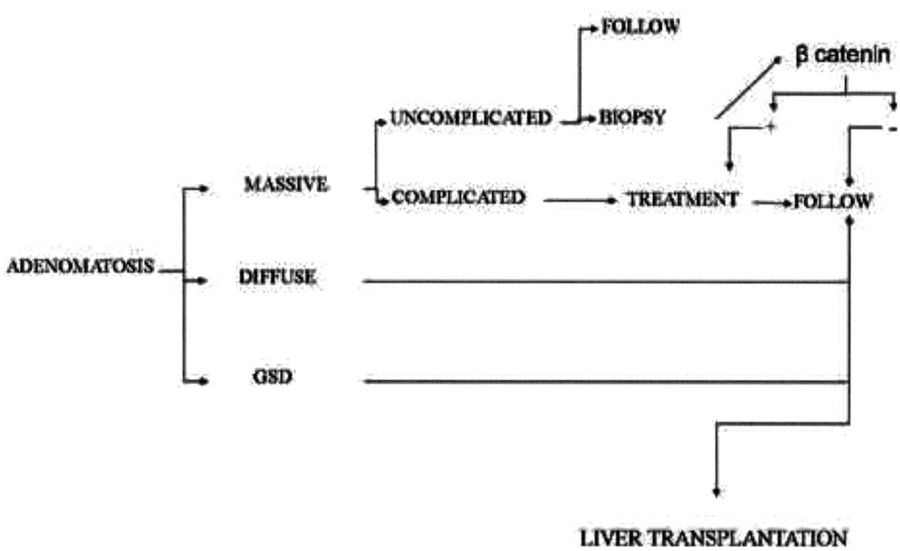

Even the resection of only the complicated nodule (i.e., hemorrhagic liver nodule) seems appropriate as the first step toward enlisting for liver transplantation. Multiple resections are the preferable options in patients with liver

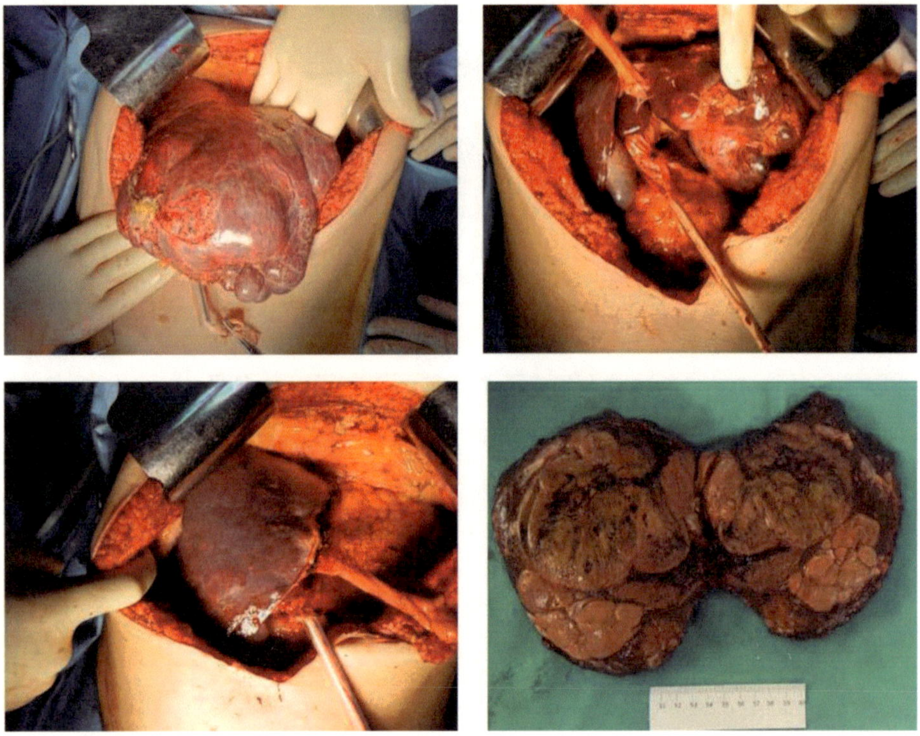

Figure 19.
Upper left: massive liver adenomatosis that deforms the contour of the left lateral sector. Upper right: a left lateral sectionectomy is planned and a cotton loop around hepatic pedicle is placed for Pringle maneuver. Lower left: intraoperative aspect after left lateral sectionectomy. Lower right: sectioned surgical specimen with evidence of the largest HA.

adenomatosis, unless technically impossible or unsafe. Radiofrequency ablation or embolization in these patients was successful in some authors' experience [74]. Liver adenomatosis becomes an indication for liver transplantation if there is evidence of malignant transformation or complications [75]. Observing these changes is possible only if patients are carefully followed on a regular basis with imaging. Liver transplantation should be considered as the last resort for patients with adenomatosis. Patients with GSD should undergo transplantation earlier than other patients with HA because the literature considers this underlying disease as a risk factor for malignant transformation of adenomas [72]. Like in transplantation for HCC, imaging diagnosis of vascular invasion should be considered an absolute contraindication to transplantation. So all the efforts are directed to early diagnose a malignant transformation of HA, and any suspicion of malignancy has to be rapidly confirmed by biopsy. Discussion with the patients with liver adenomatosis about liver transplantation must be initiated when a major criterion or at least 3 minor criteria are identified. The only major criterion is the histological proof of malignancy in at least one adenoma. The minor criteria are: (1) more than 2 serious (life-threatening) hemorrhages, (2) more than 2 previous hepatectomies, (3) β mutated or inflammatory adenomas, (4) underlying liver disease (major steatosis and vascular abnormalities), and (5) age > 30 years [72] (**Figure 20**).

7.4 Alternative treatment of HA

Other options of treatment include: transarterial embolization or ablation and radiofrequency ablation. TAE is considered as a safe and effective mini-invasive

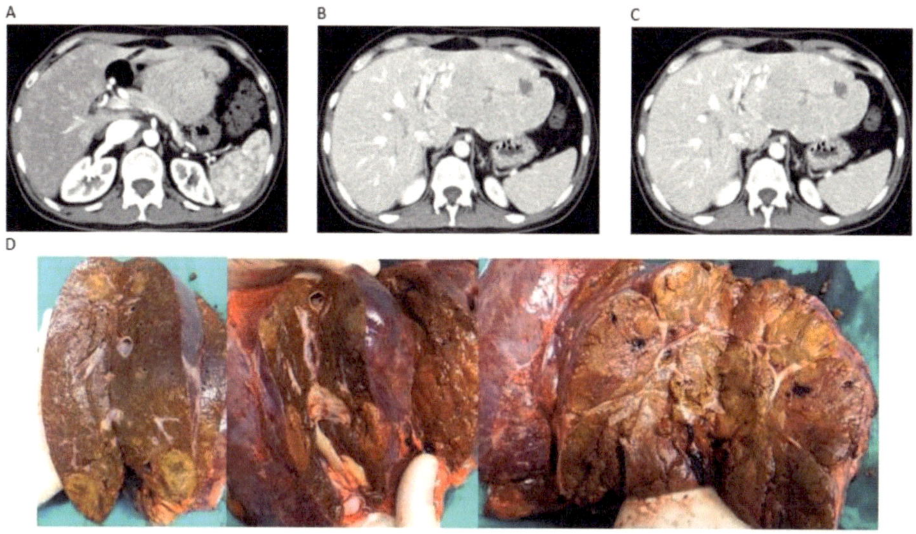

Figure 20.
Liver adenomatosis with a voluminous adenoma of the left liver in a 47-year-old male patient who had a liver transplantation. A-C. CECT of the liver with adenomatosis. D. Total hepatectomy specimen with numerous adenomas of various sizes, a voluminous adenoma in the left liver, and blood clots due to intratumoral bleeding.

procedure to be used in both elective and emergency conditions. For small lesions, TAE can achieve complete resolution and thus avoidance of liver surgery entirely. TAE may be also used as means to shrink the tumors to a size that renders them approachable for subsequent surgical resection [76]. TAE can reduce the size of large adenomas, multiple adenomas, or adenomas that are in a surgical inaccessible localization alleviating the symptoms and reducing the risk of perioperative bleeding. It has a low rate of complications (8%). These complications associated with TAE include post-embolization syndrome, temporary renal failure, and cyst formation [77]. One pyogenic abscess after TAE was also reported as a complication after TAE for a large HA. No sufficient data exist until now to conclude that TAE reduces the risk of hemorrhage or malignant transformation of residual HA, despite reports of a reduction in tumor size.

Radiofrequency ablation has its shortcomings, such as the need of many sessions in order to destruct the tumor completely, but it may be a very good option for tumors that cannot be operated [78].

Medical treatment such as administration of the SRC inhibitor dasatinib or JAK1/2 inhibitor ruxolitinib could be a new alternative in the future [79].

7.5 Management of pregnant patient

Pregnancy is no longer considered a contraindication in hepatocellular adenoma less than 5 cm. Given the fact that the HA behaves as a hormone-dependent tumor that seems to grow or regress according to estrogen level increase or decrease, respectively, it is advised that patients with adenomas who contemplate pregnancy firstly resolve the liver tumor prior to remaining pregnant [80]. If HA was diagnosed in a fertile but nonpregnant woman, and if the tumor is greater than 5 cm or she has experienced adenoma-related complications, resection is indicated before pregnancy. If HA is incidentally identified during pregnancy, the best management varies from case to case. For the smaller lesions, a conservatory approach is feasible on the condition of ultrasound follow-up every 6 weeks.

Adenomas greater than 5 cm that are discovered during pregnancy need individualized approach. Surgery is recommended during second trimester to minimalize the risks for both the mother and the fetus. Radiofrequency has been an option performed during the first and second trimester [18]. Angioembolization poses the radiation risk to the fetus early in pregnancy and must be avoided in the first trimester.

Pregnancy induces not only an increased level of endogenous hormones but also an increased liver vascularity that puts the patient at risk for adenoma rupture especially in the third trimester [81]. However, a ruptured HA discovered during pregnancy should be immediately resected by laparotomy or laparoscopy [28, 82, 83].

7.6 Follow-up of the patients

The great majority of nonresected uncomplicated HA remains stable, in few cases disappear, and in general do not grow. There is an observation that IHA may disappear more rapidly.

The follow-up of the patients with H-HA and IHA with complete resection can be stopped few years after surgery. In case of incomplete resection and with no significant change in HA size during the first years, the follow-up must be continued but at longer intervals.

Instead, the patients with β-HA resected or RF ablated must be followed-up very closely with AFP serum level check and repeated alternating imaging (US, CEUS, CT, and MRI) in order to early diagnose a possible recurrence and, in a much worse scenario, a possible malignancy with the same positioning in the liver [84].

8. Conclusions

The incidence of hepatic adenoma has increased lately as a result of more frequent imaging investigations performed for reasons not necessarily related to the presence of this benign tumor. The classical profile of the patient with adenoma has changed as a result of the emergence of new risk factors. As a result of research into phenotype, genotype, and imaging and the correlations of these results with clinical data, it is advisable that the diagnosis of hepatic adenoma include the subgroup of classification, which indicates the appropriate management of the case. The means of fitting the liver adenoma into the four subgroups are primarily imagistic, of which MRI has an essential role. In the case of insufficient data for the correct and complete diagnosis of hepatic adenoma, tumor biopsy is needed percutaneously or after tumor resection. Management of hepatic adenoma may mean on the one hand careful monitoring to recognize one of the two worrisome complications—hemorrhage and malignancy—and on the other hand, the treatment of the tumor, which may be asymptomatic or symptomatic, uncomplicated or complicated. In the elective cases, surgical resection remains the gold standard with a clear tendency toward laparoscopic approach in specialized centers, but in emergency cases caused by adenoma rupture, interventional arteriography has gained a net advantage over surgery. For rare cases of recurrent or extremely bulky hepatic adenomas, for which surgery is not feasible, but also for cases of liver adenomatosis on certain criteria, liver transplantation from cadaveric or living donor has become a reality. Careful monitoring of post-treatment patients should be continued and adapted according to the therapeutic outcomes and histopathology of the hepatic adenoma.

Thanks

We thank our mentor Prof. Dr. Irinel Popescu, MD, PhD, FACS, for giving us the possibility to use data and iconography of patients that he operated on, in order to complete writing this chapter.

Author details

Mirela Patricia Sîrbu Boeți[1,2*], Beatrice Tivadar[2], Ioana G. Lupescu[1,3], Vlad Herlea[4,5], Mirela Boroș[3], Dana Tomescu[1,6] and Vladislav Brașoveanu[2,5]

1 'Carol Davila' University of Medicine and Pharmacy, Bucharest, Romania

2 Department of General Surgery and Liver Transplantation, Fundeni Clinical Institute, Bucharest, Romania

3 Radiology Medical Imaging and Interventional Radiology Department, Fundeni Clinical Institute, Bucharest, Romania

4 Department of Anatomopathology, Fundeni Clinical Institute, Bucharest, Romania

5 'Titu Maiorescu' University of Medicine and Pharmacy, Bucharest, Romania

6 Department of Anesthesiology and Intensive Care, Fundeni Clinical Institute, Bucharest, Romania

*Address all correspondence to: patriciaboeti@gmail.com

IntechOpen

© 2019 The Author(s). Licensee IntechOpen. This chapter is distributed under the terms of the Creative Commons Attribution License (http://creativecommons.org/licenses/by/3.0), which permits unrestricted use, distribution, and reproduction in any medium, provided the original work is properly cited.

References

[1] Whitmer B. Hepatocellular adenoma. Available from: http://emedicine.medscape.com/article/170205-overview. [8-11-2015]

[2] Vijay A, Elaffandi A, Khalaf H. Hepatocellular adenoma: An update. World Journal of Hepatology. 2015;7:2603-2609. DOI: 10.4254/wjh.v7.i25.2603

[3] Bioulac-Sage P, Sempoux C, Balabaud C. Hepatocellular adenoma: Classification, variants and clinical relevance. Seminars in Diagnostic Pathology. 2017;**34**:112-125. DOI: 10.1053/j.semdp.2016.12.007

[4] Barthelmes L, Tait IS. Liver cell adenoma and liver cell adenomatosis. HPB: The Official Journal of the International Hepato Pancreato Biliary Association. 2005;**7**:186-196. DOI: 10.1080/13651820510028954

[5] Grazioli L, Federle MP, Brancatelli G, Ichikawa T, Olivetti L, Blachar A. Hepatic adenomas: Imaging and pathologic findings. Radiographics. 2001;**21**:877-892. DOI: 10.1148/radiographics.21.4.g01jl04877

[6] Torbenson M. Hepatic adenomas: Classification, controversies, and consensus. Surgical Pathology Clinics. 2018;**11**:351-366. DOI: 10.1016/j.path.2018.02.007

[7] Paulson EK, McClellan JS, Washington K, Spritzer CE, Meyers WC, Baker ME. Hepatic adenoma: MR characteristics and correlation with pathologic findings. AJR. American Journal of Roentgenology. 1994;**163**:113-116. DOI: 10.2214/ajr.163.1.8010195

[8] Chang CY, Hernandez-Prera JC, Roayaie S, Schwartz M, Thung SN. Changing epidemiology of hepatocellular adenoma in the United States: Review of the literature. International Journal of Hepatology. 2013;**2013**:604860. DOI: 10.1155/2013/604860

[9] Antoniades K, Brooks CE Jr. Hemoperitoneum from liver cell adenoma in a patient on oral contraceptives. Surgery. 1975;**77**:137-139

[10] Baek S, Sloane CE, Futterman SC. Benign liver cell adenoma associated with use of oral contraceptive agents. Annals of Surgery. 1976;**183**:239-242

[11] Baum JK, Bookstein JJ, Holtz F, Klein EW. Possible association between benign hepatomas and oral contraceptives. Lancet. 1973;**2**:926-929

[12] Klatskin G. Hepatic tumors: Possible relationship to use of oral contraceptives. Gastroenterology. 1977;**73**:386-394

[13] Dokmak S, Belghiti J. Will weight loss become a future treatment of hepatocellular adenoma in obese patients? Liver International. 2015;**35**:2228-2232. DOI: 10.1111/liv.12925

[14] Gevers TJG, Marcel Spanier BW, Veendrick PB, Vrolijk JM. Regression of hepatocellular adenoma after bariatric surgery in severe obese patients. Liver International. 2018;**38**:2134-2136. DOI: 10.1111/liv.13934

[15] Haring MPD, Gouw ASH, de Haas RJ, Cuperus FJC, de Jong KP, de Meijer VE. The effect of oral contraceptive pill cessation on hepatocellular adenoma diameter: A retrospective cohort study. Liver International. 2019;**39**:905-913. DOI: 10.1111/liv.14074

[16] Masood S, West AB, Barwick KW. Expression of steroid hormone receptors in benign hepatic tumors. An immunocytochemical study. Archives

of Pathology & Laboratory Medicine. 1992;**116**:1355-1359

[17] Kent DR, Nissen ED, Nissen SE, Chambers C. Maternal death resulting from rupture of liver adenoma associated with oral contraceptives. Obstetrics and Gynecology. 1977;**50**:5s-6s

[18] Noels JE, van Aalten SM, van der Windt DJ, et al. Management of hepatocellular adenoma during pregnancy. Journal of Hepatology. 2011;**54**:553-558. DOI: 10.1016/j.jhep.2010.07.022

[19] van Aalten SM, Broker ME, Busschbach JJ, et al. Pregnancy and liver adenoma management: PALM-study. BMC Gastroenterology. 2012;**12**:82. DOI: 10.1186/1471-230X-12-82

[20] Shanbhogue AK, Prasad SR, Takahashi N, Vikram R, Sahani DV. Recent advances in cytogenetics and molecular biology of adult hepatocellular tumors: Implications for imaging and management. Radiology. 2011;**258**:673-693. DOI: 10.1148/radiol.10100376

[21] Bioulac-Sage P, Balabaud C, Zucman-Rossi J. Subtype classification of hepatocellular adenoma. Digestive Surgery. 2010;**27**:39-45. DOI: 10.1159/000268406

[22] Katabathina VS, Menias CO, Shanbhogue AK, Jagirdar J, Paspulati RM, Prasad SR. Genetics and imaging of hepatocellular adenomas: 2011 update. Radiographics. 2011;**31**:1529-1543. DOI: 10.1148/rg.316115527

[23] Fievet P, Sevestre H, Boudjelal M, et al. Systemic AA amyloidosis induced by liver cell adenoma. Gut. 1990;**31**:361-363. DOI: 10.1136/gut.31.3.361

[24] van Aalten SM, Verheij J, Terkivatan T, Dwarkasing RS, De Man RA, Ijzermans JN. Validation of a liver adenoma classification system in a tertiary referral Centre: Implications for clinical practice. Journal of Hepatology. 2011;**55**:120-125. DOI: 10.1016/j.jhep.2010.10.030

[25] Sempoux C, Bisig B, Couchy G, Balabaud C, Zucman-Rossi J, Bioulac-Sage P. Malignant transformation of a beta-catenin inflammatory adenoma due to an S45 beta-catenin-activating mutation present 12 years before. Human Pathology. 2017;**62**:122-125. DOI: 10.1016/j.humpath.2016.10.004

[26] Vij M, Patra S, Rela M. Pigmented hepatocellular adenoma with complete CD34 immunostaining pattern: A diagnostic dilemma. Indian Journal of Pathology & Microbiology. 2012;**55**:528-530. DOI: 10.4103/0377- 4929.107801

[27] Flejou JF, Barge J, Menu Y, et al. Liver adenomatosis. An entity distinct from liver adenoma? Gastroenterology. 1985;**89**:1132-1138

[28] Ribeiro A, Burgart LJ, Nagorney DM, Gores GJ. Management of liver adenomatosis: Results with a conservative surgical approach. Liver Transplantation and Surgery. 1998;**4**:388-398

[29] Chiche L, Dao T, Salame E, et al. Liver adenomatosis: Reappraisal, diagnosis, and surgical management: Eight new cases and review of the literature. Annals of Surgery. 2000;**231**:74-81. DOI: 10.1097/00000658-200001000-00011

[30] Grazioli L, Federle MP, Ichikawa T, Balzano E, Nalesnik M, Madariaga J. Liver adenomatosis: Clinical, histopathologic, and imaging findings in 15 patients. Radiology. 2000;**216**:395-402. DOI: 10.1148/radiology.216.2.r00jl38395

[31] Descottes B, Kalfon M, Rousseau D, Grousseau D, Catanzano G. Benign tumors of the liver. Hemoperitoneum

caused by rupture of a hepatic adenoma. Chirurgie. 1981;**107**:176-177

[32] Klompenhouwer AJ, De Man RA, Thomeer MG, IJzermans JN. Management and outcome of hepatocellular adenoma with massive bleeding at presentation. World Journal of Gastroenterology. 2017;**23**:4579-4586. DOI: 10.3748/wjg.v23.i25.4579

[33] Bieze M, Phoa SS, Verheij J, van Lienden KP, van Gulik TM. Risk factors for bleeding in hepatocellular adenoma. The British Journal of Surgery. 2014;**101**:847-855. DOI: 10.1002/bjs.9493

[34] Addeo P, Cesaretti M, Fuchshuber P, et al. Outcomes of liver resection for haemorrhagic hepatocellular adenoma. International Journal of Surgery. 2016;**27**:34-38. DOI: 10.1016/j.ijsu.2016.01.041

[35] Mizejewski GJ. Alpha-fetoprotein structure and function: Relevance to isoforms, epitopes, and conformational variants. Experimental Biology and Medicine (Maywood.). 2001;**226**:377-408

[36] Sandler MA, Petrocelli RD, Marks DS, Lopez R. Ultrasonic features and radionuclide correlation in liver cell adenoma and focal nodular hyperlasia. Radiology. 1980;**135**:393-397. DOI: 10.1148/radiology.135.2.6245428

[37] Golli M, Mathieu D, Anglade MC, Cherqui D, Vasile N, Rahmouni A. Focal nodular hyperplasia of the liver: Value of color Doppler US in association with MR imaging. Radiology. 1993;**187**:113-117. DOI: 10.1148/radiology.187.1.8451397

[38] Golli M, Van Nhieu JT, Mathieu D, et al. Hepatocellular adenoma: Color Doppler US and pathologic correlations. Radiology. 1994;**190**:741-744. DOI: 10.1148/radiology.190.3.8115621

[39] Ichikawa T, Federle MP, Grazioli L, Nalesnik M. Hepatocellular adenoma: Multiphasic CT and histopathologic findings in 25 patients. Radiology. 2000;**214**:861-868. DOI: 10.1148/radiology.214.3.r00mr28861

[40] Denecke T, Steffen IG, Agarwal S, et al. Appearance of hepatocellular adenomas on gadoxetic acid-enhanced MRI. European Radiology. 2012;**22**:1769-1775. DOI: 10.1007/s00330-012-2422-5

[41] van Aalten SM, Thomeer MG, Terkivatan T, et al. Hepatocellular adenomas: Correlation of MR imaging findings with pathologic subtype classification. Radiology. 2011;**261**:172-181. DOI: 10.1148/radiol.11110023

[42] Grazioli L, Olivetti L, Mazza G, Bondioni MP. MR imaging of hepatocellular adenomas and differential diagnosis dilemma. International Journal of Hepatology. 2013;**2013**:374170. DOI: 10.1155/2013/374170

[43] Guo Y, Li W, Xie Z, et al. Diagnostic value of Gd-EOB-DTPA-MRI for hepatocellular adenoma: A meta-analysis. Journal of Cancer. 2017;**8**:1301-1310

[44] Cuervo C, Gómez DV, Catrillón GA. Hepatocellular adenomas: Current findings in images which allow their characterization and management. Revista Colombiana de Entomología. 2014;**25**:3934-3941

[45] Mohajer K, Frydrychowicz A, Robbins JB, Loeffler AG, Reed TD, Reeder SB. Characterization of hepatic adenoma and focal nodular hyperplasia with gadoxetic acid. Journal of Magnetic Resonance Imaging. 2012;**36**:686-696. DOI: 10.1002/jmri.23701

[46] McInnes MD, Hibbert RM, Inacio JR, Schieda N. Focal nodular hyperplasia and hepatocellular adenoma: Accuracy of Gadoxetic acid-enhanced MR imaging--a systematic

review. Radiology. 2015;**277**:413-423. DOI: 10.1148/radiol.2015142986

[47] Chaib E, Gama-Rodrigues J, Ribeiro MA Jr, Herman P, Saad WA. Hepatic adenoma. Timing for surgery. Hepato-Gastroenterology. 2007;**54**:1382-1387

[48] Rubin RA, Lichtenstein GR. Hepatic scintigraphy in the evaluation of solitary solid liver masses. Journal of Nuclear Medicine. 1993;**34**:697-705

[49] Zucman-Rossi J, Jeannot E, Nhieu JT, et al. Genotype-phenotype correlation in hepatocellular adenoma: New classification and relationship with HCC. Hepatology. 2006;**43**:515-524. DOI: 10.1002/hep.21068

[50] Tokoro T, Kato Y, Sugioka A, Mizoguchi Y. Malignant transformation of hepatocellular adenoma over a decade. BMJ Case Reports. 2014;**2014**:bcr2014205261. DOI: 10.1136/bcr-2014-205261

[51] Nagy G, Dezso K, Kiss G, Gerlei Z, Nagy P, Kobori L. Benign liver tumours—Current diagnostics and therapeutic modalities. Magyar Onkologia. 2018;**62**:5-13

[52] Buhler H, Pirovino M, Akobiantz A, et al. Regression of liver cell adenoma. A follow-up study of three consecutive patients after discontinuation of oral contraceptive use. Gastroenterology. 1982;**82**:775-782

[53] Foster JH, Berman MM. The malignant transformation of liver cell adenomas. Archives of Surgery. 1994;**129**:712-717

[54] Sherlock S. Hepatic reactions to drugs. Gut. 1979;**20**:634-648. DOI: 10.1136/gut.20.7.634

[55] Belghiti J, Pateron D, Panis Y, et al. Resection of presumed benign liver tumours. The British Journal of Surgery. 1993;**80**:380-383

[56] Popescu I, Câmpeanu I. Surgical anatomy of the liver and liver resection. Brisbane 2000 terminology. Chirurgia (Bucur.). 2009;**104**:7-10

[57] Lang H, Sotiropoulos GC, Fruhauf NR, Radtke A, Malago M, Broelsch C. Mesohepatectomy—An alternative to extended hepatectomy in the treatment of central liver tumors. Der Chirurg. 2004;**75**:424-429. DOI: 10.1007/s00104-003-0803-7

[58] Sivula A, Lempinen M. A benign hepatocellular adenoma treated by extended right lobectomy. Annales Chirurgiae et Gynaecologiae. Supplementum. 1976;**65**:46-51

[59] Herman P, Coelho FF, Perini MV, Lupinacci RM, D'Albuquerque LA, Cecconello I. Hepatocellular adenoma: An excellent indication for laparoscopic liver resection. HPB: The Official Journal of the International Hepato Pancreato Biliary Association. 2012;**14**:390-395. DOI: 10.1111/j.1477-2574.2012.00463.x

[60] Popescu I, Vasile S, Sgarbură O, Hrehoreț D, Tomulescu V. Laparoscopic left lateral segmentectomy of the liver: Indications, technique, results. Chirurgia (Bucur.). 2008;**103**:17-22

[61] Abu HM, Di FF, Wiltshire RD, Hamdan M, Layfield DM, Pearce NW. Laparoscopic liver resection for hepatocellular adenoma. World Journal of Gastrointestinal Surgery. 2011;**3**:101-105. DOI: 10.4240/wjgs.v3.i7.101

[62] Ferzli G, David A, Kiel T. Laparoscopic resection of a large hepatic tumor. Surgical Endoscopy. 1995;**9**:733-735

[63] Azagra JS, Goergen M, Gilbart E, Jacobs D. Laparoscopic anatomical (hepatic) left lateral segmentectomy—Technical aspects. Surgical Endoscopy. 1996;**10**:758-761

[64] Buell JF, Cherqui D, Geller DA, et al. The international position on laparoscopic liver surgery: The Louisville statement, 2008. Annals of Surgery. 2009;**250**:825-830. DOI: 10.1097/sla.0b013e3181b3b2d8

[65] Herman P, Kruger J, Lupinacci R, Coelho F, Perini M. Laparoscopic bisegmentectomy 6 and 7 using a Glissonian approach and a half-Pringle maneuver. Surgical Endoscopy. 2013;**27**:1840-1841. DOI: 10.1007/s00464-012-2681-x

[66] Popescu I, Ciurea S, Romanescu D, Boroş M. Isolated resection of the caudate lobe: Indications, technique and results. Hepato-Gastroenterology. 2008;**55**:831-835

[67] Ribeiro Junior MA, Chaib E, Saad WA, D'Albuquerque LA, Cecconello I. Surgical management of spontaneous ruptured hepatocellular adenoma. Clinics (São Paulo, Brazil). 2009;**64**:775-779. DOI: 10.1590/S1807- 59322009000800011

[68] Rooks JB, Ory HW, Ishak KG, et al. Epidemiology of hepatocellular adenoma. The role of oral contraceptive use. JAMA. 1979;**242**:644-648

[69] Mueller J, Keeffe EB, Esquivel CO. Liver transplantation for treatment of giant hepatocellular adenomas. Liver Transplantation and Surgery. 1995;**1**:99-102

[70] Vennarecci G, Santoro R, Antonini M, et al. Liver transplantation for recurrent hepatic adenoma. World Journal of Hepatology. 2013;**5**:145-148. DOI: 10.4254/wjh.v5.i3.145

[71] Colle I, Laureys G, Raevens S, et al. Living related liver transplantation in an adult patient with hepatocellular adenoma and carcinoma 13 years after bone marrow transplantation for Fanconi anemia: A case report. Hepatology Research. 2013;**43**:991-998. DOI: 10.1111/hepr.12043

[72] Chiche L, David A, Adam R, et al. Liver transplantation for adenomatosis: European experience. Liver Transplantation. 2016;**22**:516-526. DOI: 10.1002/lt.24417

[73] Govender M, Matsevych OY. Laparoscopic left lateral sectionectomy at Dr George Mukhari academic hospital. South African Journal of Surgery. 2017;**55**:84

[74] Ahn SY, Park SY, Kweon YO, Tak WY, Bae HI, Cho SH. Successful treatment of multiple hepatocellular adenomas with percutaneous radiofrequency ablation. World Journal of Gastroenterology. 2013;**19**:7480-7486. DOI: 10.3748/wjg.v19.i42.7480

[75] Donato M, Hamidian JA, Andrade AI, Kim R, Chaudhery SI, Sangster G. Hepatic adenomatosis: A rare but important liver disease with severe clinical implications. International Surgery. 2015;**100**:903-907. DOI: 10.9738/INTSURG-D-14 -00161.1

[76] Sinkler MA, Bosley M. Massive hepatic adenoma response to bland embolization: A case study. Radiology Case Reports. 2019;**14**:48-51. DOI: 10.1016/j.radcr.2018.09.016

[77] van Rosmalen BV, Coelen RJS, Bieze M, et al. Systematic review of transarterial embolization for hepatocellular adenomas. The British Journal of Surgery. 2017;**104**:823-835. DOI: 10.1002/bjs.10547

[78] van Vledder MG, van Aalten SM, Terkivatan T, De Man RA, Leertouwer T, IJzermans JN. Safety and efficacy of radiofrequency ablation for hepatocellular adenoma. Journal of Vascular and Interventional Radiology. 2011;**22**:787-793. DOI: 10.1016/j.jvir.2011.02.024

[79] Blanc JF, Frulio N, Chiche L, Bioulac-Sage P, Balabaud C. Hepatocellular adenoma management: Advances but still a long way to go. Hepatic Oncology. 2015;**2**:171-180. DOI: 10.2217/hep.14.41

[80] Estebe JP, Malledant Y, Guillou YM, et al. Spontaneous rupture of an adenoma of the liver during pregnancy. Journal de Chirurgie (Paris). 1988;**125**:654-656

[81] Cobey FC, Salem RR. A review of liver masses in pregnancy and a proposed algorithm for their diagnosis and management. American Journal of Surgery. 2004;**187**:181-191. DOI: 10.1016/j.amjsurg.2003.11.016

[82] Broker ME, Ijzermans JN, van Aalten SM, De Man RA, Terkivatan T. The management of pregnancy in women with hepatocellular adenoma: A plea for an individualized approach. International Journal of Hepatology. 2012;**2012**:725735, 10.1155/2012/725735

[83] Gryspeerdt F, Aerts R. Laparoscopic liver resection for hemorrhagic hepatocellular adenoma in a pregnant patient. Acta Chirurgica Belgica. 2018;**118**(5):322-325. DOI: 10.1080/00015458.2017.1379790

[84] Federle MP. Hepatic adenoma in speciality imaging - hepatobiliary and pancreas. In: Federle, Jeffrey, Tublin, editors. 1st edition. Amyrsis; 2013. p. I-262-I-270. ISBN: 978-1-931884-67-9

Chapter 8

Surgical Treatment of Hepatic Hydatidosis

Luis Burgos San Juan, Hector Losada Morales, Jorge Silva Abarca, Cesar Muñoz Castro, Marcelo Klein Diaz and Pablo Guzmán González

Abstract

Hepatic hydatid disease has been reported from ancient times. It is a zoonotic infection caused by nine recognized species of tapeworms of the genus *Echinococcus*. Some of them are known to cause human echinococcosis, and there is reasonable doubt regarding the others. Diagnosis is supported by epidemiological history, clinical presentation, radiological imaging, and serological tests. Various pathological forms may become life-threatening, and in those cases, the treatment is extremely complex. The main objective of the treatment is to completely cure the illness in order to avoid further complications and recurrences. Hepatic surgery, using different techniques, achieves best results with acceptable morbidity and mortality rates. In the South of Chile, the geographical location in which we work, this illness is endemic with high incidence and prevalence. The hepatobiliopancreatic units of the regional surgical centers of Temuco have plenty of experience treating liver hydatid disease. In this chapter we shall focus especially on epidemiology, etiopathogenesis, diagnosis, and surgical treatment of hepatic hydatidosis.

Keywords: hepatic hydatidosis, epidemiology, etiopathogeny, diagnosis, surgical treatment

1. Introduction

Human echinococcosis, also called hydatidosis, is a zoonosis which has been known from ancient times. There are mentions about hydatid disease both in humans and animals in documents as old as the Ebers Papyrus and the Babylonian Talmud [1, 2]. Around the mid-nineteenth century, a significant breakthrough happened when the etiology and the life cycles of different *Echinococcus* species were defined, although there are still many related questions pending to resolve [3]. Hydatid disease is caused by nine recognized species of tapeworm of the genus *Echinococcus* (*E.*). Seven of them cause different forms of human echinococcosis, and the remaining two are being studied for a possible human affectation. Some of the life cycles of these tapeworms have domestic animals as hosts, e.g., dogs as definitive hosts and sheep as intermediate hosts. Humans are accidental intermediate hosts. Other species of these parasites have wild life cycles, infecting almost exclusively wild animals and rarely humans. Additionally, more complex cycles with interaction of wild and domestic animals have been described as well. There are reported variants of these cycles depending on geographical location [4].

Cystic echinococcosis, the most common form of hydatidosis, is an endemic zoonosis caused by the larval stage (metacestodes) of the tapeworm *E. granulosus*. In relation to the geographical distribution, the disease is present in many countries around the world [5]. The diagnosis is supported by epidemiological history, anamnestic data, clinical presentation, radiological imaging, and serological tests. Surgical treatment employs different techniques, aiming for the best outcome for the patient. Partial cystectomy, pericystectomy, and hepatic resection are performed by either open or laparoscopic surgical access, with or without neoadjuvant or adjuvant medical therapy. There are also different procedures for the evacuation of the parasite, using percutaneous or endoscopic access. In selected cases, antiparasitic drug therapy is employed as the only treatment for this illness [6]. The prognosis for these patients will depend on the selection of the most adequate therapy according to several factors mainly related to the physical status of the patient and the larval stage of the parasite and its location [7]. Complicated cases must be treated in reference centers by well-trained and experienced hepatobiliary surgeons. This zoonosis has not yet been completely eradicated, and if affected countries do not apply epidemiological control policies, a great amount of resources will have to be allocated to the treatment of this illness. Cystic echinococcosis of the liver is endemic, especially in the South of Chile [8]. For this reason, the main theme of this chapter will be centered in topics concerning this form of hydatidosis.

2. Epidemiology

The most common form of hydatidosis is cystic echinococcosis caused by *E. granulosus*; it is present in several countries around the world and represents a major public health problem in some regions [9, 10]. It is considered endemic in areas such as Peru, Chile, Argentina, Uruguay, southern Brazil, the Mediterranean region, Central Asia, Western China, and East Africa [11]. Antarctica is the only continent free of this parasitic disease, and it has also been eradicated through efficient epidemiological control programs in Iceland, New Zealand, Tasmania, Falkland Islands, and Cyprus [12]. This pathology affects different organs, although the liver is the most commonly compromised, accounting for 70–75% of the cases. Alveolar echinococcosis caused by *E. multilocularis* is restricted to the Northern Hemisphere and might determine high morbidity and mortality [13]. Polycystic echinococcosis is caused by *E. vogeli* and only reported in Central and South America with low incidence rates [14]. Unicystic echinococcosis, caused by *E. oligarthrus*, is extremely rare in humans, and the only localization in which it has been reported is the orbit of the eye and the myocardium [15]. Other two species of the genus *Echinococcus*, *E. shiquicus* [16] and *E. felidis* [17], are present in the Tibetan Plateau and Africa, respectively, and there are investigations about risks of human affectation. In the South of Chile, cystic echinococcosis is an endemic zoonosis with an average incidence of 1.9/100,000 and a mortality rate of 0.2/100,000 inhabitants. The hospital discharge rate corresponds to 6.3/100,000, and this figure rises to 28.1/100,000 in our Araucanía Region [8].

3. Etiopathogeny

Hydatidosis is caused by the larval stages of taeniid cestodes of the genus *Echinococcus*. There are nine species of this tapeworm currently identified, eight well-defined species and one genotypic cluster, that in future investigations could be defined as one to three different species. These nine species of *Echinococcus* are as follows: *E. granulosus* sensu stricto, *E. equinus*, *E. ortleppi*, *E. multilocularis*, *E. vogeli*, *E. oligarthrus*, *E. canadensis* cluster, *E. shiquicus*, and *E. felidis*. Each of them has a different life cycle, transmission routes, pathology forms of clinical presentation, possible human affectation, different geographical location, and biological behavior. Some of these species may affect humans, others only animals, and in others this is still unclear [18]. For example, regarding *E. shiquicus* and *E. felidis*, although they were known to infect only animals, there is growing apprehension about an eventual human affectation, and there is an ongoing research to support this with molecular and genomic studies [19, 20]. Other species of these parasites have exclusively wild life cycles. The study of their complex genotypic diversity aims to successfully prevent the transmission of this infection to humans [21]. The life cycle of these parasites starts with adult taeniid cestodes living in the small intestine of canids or felids (definitive host). Next, the adult tapeworms release their eggs, thus contaminating the feces, which are then ingested by rodents, ungulates, other herbivores, and occasionally humans (intermediate hosts). When humans are infected, the eggs reach the small intestine, and larval oncospheres hatch, which adhere and penetrate the intestinal mucosa by using their hooks and then migrate through the portal circulation to reach their first fixed location in the liver (50–70% of the cases). This happens most commonly in the right hepatic lobe due to the anatomical distribution of the portal venous system. The lungs are affected in 20–30% of the cases and much less frequently the spleen, kidneys, heart, muscles, bone, and central nervous system. For example, once located in the liver, the metacestodes begin their development and growth giving place to the formation of the hydatid cyst [22].

The anatomical structure of the cyst has an outer acellular laminated membrane that allows the entry of nutrients from the host. Then there is the inner nucleated germinal membrane, in which the daughter vesicles are produced. In an asexual form, the protoscoleces are formed inside the daughter vesicles. The immunological system of the intermediate host reacts to isolate the parasite, forming a fibrous layer called adventitia, which can calcify with the passage of time (**Figure 1A**, **B**). The life cycle closes when the animal's definitive host is fed by contaminated viscera, and each protoscolece can develop an adult tapeworm in its small intestine [23] capsules and scolices.

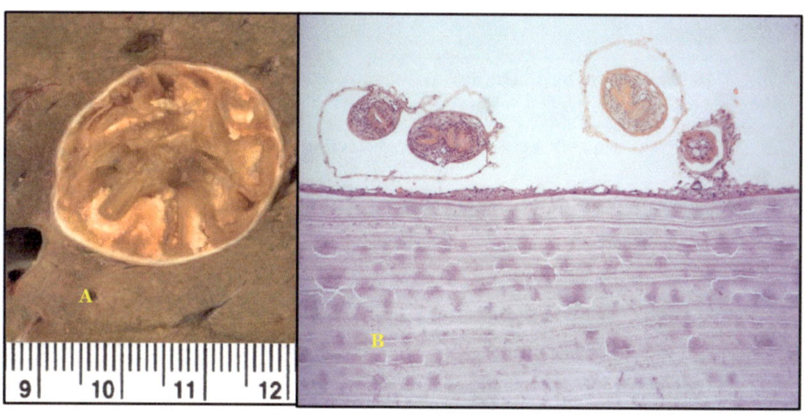

Figure 1.
(a) Hepatic solitary cyst, rounded, whitish external wall of uniform thickness. The cyst contains turbid liquid color upon formalin fixation and whitish yellowish germinal and laminated layer floating within the cyst. (b) The wall of the hydatid cyst has a laminated acellular membrane and a germinal layer with brood.

4. Diagnosis

Currently, the diagnosis must always consider the epidemiological background. The definitive diagnosis is reached through the use of imaging and in some cases with the additional contribution of serology. In the near future, earlier stages of the parasitosis will be diagnosed by means of advances in immunological tests [24, 25].

4.1 Clinical features

Humans remain asymptomatic for a prolonged period of time after being infected due to the slow growth of the hydatid cyst in the liver (1–5 mm per year). Small and medium cysts of central hepatic location are usually asymptomatic, or a slight pain in the epigastrium and right hypochondrium might be reported by the patient, together with a sensation of abdominal discomfort. Besides, the previous immune status of the patient and the anatomical location of the cyst could determine a late manifestation of the first symptoms [26]. When the cysts grow and reach a significant size, the mass effect on the bile tree and hepatic vasculature determine other clinical manifestations derived from biliary obstruction, portal hypertension, and Budd-Chiari syndrome. The magnitude of this effect will determine different degrees of jaundice and portal hypertension, which may range from a slight increase of bilirubinemia and the appearance of venous collaterals of the abdominal wall to very severe jaundice, ascites, and upper digestive hemorrhage secondary to rupture of the gastroesophageal varices [27].

4.2 Imaging

In 1981, Gharbi reported an ultrasonography classification of the hepatic hydatidosis, describing five categories in relation to the morphological findings of the cysts, according to their stage of evolution [28]. In 2002, based on this classification, the World Health Organization Informal Working Group on Echinococcosis (WHO-IWGE) formulated a new classification adding two more categories, with the aim of guiding in the selection of the best treatment and follow-up of the results obtained (**Tables 1** and 2) [29–31]. Current imaging offers several tools to

WHO-IWGE	Radiologic characteristics	Definition of cyst
CL	Unilocular cystic lesion with uniform anechoic content, cyst wall not visible	Cystic lesion
CE1	Unilocular cystic lesion with uniform anechoic content, cyst wall visible, snowflake sign	Active cyst
CE2	Multivesicular, multiseptated cysts, daughter cysts present, honeycomb sign	Active cyst
CE3A	Unilocular cyst containing liquid with a floating membrane inside, water-lily sign	Transitional cyst
CE3B	Cysts with daughter cysts in solid matrix	
CE4	Cysts with heterogeneous hypoechoic or hyperechoic degenerative contents, no daughter cysts	Inactive cyst
CE5	Cysts characterized by a thick calcified wall, which is arch shaped, producing a cone-shaped shadow; degree of calcification varies from partial to complete	Inactive cyst

Table 1.
WHO-IWGE ultrasound classification.

WHO	Surgery	PAIR	Drug therapy	Suggestion	Resource setting
CE1		✓	✓	<5 cm ABZ PAIR PAIR >5 cm PAIR+ALB PAIR	Optimal Minimal Optimal Minimal
CE2	✓	✓	✓	Other PT + ALB Other PT	Optimal Minimal
CE3a		✓	✓	Other PT < 5 cm ABZ PAIR >5cmPAIR+ ABZ PAIR	Optimal Minimal Optimal Minimal
CE3b	✓	✓	✓	Non-PAIR PT + ABZ Non-PAIR PT	Optimal Minimal
CE4				Watch and wait	Optimal
CE5				Watch and wait	Optimal

Table 2.
Suggested stage-specific approach to uncomplicated cystic echinococcosis of the liver.

guide a better management of this disease. Usually, the imaging diagnostic begins with the use of ultrasonography (US), and then other imaging tests could also be used to achieve a better diagnosis of the most complex forms of parasitosis, such as contrast-enhanced ultrasound (CEUS), computed tomography (CT), magnetic resonance imaging (MRI), magnetic resonance cholangiography (MRC), endoscopic retrograde cholangiography (ERC), and conventional X-rays.

4.2.1 Ultrasonography

The US is widely used due to its low cost and high-definition images, which allow to define the pathological characteristics of hepatic hydatid cysts and other locations in the peritoneal cavity (**Figures 2–4**). It is also useful for the differential diagnosis of hydatid cyst with other liver tumors. The use of mobile devices allows having a portable tool for the screening of populations in endemic

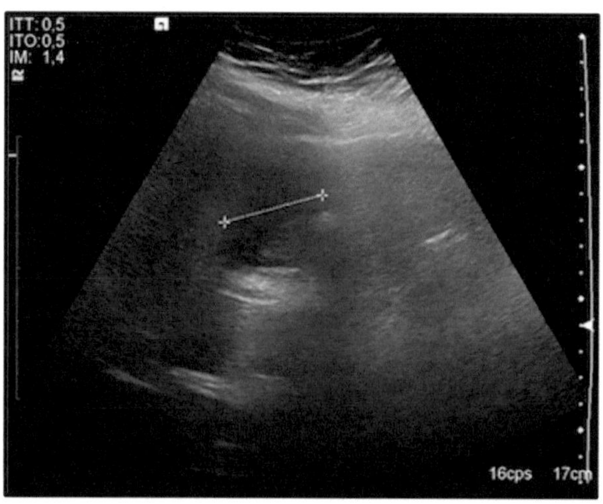

Figure 2.
Cyst of solid appearance (CE4).

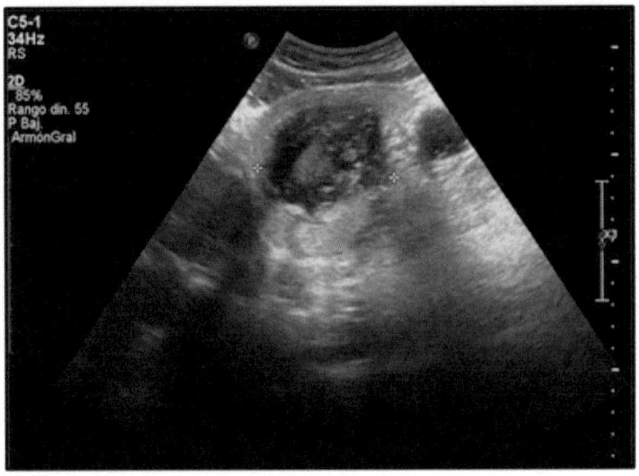

Figure 3.
Heterogeneous matrix. Ball of wool sign (CE4).

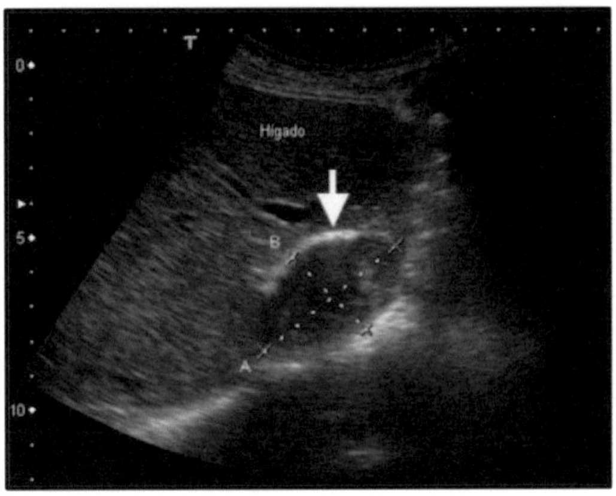

Figure 4.
Calcified anterior wall of cyst. Arciform image (white arrow).

areas with high risk of affectation [30, 32, 33]. Due to the difficult differentiation of certain forms of alveolar echinococcosis from other kinds of hepatic tumors, CEUS is being increasingly used in certain regions with endemic affectation of this pathology [34].

4.2.2 Computed tomography

Sometimes, the ultrasound does not help much in the diagnosis of liver hydatidosis for different reasons, such as obesity, presence of abundant intestinal gas, hydatid recurrence, or residual cavities secondary to previous surgery. When that is the case, CT is used, taking advantage of its higher sensitivity and specificity. Unenhanced CT allows to have a better radiological diagnosis of the different forms of cyst calcification [33]. The contrast-enhanced CT aids in choosing the best surgical techniques according to the different forms of presentation or complications related to the disease, e.g., by allowing a more accurate appreciation of the involvement of the vasculature and biliary tree. CT also aids in diagnosing the cystic migration to the thorax and the biliary tree [35, 36]. Another advantage of the use of contrast-enhanced CT is to achieve a better differential diagnosis from other focal liver lesions [37] (**Figures 5–11A, B**).

4.2.3 Magnetic resonance imaging

MRI is useful for diagnosis of cases of cholangiohydatidosis. Compared to US and CT, the MRI T2-weighted sequence is better at defining the internal structure of the cyst. In general, it is indicated for patients that present difficulties when performing ultrasound, such as bowel gas excess, previous surgeries, disseminated hydatidosis, and obesity. In addition, MRI is recommended when CT is contraindicated due to comorbidities. MRC is used to determine the existence of cysto-biliary fistula and the presence of hydatid material in the biliary tree. It also visualizes the cysto-biliary fistula both toward the bronchi and to the biliary tree [38, 39] (**Figures 11a**, **b–17**).

4.2.4 Endoscopic retrograde cholangiography

The rupture of a hydatid cyst in the intrahepatic bile duct can initiate some complications, which might become serious mainly due to the development of

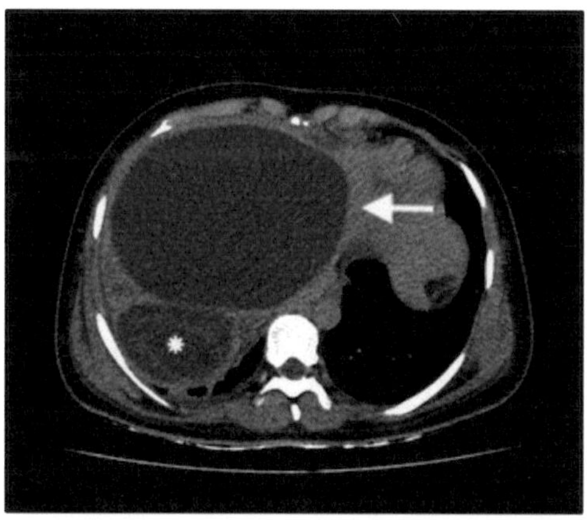

Figure 5.
Unilocular cyst (CE1, white arrow). Detached membrane. Cyst (CE2, white star).

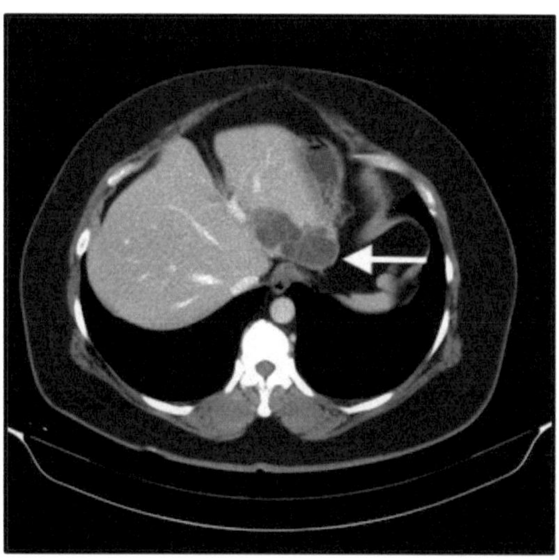

Figure 6.
Contrast-enhanced CT. Septated cyst (white arrow).

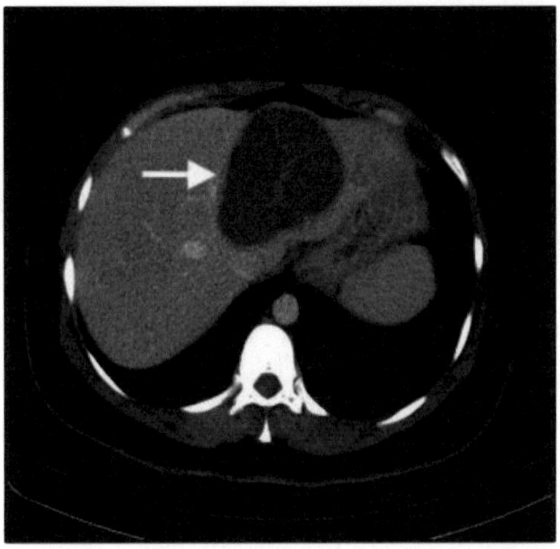

Figure 7.
Daughter vesicles in mother cyst (white arrow).

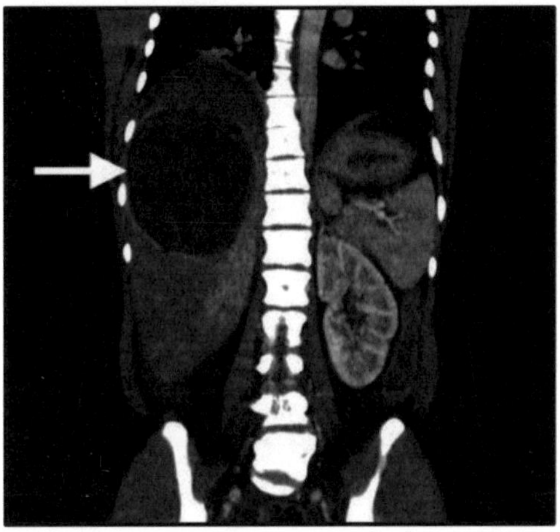

Figure 8.
Coronal contrast-enhanced CT. CE3 A, water-lily sign (white arrow).

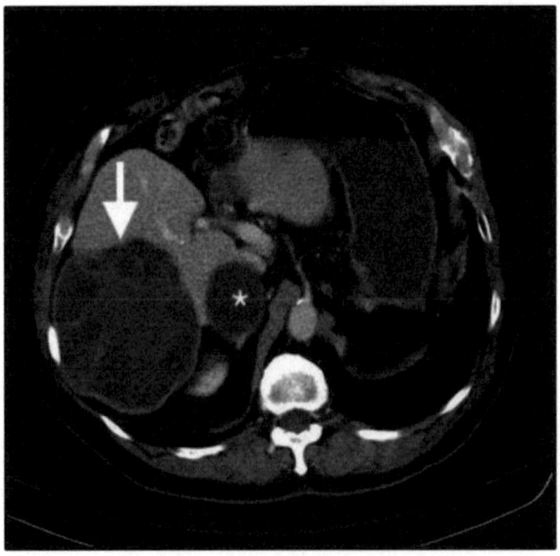

Figure 9.
Central matrix. Daughter vesicles. Cartwheel sign (white arrow).

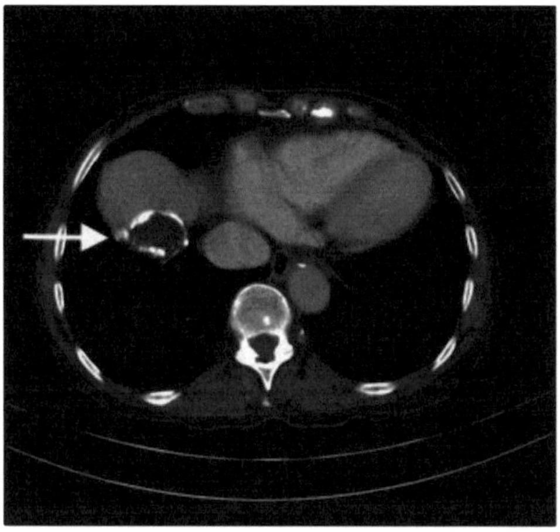

Figure 10.
Dome location with annular calcification (CE 5, white arrow).

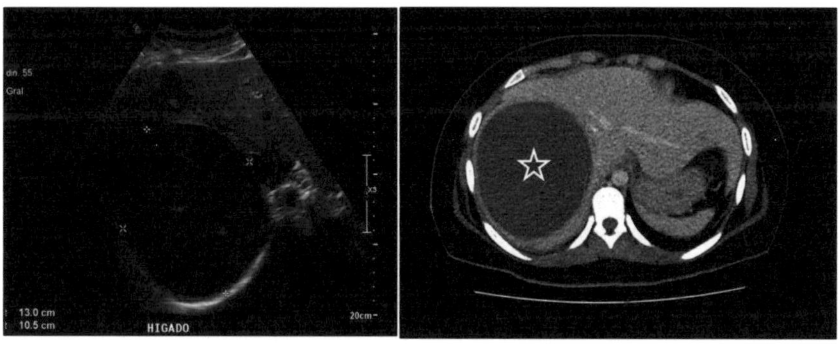

A B

Figure 11.
(A) US content, heterogeneous with a solid appearance (CE4). (B) In the same patient, the contrast-enhanced CT diagnoses an unilocular hydatid cyst (CE1).

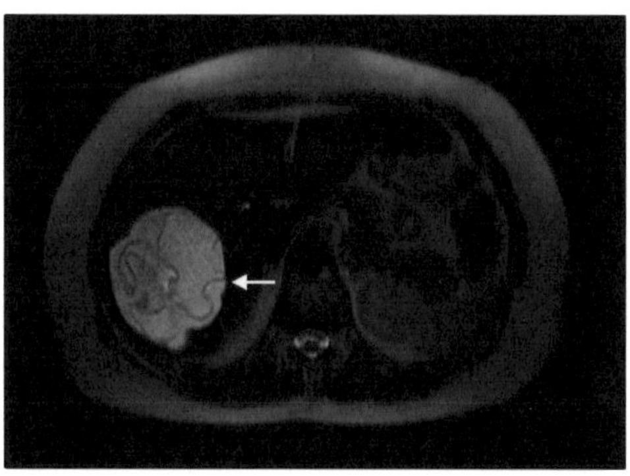

Figure 12.
MRI T2 axial. Detached membranes. Hypointense pericyst (white arrow). Water-lily sign.

cholangitis and septicemia. In these cases, the ERC provides the diagnosis and performs the removal of hydatid material, with the objective of improving the general conditions of the patient before carrying out the definitive surgical treatment [40].

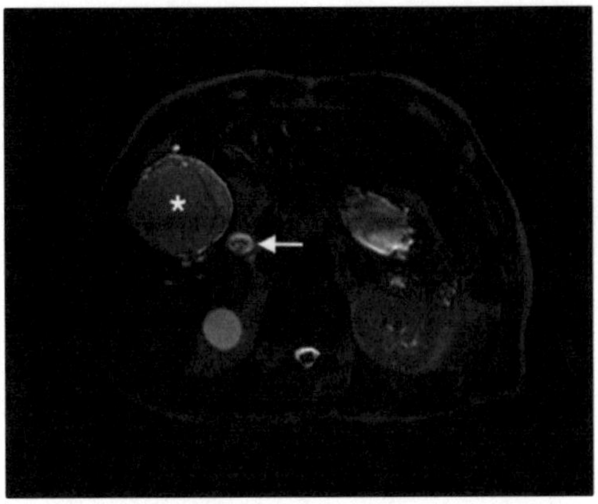

Figure 13.
MRI T2 axial. Detached membranes (white star). Hydatid membranes in bile duct (white arrow).

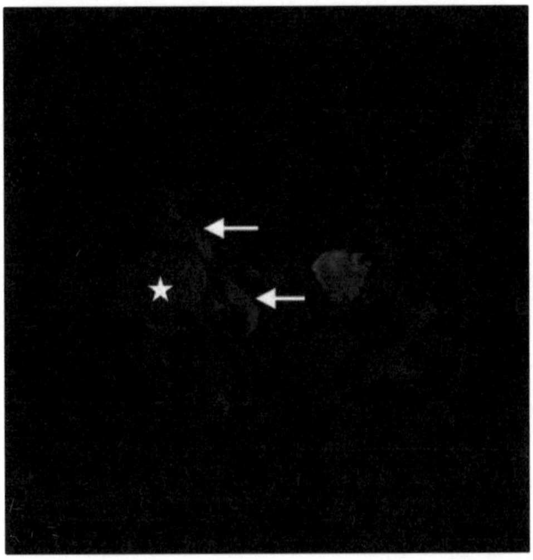

Figure 14.
MRI coronal. Detached membranes. Bile duct with membranes (white arrow).

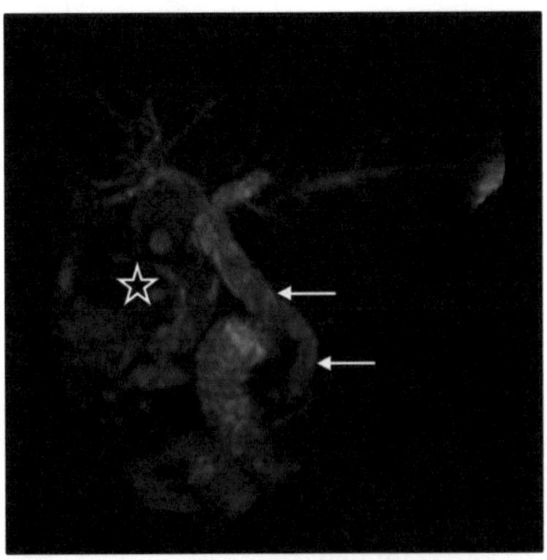

Figure 15.
MR cholangiography. Residual cyst membranes (white star). Cholangiohydatidosis.

4.3 Serology

Currently, diagnosis and follow-up of patients with cystic echinococcosis are achieved especially through imaging. Serology is used for the same purpose, using the detection of IgG-specific antigens. However, low sensitivity and specificity rates have been reported. In addition, false positives appear during follow-up due to the persistence of antibodies over time. There is a lot of research (recombined proteins, isotopic antibodies, subisotopic IgG, synthetic peptides), which seek to develop new antibodies by means of the molecular technique, allowing a better diagnosis of this parasitosis [41, 42].

5. Complications

Frequently, there are complications secondary to the hepatic location of the cyst or by involvement of adjacent organs, in which case symptoms and signs of greater intensity will appear. Among them, the following should be mentioned:

- More intense pain might appear when the Glisson capsule is stressed by larger cysts. In these cases, an abdominal mass mobilizing together with the respiratory movements is visualized during the physical examination. These giant cysts are easily visualized with the ultrasound. CT allows to define in more detail the elevated right hemidiaphragm and the development of secondary pulmonary basal atelectasis.

- Another complication of large cysts occurs when there is an intrahepatic breach or rupture of the cyst to the peritoneum either spontaneously or by trauma. The discharge of fertile hydatid fluid in the liver or peritoneal cavity causes anaphylaxis of a different magnitude and new hydatid implants [43]. These complications are better visualized with the use of CT.

- Cyst rupture and emptying of hydatid fluid or membranes into the biliary tree lead to obstructive jaundice, many times accompanied by severe acute cholangitis [44, 45]. The cysts can become infected as well and determine the formation of liver abscesses, which can sometimes lead to septicemia. In these cases, CT and MRC allow to achieve a better definition of the characteristics of the abscess and whether there is emptying of hydatid material into the biliary tree.

- The chronic inflammatory process of hepatic cysts located in segments of the liver dome determines firm adhesions to the right hemidiaphragm and even transits toward the pleuropulmonary space. As a result of this transphrenic transit, patients may present pleural empyemas or bronchopneumonia [46]. CT and MRC help to achieve a better definition and provide the most appropriate and safe management.

- There are occasions in which large cysts may be more complicated due to the simultaneous rupture and emptying of hydatid material to the biliary tree and bronchi. A bilio-pleuro-bronchial fistula is established with the occurrence of the pathognomonic sign of bilioptysis, i.e., the expectoration of the bile. These patients present a fairly severe septic episode with hepatic and respiratory functional compromise [47]. The thorax-abdominal CT and MRC are useful to diagnose this complication [39].

- Rarely, cysts located adjacent to the retrohepatic vena cava can rupture and cause severe cardiorespiratory failure due to bilateral pulmonary arterial embolism with multiple pulmonar hydatid dissemination [48]. In that case, a CT angiography (CTA) is used to better diagnose this serious complication.

6. Surgical treatment

The main objective of the treatment of hepatic hydatidosis is the eradication of the parasite and avoidance of recurrence. There is consensus, in considering surgery as the best option to achieve this purpose. It is currently possible to perform different surgical techniques with acceptable rates of morbidity and mortality, which are applied according to the pathological conditions of cysts. In cases of greater complexity, surgery can be complemented with other therapies such as minimally invasive procedures and chemotherapy. Surgical treatment has indications and contraindications depending on the patient's condition and the forms of disease presentation [6].

At the dawn of the surgery to treat hepatic hydatidosis, only conservative techniques were used. Among them, marsupialization consisted in the opening and extraction of the parasite followed by externalizing the residual cavity toward the abdominal wall, waiting for the closure by secondary intention. Cysto-enteroanastomosis was also performed, anastomosing the hepatic residual cavity into the duodenum or a defunctionalized jejunal loop. Currently, these conservative techniques are not indicated due to the high risk of complications such as recurrences, liver abscesses, intestinal obstruction, biliary fistulas, biliomas, biliary peritonitis, cholangitis, and septicemia. However, there are surgical centers that report good results in cases with large cysts treated by laparoscopic cystojejunostomy [49].

There are various procedures of resective surgery performed in different surgical centers. When indicated, it is necessary to consider age, general condition of the patient, pathological state of the cysts and location in other organs, and the existence of important comorbidities difficult to control. Despite being a benign pathology, its evolution can sometimes be very complicated, requiring multiple surgeries and leading to a poor prognosis. The surgical resections are performed either through open or laparoscopic surgery. The following are the most used techniques from least to greatest complexity.

6.1 Subtotal cystectomy by open surgery

This technique, performed by open surgery, follows the steps below according to the location of the cysts (**Figures 18–21**):

- Right or bilateral subcostal laparotomy.

- In order to obtain a good access to the cyst, the section of the round ligament and the dissection of adhesions to the diaphragm or adjacent organs might be required. The use of intraoperative ultrasound is useful in posterior and central cyst locations, to avoid injuring the retrohepatic cava vein or hepatic veins.

- During puncture and removal of the fluid and hydatid membrane, it is necessary to isolate the surgical field with compresses embedded in scolicidal agents (20% hypertonic saline solution or diluted povidone iodine).

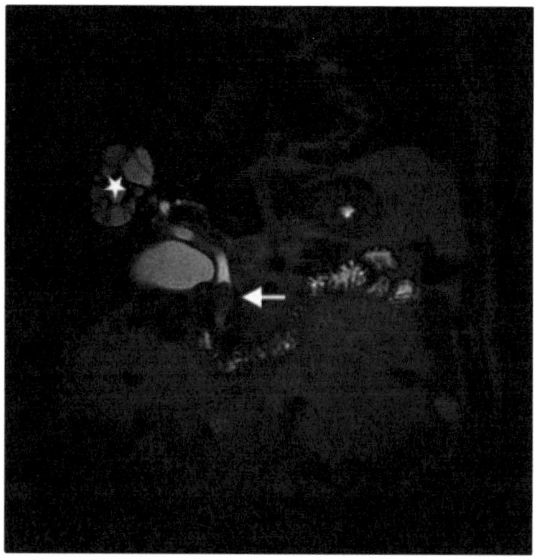

Figure 16.
MRI T2 coronal septated cysts. Multiple daughter vesicles (white star). Membranes in bile duct (white arrow).

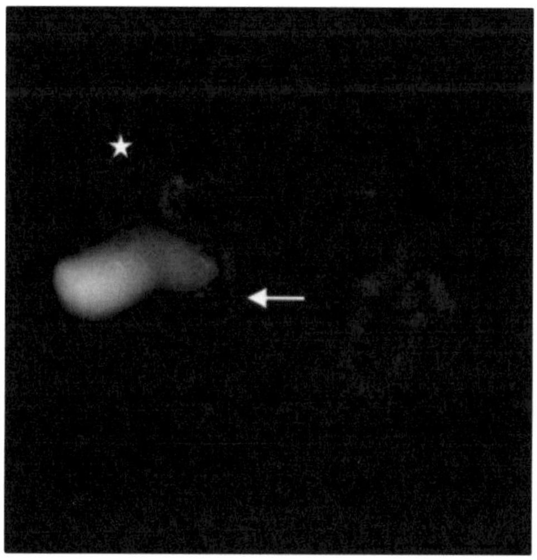

Figure 17.
MR cholangiography. Same findings as demonstrated in **Figure 15**.

- Wide resection of the adventitia and further revision to eliminate daughter vesicles in cavities located in the remaining adventitia.

- Identification and suture of biliary communications.

- Closure of the residual cavity by means of capitonnage or omentoplasty. In giant cysts, capitonnage is not recommended to avoid distortion of the biliary tree and intrahepatic vasculature with subsequent functional sequelae.

- In some cases, to prevent postoperative biliary fistulae, a drain is placed in the residual cavity, or a choledocostomy with a Kehr tube is performed.

- When the cyst is close to the main bile duct or to the subhepatic and cava vein, the adjacent adventitia should be left in situ to prevent biliary fistulae or bleedings.

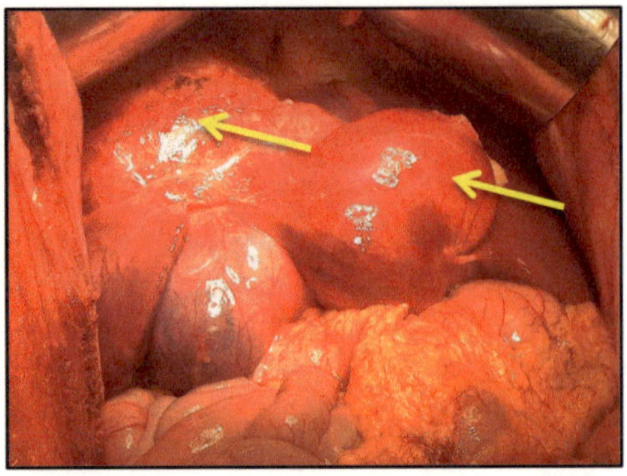

Figure 18.
Open surgery. Multiple cysts (yellow arrow).

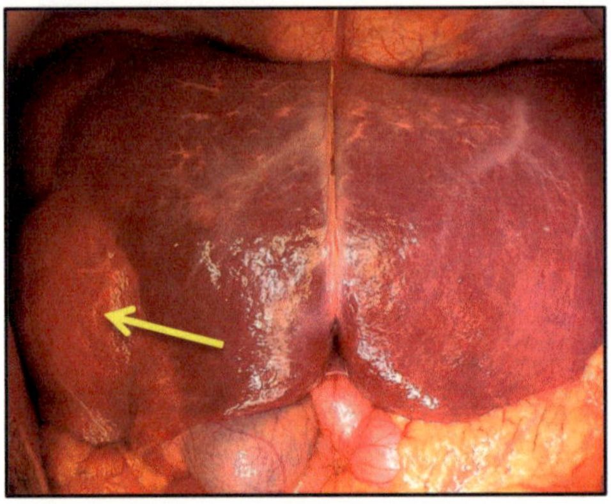

Figure 19.
Hepatic mobilization. Subcostal laparotomy.

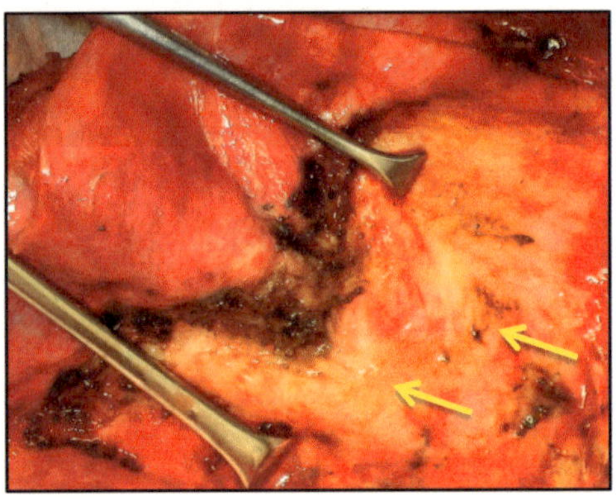

Figure 20.
Open surgery. Subtotal cystectomy biliary communications (yellow arrow).

6.2 Laparoscopic subtotal cystectomy

Laparoscopic subtotal hepatic cystectomy has all the advantages of minimally invasive procedures (**Figures 22–24**). It offers magnified vision with better appreciation of the cyst, residual cavity, and biliary communications. In addition, it presents less postoperative pain and earlier discharge. Comparative studies are reported

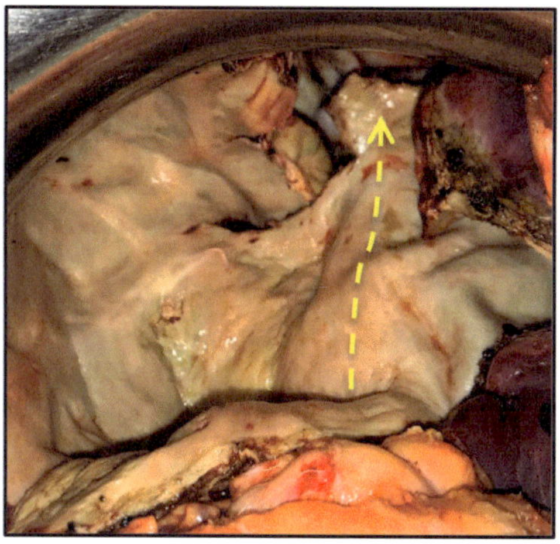

Figure 21.
Subtotal cystectomy. Giant hydatid cyst. Retrohepatic cava vein (yellow-dotted arrow).

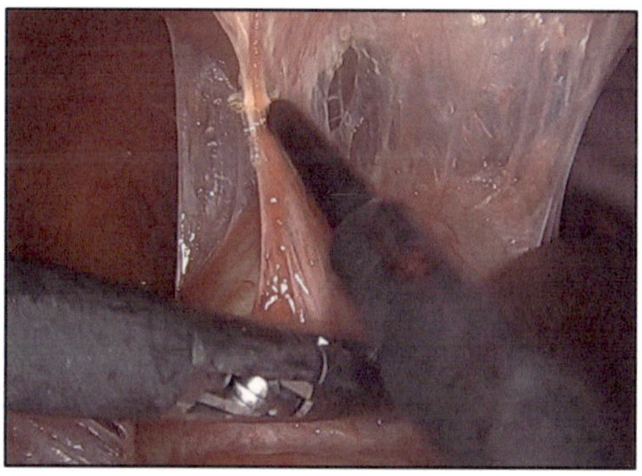

Figure 22.
Laparoscopic subtotal pericystectomy. Dissection of diaphragm adhesion.

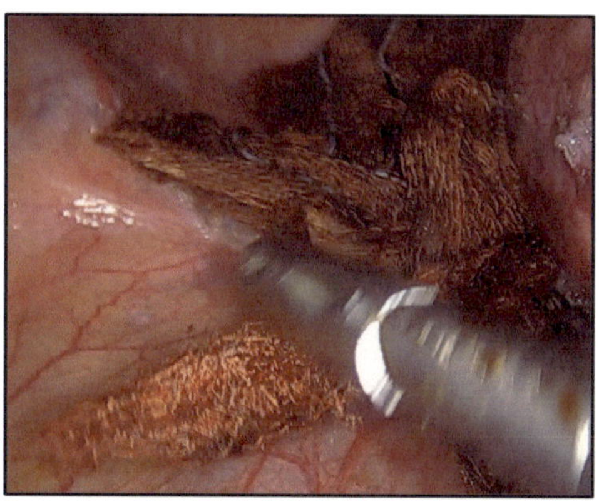

Figure 23.
Protection of the surgical field, iodine povidone.

between the two techniques, and the future trend seems to prefer laparoscopic technique [50]. However, technical difficulties currently persist to avoid the spillage of fertile hydatid material into the peritoneal cavity with anaphylactic reactions and secondary hydatid implants. For this reason, and to prevent this complication and

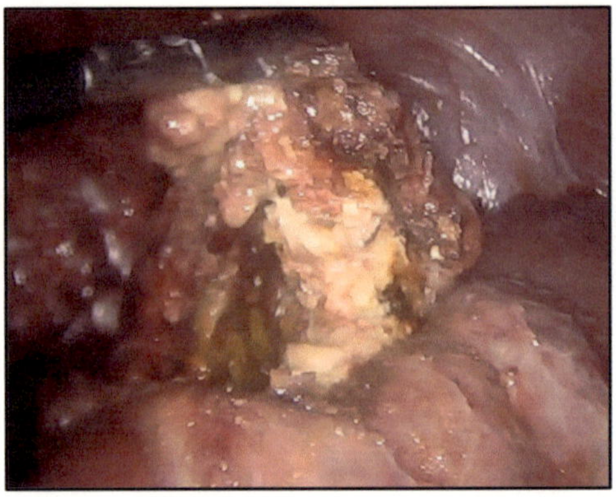

Figure 24.
Partial resection of adventitia.

a possible uncontrollable bleeding, the laparoscopic approach is contraindicated in the following situations:

- Cyst diameter more than 10 cm
- More than three cysts and/or presence of peritoneal cysts or in other organs
- Very thin or calcified adventitia
- Cysts located in the dome and central locations of the liver
- Complicated cysts with rupture and emptying on the biliary tree or peritoneum
- Imaging signs of accentuated pericystic inflammation
- Cysts with fibrous adhesions to the diaphragm on the way to a thoracic migration

Following the rules of laparoscopic liver surgery, the location of the entrance ports depends on the anatomical location of the cysts. To prevent the spillage of hydatid material into the peritoneal cavity, it is necessary to have a good puncture and aspiration system, similar to Perforator-Grinder [51].

6.3 Pericystectomy

Open or laparoscopic pericystectomy is based on the concept of complete parasite removal. This technique consists of resecting the cyst by a plane through the hepatic parenchyma adjacent to the adventitia, thus achieving avoidance of recurrence due to the presence of daughter vesicles in the adventitia or in the surrounding hepatic parenchyma [52]. In cases of complicated cysts, pericystectomy is not recommended due to the risk of further bleeding or bile duct injuries. Previous radiological studies are crucial to determine the relationship of these structures with the cysts. Currently, laparoscopic pericystectomy helps to prevent the aforementioned risks thanks to its magnified vision, more efficient hepatic transection instruments, and widespread access (**Figure 25**). Well-trained surgeons in laparoscopic hepatic surgery have a better chance of successfully performing this technique [53].

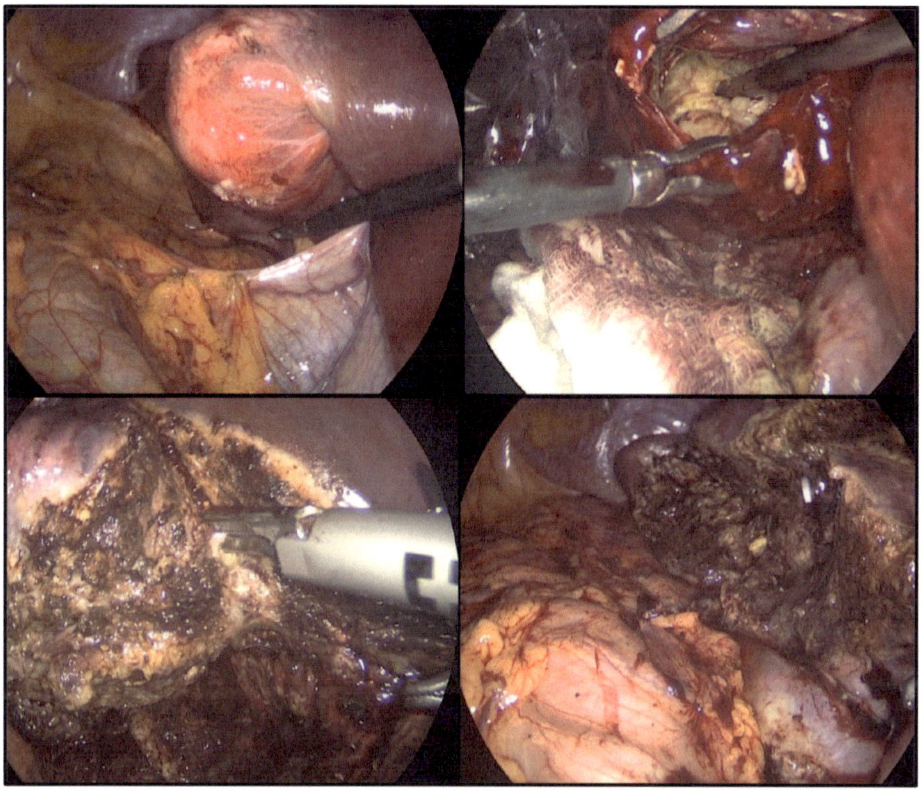

Figure 25.
Steps of laparoscopic pericystectomy.

6.4 Hepatic resection

Sometimes it is necessary to carry out liver resections, e.g., when there are hydatid recurrences in the same lobe previously operated or in residual cavities, which have the risk of subsequent infection with development of liver abscesses and cholangitis. When the infection is controlled by antibiotic therapy or percutaneous drainages, it is recommended to resect the compromised lobe, which is usually more atrophic. This surgery will be consequently more laborious. Nevertheless, the compensatory hypertrophy of the unaffected lobe determines a lower risk of postoperative hepatic failure. With the aim of completely eradicating the parasite and preventing recurrence, several surgical centers perform hepatic resection more frequently by both open and laparoscopic surgeries with acceptable morbidity and very low mortality. Liver resection is more indicated in alveolar echinococcosis by higher frequency of recurrence and infiltrative behavior similar to malignant neoplasms. There are recent reports of liver transplantation and also ex vivo resection surgery with autotransplantation for this type of echinococcosis [54]. Summarizing, hepatic resection, not very used in the past, now appears as a viable alternative for selected cases carried out in specialized reference centers.

The morbidity of resective surgery depends on the complexity of the hydatidosis and the magnitude of the surgery performed. Among the most difficult to treat are biliary fistulas, bleeding, and infections. For example, for patients with fistulization of the cyst toward the bile duct and thorax, it is advisable to work in stages, e.g., treating cholangitis first, and then, when the patient is stabilized, a pleural empyema is drained. Once general conditions have been recovered, the resective surgery is indicated. In relation to morbidity and mortality rates, what has been reported so far shows a great disparity of figures. A surgeon from our university conducted a study of the risk factors that determine the postoperative morbidity in a significant number of international publications. The results indicate a fairly low level of evidence [55]. The challenge is to perform a prospective series, to achieve consensus on the indications of surgery to treat this complex disease.

7. Percutaneous treatment

This therapy is carried out by means of puncture, aspiration, injection of scolicidal agents, and reaspiration of fluid and hydatid membranes (PAIR). The procedure is performed under ultrasonographic guidance in selected cases. This procedure was developed by a Tunisian team in 1986. The WHO recommends this procedure because it is less invasive when compared to surgery, allows a good evacuation of the parasite, reduces the time of hospitalization, and is less expensive. The following guidelines contain indications and contraindications for this procedure (**Tables 3** and **4**) [56]. It is necessary to have anesthesiological support to treat an eventual anaphylaxis crisis due to hydatid fluid spillage while PAIR is performed [57].

1. Non-echoic lesion 5 cm in diameter
2. Cysts with daughter cysts and/or membrane detachment
3. Multiple cysts if accessible to puncture
4. Infected cysts
5. Patients who fail to respond to chemotherapy alone
6. Patients in whom surgery is contraindicated
7. Patient who refuse surgery
8. Patients who relapse after surgery
9. Children >3 years old
10. Pregnant women

Table 3.
Indications for PAIR.

1. Noncooperative patient
2. Inaccessible or risky location of the liver cyst
3. Cyst in the spine, brain, and/or heart
4. Inactive or calcified lesion
5. Cyst communicating with the biliary tree

Table 4.
Contraindications for PAIR.

8. Chemotherapy

The use of treatments with drugs capable of penetrating and collapsing hepatic hydatid cysts is reported in numerous publications. These drugs are prescribed alone or together with surgery and less-invasive therapies such as PAIR. Currently, albendazole has shown effectiveness in reducing the size or even causing the death of the parasite. For this reason, it is employed to prevent recurrence after surgery. It is also used as the only therapy in patients who refuse surgery or who are inoperable due to disseminated hydatidosis or because of other comorbidities [58]. In Chile, it is indicated preoperatively in doses of 10 mg/kg of weight for one cycle of 14 or 21 days and postoperatively from one to three cycles according to eventual appearance of hepatic dysfunction.

9. Conclusion

Hepatic hydatidosis is still a disease that spreads without epidemiological control in many parts of the world. Also, a continuous biological adaptation of the parasite to subsist in the intermediate host has been demonstrated, which would explain the great difficulties in eradicating this zoonosis. The permanent and even increasing incidence of this disease determines very high health costs necessary to treat patients, sometimes with complex pathological presentations. Efforts are being made to find new alternatives to diagnose early stages of the parasitosis. The creation of new vaccines with the intention of immunizing the intermediate host would determine a better control of human hydatidosis. Surgical advances are allowing for more and more radical surgical procedures with acceptable rates of morbidity and mortality. However, the implementation of minimally invasive surgeries presents significantly higher costs. Logic would dictate that the best path is to minimize the number of new patients affected through successful epidemiological control.

Author details

Luis Burgos San Juan[1,2,3*], Hector Losada Morales[1,2,3], Jorge Silva Abarca[1,2,3], Cesar Muñoz Castro[4,5], Marcelo Klein Diaz[6] and Pablo Guzmán González[7]

1 Hepatobiliopancreatic Surgery Unit, Surgery Service, Hospital Dr. Hernán Henríquez, Temuco, Chile

2 Surgery Department, Universidad de la Frontera, Temuco, Chile

3 Surgery Department, Clínica Alemana de Temuco, Chile

4 Digestive Surgery and Hepatobiliopancreatic Surgery Unit, Surgery Service, Hospital Regional, Talca, Chile

5 Department of Surgery, Universidad Católica del Maule, Talca, Chile

6 Interventional Radiology Unit, Imaging Service, Hospital Dr. Hernán Henríquez, Temuco, Chile

7 Pathological Anatomy Department, Hospital Dr. Hernán Henríquez Aravena, Temuco, Chile

*Address all correspondence to: luis.burgos.s@ufrontera.cl

IntechOpen

© 2019 The Author(s). Licensee IntechOpen. This chapter is distributed under the terms of the Creative Commons Attribution License (http://creativecommons.org/licenses/by/3.0), which permits unrestricted use, distribution, and reproduction in any medium, provided the original work is properly cited.

References

[1] Ebell B, Banov L Jr. The Papyrus Ebers: The Greatest Egyptian Medical Document. Copenhagen: Levin & Munksgaard; 1937

[2] Cordero del Campillo M. Notas históricas de la equinococosis/hidatidosis. In: Jornada científica de la Asociación Española de Hidatidología Parte I. León: Universidad de León. 19-X-2007

[3] Eckert J, Thompson RC. Historical aspects of Echinococcosis. Advances in Parasitology. 2017;**95**:1-64

[4] Nakao M, Lavikainen A, Yanagida T, Ito A. Phylogenetic systematics of the genus Echinococcus (Cestoda: Taeniidae). International Journal for Parasitology. 2013;**43**(12-13):1017-1029

[5] Brunetti E, Garcia HH, Junghanss T, International CE Workshop in Lima, Peru, 2009. Cystic echinococcosis: Chronic, complex, and still neglected. PLoS Neglected Tropical Diseases. 2011;**5**(7):e1146

[6] Sozuer E, Akyuz M, Akbulut S. Open surgery for hepatic hydatid disease. International Surgery. 2014;**99**:764-769

[7] Gomez i Gavara C, López-Andújar R, Belda Ibáñez T, Ramia Angel JM, Moya Herraiz Á, Orbis Castellanos F, et al. Review of the treatment of liver hydatid cysts. World Journal of Gastroenterology. 2015;**21**(1):124-131

[8] Cortes S, Valle C. Human hydatidosis: General aspects and epidemiological situation in Chile according to hospital discharge and mandatory reporting from 2001 to 2005. Revista Chilena de Infectología. 2010;**27**:329-335

[9] Deplazes P, Rinaldi L, Alvarez Rojas CA, Torgerson PR, Harandi MF, Romig T, et al. Global distribution of alveolar and cystic Echinococcosis. Advances in Parasitology. 2017;**95**:315-493

[10] Grosso G, Gruttadauria S, Biondi A, Marventano S, Mistretta A. Worldwide epidemiology of liver hydatidosis including the Mediterranean area. World Journal of Gastroenterology. 2012;**18**(13):1425-1437

[11] Brunetti E, Kern P, Vuitton DA, Writing Panel for the WHO-IWGE. Expert consensus for the diagnosis and treatment of cystic and alveolar echinococcosis in humans. Acta Tropica. 2010;**114**:1-16

[12] Christofi P, Deplazes N, Christofi I, Tanner PE, et al. Screening of dogs for Echinococcus granulosus coproantigen in a low endemic situation in Cyprus. Veterinary Parasitology. 2002;**104**:299-306

[13] Chen KF, Tang YY, Wang R, Fang D, Chen JH, Zeng Y, et al. The choose of different surgical therapies of hepatic alveolar echinococcosis: A single-center retrospective case-control study. Medicine (Baltimore). 2018;**97**(8):e0033

[14] Mayor P, Baquedano LE, Sanchez E, Aramburu J, Gomez-Puerta LA, Mamani VJ, et al. Polycystic echinococcosis in Pacas, Amazon region, Peru. Emerging Infectious Diseases. 2015;**21**(3):456-459

[15] D'Alessandro A, Rausch RL. new aspects of neotropical polycystic (*echinococcus vogeli*) and unicystic (*echinococcus oligarthrus*) echinococcosis. Clinical Microbiology Reviews. 2008;**21**(2):380-401

[16] Boufana B, Qiu J, Chen X, Budke CM, Campos-Ponce M, Craig PS. First report of echinococcus shiquicus in dogs from eastern Qinghai-Tibet plateau region, China. Acta Tropica. 2013;**127**(1):21-24

[17] Hüttner M, Nakao M, Wassermann T, Siefert L, Boomker JD, Dinkel A, et al.

Genetic characterization and phylogenetic position of echinococcus felidis (Cestoda: Taeniidae) from the African lion. International Journal for Parasitology. 2008;**38**(7):861-868

[18] Romig T, Deplazes P, Jenkins D, Giraudoux P, Massolo A, Craig PS, et al. Ecology and life cycle patterns of echinococcus species. Advances in Parasitology. 2017;**95**:213-314

[19] Xiao N, Qiu J, Nakao M, Li T, Yang W, Chen X, et al. Echinococcus shiquicus, a new species from the Qinghai-Tibet plateau region of China: Discovery and epidemiological implications. Parasitology International. 2006;**55** Suppl:S233-S236

[20] Carmena D, Cardona GA. Echinococcosis in wild carnivorous species: Epidemiology, genotypic diversity, and implications for veterinary public health. Veterinary Parasitology. 2014;**202**(3-4):69-94. DOI: 10.1016/j.vetpar.2014.03.009. Epub 2014 Mar 15

[21] Rinaldi F, Brunetti E, Neumayr A, Maestri M, Goblirsch S, Tamarozzi F. Cystic echinococcosis of the liver: A primer for hepatologists. World Journal of Hepatology. 2014;**6**:293-305

[22] Bhutani N, Kajal P. Hepatic echinococcosis: A review. Annals of Medicine and Surgery(London). 2018;**36**:99-105

[23] Pakala T, Molina M, Wu GY. Hepatic Echinococcal cysts: A review. Journal of Clinical and Translational Hepatology. 2016;**4**(1):39-46

[24] Mihmanli M, Idiz UO, Kaya C, Demir U, Bostanci O, Omeroglu S, et al. Current status of diagnosis and treatment of hepatic echinococcosis. World Journal of Hepatology. 2016;**8**(28):1169-1181

[25] Zhang W, Wen H, Li J, Lin R, McManus DP. Immunology and immunodiagnosis of cystic echinococcosis: An update. Clinical & Developmental Immunology. 2012;**2012**:101895

[26] McManus DP, Gray DJ, Zhang W, Yang Y. Diagnosis, treatment, and management of echinococcosis. BMJ. 2012;**344**:e3866

[27] Eckert J, Deplazes P. Biological, epidemiological, and clinical aspects of echinococcosis, a zoonosis of increasing concern. Clinical Microbiology Reviews. 2004;**17**(1):107-135

[28] Gharbi HA, Hassine W, Brauner MW, Dupuch K. Ultrasound examination of the hydatic liver. Radiology. 1981;**139**:459-463

[29] Group WHOIW. International classification of ultrasound images in cystic echinococcosis for application in clinical and field epidemiological settings. Acta Tropica. 2003;**85**:253-261

[30] Solomon N, Fields PJ, Tamarozzi F, Brunetti E, CNL M. Expert reliability for the World Health Organization standardized ultrasound classification of cystic echinococcosis. The American Journal of Tropical Medicine and Hygiene. 2017;**96**(3):686-691

[31] Kammerer WS, Schantz PM. Echinococcal disease. Infectious Disease Clinics of North America. 1993;7(3):605-618

[32] Macpherson CN, Bartholomot B, Frider B. Application of ultrasound in diagnosis, treatment, epidemiology, public health and control of Echinococcus granulosus and E. multilocularis. Parasitology. 2003;**127**(Suppl):S21-S35

[33] Hosch W, Junghanss T, Werner J, Dux M. Imaging methods in the diagnosis and therapy of cystic echinococcosis. Röfo. 2004;**176**:679-687

[34] Cai D, Li Y, Jiang Y, Wang H, Wang X, Song B. The role of contrast-enhanced ultrasound in the diagnosis of hepatic alveolar echinococcosis. Medicine (Baltimore). 2019;**98**(5):e14325

[35] Marrone G, Crino' F, Caruso S, Mamone G, Carollo V, Milazzo M, et al. Multidisciplinary imaging of liver hydatidosis. World Journal of Gastroenterology. 2012;**18**:1438-1447

[36] Stojkovic M, Rosenberger K, Kauczor HU, Junghanss T, Hosch W. Diagnosing and staging of cystic echinococcosis: How do CT and MRI perform in comparison to ultrasound? PLoS Neglected Tropical Diseases. 2012;**6**:e1880

[37] Hosch W, Stojkovic M, Janisch T, Heye T, Werner J, Friess H, et al. MR imaging for diagnosing cysto-biliary fistulas in cystic echinococcosis. European Journal of Radiology. 2008;**66**:262-267

[38] Tocchi A, Mazzoni G, Miccini M, Drumo A, Cassini D, Colace L, et al. Treatment of hydatid bronchobiliary fistulas: 30 years of experience. Liver International. 2007;**27**(2):209-214

[39] Muñoz C, Burgos L, Fonseca V. Fístula biliobronquial de origen hidatídico. Revista Chilena de Cirugía. 2009;**61**(6):504-506

[40] Dolay K, Akbulut S. Role of endoscopic retrograde cholangiopancreatography in the management of hepatic hydatid disease. World Journal of Gastroenterology. 2014;**20**(41):15253-15261

[41] Manzano-Román R, Sánchez-Ovejero C, Hernández-González A, Casulli A, Siles-Lucas M. Serological diagnosis and follow-up of human cystic echinococcosis: A new Hope for the future? BioMed Research International. 2015;**2015**:428205

[42] Hernández-González A, Sánchez-Ovejero C, Manzano-Román R, González Sánchez M, Delgado JM, Pardo-García T, et al. Evaluation of the recombinant antigens B2t and 2B2t, compared with hydatid fluid, in IgG-ELISA and immunostrips for the diagnosis and follow up of CE patients. PLoS Neglected Tropical Diseases. 2018;**12**(9):e0006741

[43] Atli M, Kama NA, Yuksek YN, Doganay M, Gozalan U, Kologlu M, et al. Intrabiliary rupture of a hepatic hydatid cyst: Associated clinical factors and proper management. Archives of Surgery. 2001;**136**:1249-1255

[44] Busić Z, Amić E, Servis D, Predrijevac M, Stipancić I, Busić D. Common bile duct obstruction caused by the hydatid daughter cysts. Collegium Antropologicum. 2004;**28**(1):325-329

[45] Nemati Honar B, Hayatollah G, Nikshoar M, Forootan M, Feizi AM. Liver hydatid cyst and acute cholangitis: A case report. Acta Medica Iranica. 2016;**54**(4):286-288

[46] Msaad S, Yangui I, Ketata W, Abid N, Feki W, Abid H, et al. Hydatid cysts of the liver ruptured into the thorax (about five cases). Revue de Pneumologie Clinique. 2015;**71**(5):255-263

[47] Bel Haj Salah R, Triki W, Bourguiba MB, Ben MM, Zaouche A. Rupture aiguë d'un kyste hydatique foie dans la plèvre droite À propos de deux observations. Chirurgie Thoracique et Cardio-Vasculaire. 2011;**15**(3): 182-184

[48] Bayaroğullari H, Davran R, Cavuş Y, Yetim TD, Evirgen Ö. Liver hydatid cyst leading to bilateral pulmonary artery embolism and bilateral multiple pulmonar echinococcosis via inferior vena cava: Report of a case. Clinical Imaging. 2013;**37**(2):374-378

[49] Yilmaz H, Sahin M, Ece I, Yormaz S, Alptekin H. A new approach to the complicated liver Hydatid cyst-laparoscopic roux-en-Y Cystojejunostomy. Prague Medical Report. 2015;**116**(3):233-238

[50] Jabbari Nooghabi A, Mehrabi Bahar M, Asadi M, Jabbari Nooghabi M, Jangjoo A. Evaluation and comparison of the early outcomes of open and laparoscopic surgery of liver Hydatid cyst. Surgical Laparoscopy, Endoscopy & Percutaneous Techniques. 2015;**25**(5):403-407

[51] Sormaz IC, Avtan L. Minimally-invasive treatment of hepatic hydatid disease with perforator-grinder-aspirator apparatus and follow-up of 42 patients. Acta Gastroenterologica Belgica. 2017;**80**(4):477-480

[52] Peng X, Zhang S, Niu JH. Total subadventitial cystectomy for the treatment of 30 patients with hepatic hydatid cysts. Chinese Journal of General Surgery. 2002;**17**:529-530

[53] Tai QW, Tuxun T, Zhang JH, Zhao JM, Cao J, Muhetajiang M, et al. The role of laparoscopy in the management of liver hydatid cyst: A single-center experience and world review of the literature. Surgical Laparoscopy, Endoscopy & Percutaneous Techniques. 2013;**23**(2):171-175

[54] Wen H, Vuitton L, Tuxun T, Li J, Vuitton DA, Zhang W, et al. Echinococcosis: Advances in the 21st century. Clinical Microbiology Reviews. 2019;**32**(2)

[55] Manterola C, Otzen T, Muñoz G, Alanis M, Kruuse E, Figueroa G. Surgery for hepatic hidatidosis. Risk factors and variables associated with postoperative morbidity. Overview of the existing evidence. Cirugía Española. 2017;**95**(10):566-576

[56] PAIR: Puncture, Aspiration, Injection, Re-Aspiration- An option for the treatment of Cystic Echinococcosis World Health Organization. WHO/CDS/CSR/APH/2001.6

[57] Kabaalioğlu A, Ceken K, Alimoglu E, Apaydin A. Percutaneous imaging-guided treatment of hydatid liver cysts: Do long-term results make it a first choice? European Journal of Radiology. 2006;**59**(1):65-73

[58] Dehkordi AB, Sanei B, Yousefi M, Sharafi SM, Safarnezhad F, Jafari R, et al. Albendazole and treatment of hydatid cyst, review of literature. Infectious Disorders Drug Targets. 2018. [Epub ahead of print]

Chapter 9

How to Treat Bilobar Liver Metastases: New Surgical Challenges

Fabio Uggeri, Enrico Pinotti, Mattia Garancini, Mauro Scotti, Marco Braga and Fabrizio Romano

Abstract

To date, the improvements in survival of patients with liver metastases and advances in technology allowed the surgical indications to be extended. In complex cases, however, the possibility of performing a curative hepatic resection collides with the need to preserve a sufficient liver volume to avoid a postoperative hepatic failure. Currently postoperative liver failure is the major cause of death for these patients. In the attempt to overcome this limit in the last decades, we tried to introduce new measures and develop new surgical techniques. From the introduction by Makuuchi in the 1980s of the preoperative portal embolization, many surgical techniques have been proposed and perfected. The aim of this chapter is to describe the new surgical techniques for the approach of complex hepatic metastases.

Keywords: hepatic liver metastases, hepatectomy, liver failure, two-stage hepatectomy, ALPPS

1. Introduction

In the recent decades, the improvement of technology associated with a refinement of preoperative imaging allowed to expand surgical indications, leading to treat patients until a few years ago judged unresectable. These improvements have made major liver surgery more feasible and sure with a clean reduction of morbidity and mortality rate. Today after major hepatectomy, mortality ranges from 0.5 and 4%, making surgery a therapeutic option even in case of advanced disease.

Beyond the extension of surgical indications, the pivotal point remains the possibility to perform a curative resection (R0). Unfortunately, situations such as chronic liver diseases or an extensive disease do not let to achieve a radical resection for the inability to maintain a suitable remnant liver after resection for an adequate postoperative function. Nowadays this is the limits to overcome.

At the current state of knowledge, the future liver remnant (FLR) estimated before surgical resection should be more of 25% of the total liver volume in patients without hepatic disease and of around 40% in the patients with history of liver pathologies (viral chronic hepatitis, alcoholic, nonalcoholic steatohepatitis (NASH), chemotherapeutic damage).

IntechOpen

An effective and safe surgery can only be achieved with a perfect knowledge of the surgical anatomy. This anatomy corresponds to a functional liver vascular distribution based on the concept of the anatomical division of the liver proposed by Claude Couinaud, Ton That Tung, and Henri Bismuth, which divides the liver into independent portions that can be handled separately without compromising the function of the remnant liver.

Unfortunately, today it is not uncommon to evaluate patients at the first instance inoperable due to the disseminated hepatic spread. The research of new surgical strategies to effectively extend the number of liver resections and the concept of "resectability" were one of the biggest challenges in oncologic surgery over the last 30 years.

To overcome this limit, new surgical techniques have been proposed with the clear intention of promoting liver regeneration by modifying the procedures first performed in a single procedure in more steps. Moreover in the case of large and complex surgical resections, an accurate study of the liver is recommended to evaluate the postoperative functional reserve with a volumetric and functional assessment (clearance of indocyanine green, scintigraphy, CT, MR).

Laboratory tests on animals and clinical data showed that the closure of portal flow toward a hemiliver induces contralateral lobe hypertrophy. Portal flow redistribution can be achieved with surgical ligation (PVL) or percutaneous embolization (portal vein embolization (PVE)). The purpose of PVE is to increase preoperatively the volume of the future remnant liver to allow the surgery and reduce postoperative morbidity, when the only contraindication to surgery is represented by the initial insufficient remnant liver. The first to propose this technique in the 1980s was Makuuchi, and since then huge progress has been made. Makuuchi and his group [1] first used this technique in 14 patients with cholangiocarcinoma to minimize the possibility of postoperative hepatic dysfunction. The results obtained were encouraging without showing major complications and being able to perform surgical resection in 85% of patients in a timing from 4 to 41 days after embolization.

The experience of Makuuchi marked a crossroad for the birth of a new surgical attitude to approach extended right-side hepatectomy, in fact the procedure was shortly adopted by several surgeons [2–4].

Once the new technique was universally accepted, some surgeons proposed during the next decade a technical progress describing a sequential surgical procedure called "two-stage hepatectomy (TSH)" [5]. To achieve the goal of radical resection in patients with colorectal hepatic metastases, the authors outline a previously therapeutic approach [6]. A procedure includes a first surgical step in which the removal of the lesions of the left lobe associated with the closure of the right portal branch is performed. Liver hypertrophy associated with chemotherapy limits the growth and spread of residual lesions and then allows the patients to undergo surgery in the absence of disease progression and in the presence of a residual volume adequate to prevent postoperative hepatic failure. The feasibility of the procedure was 81% with a mortality rate of 15% for the second stage. At the beginning the technique did not provide for all patients portal embolization, and then the routine use of the latter led to a higher rate of hypertrophy and therefore with a greater rate of patient treated with curative intent [7]. Although the first results were encouraging, the drawback of TSH led to the impossibility of achieving sufficient hypertrophy in an acceptable time to avoid a progression of the disease that in some studies did not allow up to 28% of treated patients to undergo second surgical phase [8]. The reasons of technique failure were due to disease progression inherent to long time to reach the proper hypertrophy or the impossibility to achieve the desired liver hypertrophy in consideration of the unsuitable size of the remnant liver.

In the attempt to overcome these limits, in 2012 Schnitzbauer [9] proposed a new surgical approach, named subsequently by Santibanes [10] "*associating liver partition and portal vein ligation for staged hepatectomy* (ALPPS)." The procedure involves the separation of the future remnant liver from diseased liver through "split" in situ of the hepatic parenchyma in combination with ligation of the portal vein during the first phase. Schnitzbauer [9] reported a hypertrophy of the remnant liver achieved in a very short time (average future remnant liver hypertrophy of 74% in about 9 days). The mechanism by which ALPPS leads to such a dramatic increase in hepatic hypertrophy compared to PVE still needs to be fully clarified. Initially it was thought that the stimulus to hypertrophy was related to the cessation of blood flow between the diseased segments and the FLR, but some authors have subsequently reported how step I in ALPPS leads to an increase in levels of interleukin-6 and tumor necrosis factor-α in liver tissue 1 hour after the procedure compared to PVL [11]. Therefore, rapid hypertrophy could be associated with a systemic increase in circulating growth factors as an inflammatory reaction to parenchymal split.

Beyond the first promising results, the high complication rate (44%) with a mortality of 12% described by Schnitzbauer led to several questions about the role and indications of the technique in the surgical community. The subsequent expedients to the original technique and the proposal of more restrictive indications based on practice have led to a significant reduction of the postoperative morbidity and mortality rate. In fact the results of the most recent ALPPS register report more encouraging data, with a 90-day mortality of 9% and serious complications of 27% [12].

Since its introduction until today, under the term ALPPS, many variations and adaptations of the original technique are grouped. The common thread of all these variants is to try to reduce morbidity and mortality while maintaining an adequate hypertrophy response from the liver.

The purpose of the chapter is to analyze which surgical techniques, to date, can be performed in the presence of diffuse liver metastases.

2. Liver failure

Within this context of extended resection, postoperative liver failure remains a real concern. The term "small for size syndrome" (SFSS) has been first used in liver transplantation to describe the development of acute liver failure, situation in which the donor's liver was too small for the given recipient. Few years later, Dahm [13] proposed a systematic definition of SFSS. Small for size syndrome was defined as the presence of two of the following criteria in the first three postoperative days: serum bilirubin >6 mg/dL, international normalized ratio (INR) > 2, and the presence of encephalopathy grade III/IV.

As in liver transplantation, the extension of surgical indications in the presence of bilobar metastases led to the concept of post-hepatectomy liver failure (PHLF). PHLF is a clinical manifestation that occurs when the remnant liver is not sufficient to provide for metabolic demand. To predict early mortality after extensive hepatectomy in 2005, Balzan [14] proposed that the persistence of either PT < 50% or a serum bilirubin >3 mg/dL on 5 postoperative days is to be considered a predictive mortality index and indicates PHLF. The result of the study demonstrated that the conjunction of these two values on 5 postoperative days could predict nearly 100% morbidity rate and 50% mortality rate.

Recently the International Study Group for Liver Surgery (ISGLS) [15] has proposed to define PHLF as a "postoperatively acquired deterioration in the ability of the liver to maintain its synthetic, excretory, and detoxifying functions, characterized by an increased INR and concomitant hyperbilirubinemia on or after postoperative five days."

PHLF incidence ranges from 0 to 2% after resection of a healthy liver but can reach 7% after major hepatectomy. Cirrhotic liver may exceed 30% [16]. PHLF is the main cause of mortality after extensive hepatic resection, and it may occur even after the 30th postoperative days [17]. In the last decades, surgical techniques in the field of hepatic surgery have focus their attention to develop and implement a series of tools to induce hypertrophy in the future remnant liver to overcome this longstanding problem.

2.1 Two-stage hepatectomy (TSH)

Patients with disseminated and large liver cancers are one of the major surgical challenges; two-stage hepatectomy with PVE or PVL, associated by subsequent hepatectomy, can represent a solution to this dilemma [7].

In the late 1990s, the studies of Bismuth [6] and Azoulay [18] had highlighted how patients with initially unresectable colorectal liver metastases could benefit by the use of PVE associated with neoadjuvant chemotherapy. Preoperative treatment led patients to surgery with survival benefits comparable to those obtained with primary liver resection (40% patients alive at 5 years).

Whereas not all patients with intrahepatic multinodular liver disease undergoing portal vein embolization were able to achieve curative surgery, approximately 20 years ago, Adam et al. [5] proposed a new surgical strategy with a possible curative intent: two-stage hepatectomy "TSH." They modified this practice by introducing an initial stage in which in addition to the ligation or portal embolization were surgically removed the highest number of metastases but not all of them. The hepatic hypertrophy and chemotherapy limiting the metastatic diffusion allowed to perform a second stage for curative purposes reducing the risk of postoperative hepatic failure (**Figure 1**). They were the first to report the results of TSH in terms of feasibility, risks, and patient outcome. The rate of completion of the procedure was 81% with a survival of 35% at 3 years. The risks related to the procedure were inherent in the possible tumor progression between the two stages. But the survival benefit of treated versus untreated patients exceeded methodical risks. The authors reported a mortality rate of 15% comparable to that of patients undergoing primary resection during the same period.

Currently TSH is indicated for multiple colorectal liver lesions judged unresectable in the first instance. As mentioned above the technique provides a first

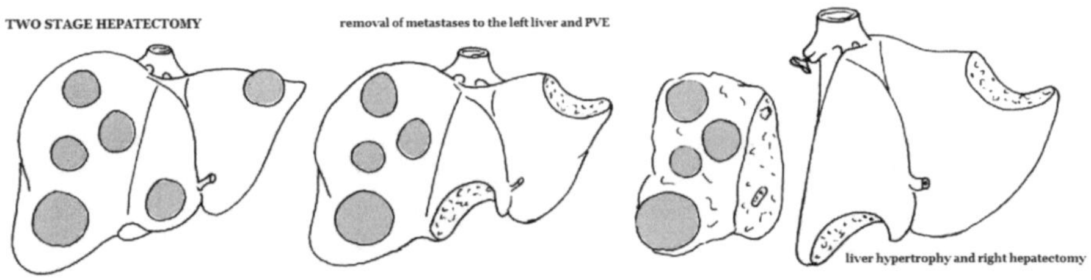

Figure 1.
Two-stage hepatectomy (surgical steps).

stage in which the future remnant liver (usually the left lobe) is surgically or by ablation reclaimed. The first step also provides the execution of PVL or PVE. Portal occlusion stimulates liver regeneration as the possible growth of occult metastases in the remnant liver. In fact the possible progression of disease is the main cause that can prevent the completion of the second surgical phase.

The success of the surgical procedure is closely related to liver regeneration between the two procedures, which avoids the possible risk of postoperative liver failure. The rate of liver regeneration is normally assessed through the execution of a CT scan between 30 and 50 days after the portal occlusion. Although portal occlusion leads to a higher rate than 40% of liver regeneration, it is not always possible to reach the second stage of treatment [19]. Disease progression and insufficient liver regeneration are the main causes leading to a failure of the treatment that ranges from 22–28% [20]. Patients who do not undergo the second stage have an extreme unfavorable prognosis compared to patients who complete the treatment. Three and five survival rates were 68% and 49%, respectively, for patients who underwent second-stage resection and 6 and 0%, respectively, for patients who did not [21, 22]. Patients enrolled to the second surgery have a median overall survival of 36 months [23]; these outcomes are comparable with those patients with resectable colorectal liver metastases at the diagnosis [24–26]. With regard to morbidity and mortality after the first and second stage, in a recent study, Passot [21] reported a morbidity rate of 26% for the second stage compared to 6% of the first. Instead the postoperative mortality at 90 days after the second surgery is around 7%, which is halved compared to the data reported by the first studies.

Considering the technique feasible in selected patients with acceptable morbidity and mortality rates, are there selection criteria to select patients? Interesting in this regard is the paper of Narita [27] which stated that the presence of three or more metastases in the FLR can be considered a negative prognostic factor. A high number of metastases in the remnant liver is correlated to an increased possibility of disease progression during the two surgical stages and may encourage the appearance of "de novo" metastases.

A possible explanation of disease progression, which manifests itself from 13 to 35% of patients [27, 28], is given by numerous experimental studies which suggested that a hypoxia-induced alteration of tumor microenvironment leads to an increased production of vascular endothelial growth factors (VEGF), which can stimulate beyond liver regeneration the growth of dormant micrometastases [22, 29].

The technique, today, should be considered in selected patients with bilobar colorectal liver metastases in whom a right hepatectomy would leave more than three metastases or any metastases of >3 cm in the FLR [30].

Chemotherapy has a key role in the success of sequential treatment. The objective response to preoperative chemotherapy has been shown to be a strong predictor of survival after resection for colorectal liver metastases [31]. Modern chemotherapy regimens using a combination of multiple drugs (5-fluorouracil, oxaliplatin, irinotecan) have achieved really satisfactory results. Some new biological agents such as bevacizumab and cetuximab promise to lead to better results [32]. Although the effectiveness of chemotherapy and its execution should be considered as mandatory for a successful surgical treatment, its use is not without risk. Hepatic chemotherapy damage expressed in terms of liver steatosis and increased postoperative bleeding should be considered when planning an extensive hepatic resection [27, 33]. In fact, several studies have shown an increase in mortality in patients undergoing preoperative chemotherapy.

In conclusion TSH can be considered in selected patients a standard surgical procedure in the treatment of diffuse liver metastases with an acceptable mortality rate. In this regard in fact, a recent study of Baumgart [34] reported a postoperative 30th mortality rate of 0% after the TSH second stage. On the contrary the rate of completion of the procedure expected at best to be about 80% associated with an insufficient liver generation reported in some studies [35, 36] can be considered a technical limit. In combination with failure to achieve an adequate residual liver volume, disease progression related to the long time needed to achieve liver regeneration may be considered the additional limitations of the surgical procedure.

2.2 Associating liver partition and portal vein ligation for two-staged hepatectomy (ALPPS)

Associating liver partition and portal vein ligation for two-staged hepatectomy (ALPPS) is a surgical procedure recently introduced in hepatobiliary surgery [9, 10] which consists of the association, during an initial surgical time, of ligation of the right portal vein and transection of the hepatic parenchyma in order to induce a rate of residual liver hypertrophy more marked in a shorter time interval than the standard techniques (PVE, TSH), and it represented a novel concept and one of the most promising advances in oncological liver surgery.

The technique, initially described in a single patient with perihilar cholangiocarcinoma and subsequently tested in a series of patients with diffuse colorectal liver metastases, involves two separate surgical stages. The new approach described by Schnitzbauer [9] in 2012 combines in situ split of the liver usually between the left lateral sector and segment IV° with ligation of the right portal branch followed by a right or extended right hepatectomy. The removal of the liver metastases in the left lateral sector can be included in the first surgical stage (**Figure 2a, b**). A significant increase in FLR was obtained about 1 week after the first operation, and in 2 weeks in healthy livers the maximum peak of regeneration is achieved [37]. Schnitzbauer [9] observed features of hepatocyte apoptosis in the diseased liver and enhanced markers of hepatocyte proliferation in the remnant liver. Although the precise pathophysiologic mechanism by which this spectacular liver regenerative response occurs has not yet been clarified in detail, it is thought that the inflammatory response due to the portal ligature associated with the complete hepatic transection, which does not allow cross portal circulation between the two parts of the liver, is the basis of this regenerative response. The benefits of rapid liver regeneration are clear enough to allow the surgeon to complete the procedure in a shorter time than previous techniques, reducing the risk of possible progression of disease. Furthermore the advantages are expressed in a shorter period of postoperative hospital stay for the patient, and from the technical point of view, the surgeons may be faced with a lower number of postoperative adhesions performing less complicated operations [10].

From the first description of the ALPPS some technical measures have been introduced. To minimize the possibility of biliary leaks on the surface of the disease liver, due to ischemia, surgeons placed the latter in a plastic bag with a drain inside; a catheter was also placed inside the cystic duct to perform a hydraulic test to highlight any biliary leak in the FLR. They performed, moreover, a portal pedicle lymphadenectomy, not only for oncological reasons but also for a better identification of the hilar structures and portal vein ligation. To facilitate the identification of hepatic veins, hepatic artery, and portal pedicle at the time of the second operation, they routinely encircled them with a strong black silk [10]. This new approach allowed to lead to surgical treatment patients with widespread disease judged unresectable with the previous techniques.

Beyond the initial enthusiasm for the new surgical procedure, to the detriment of the latter, the high mortality rate reported in the paper of Schnitzbauer [9]

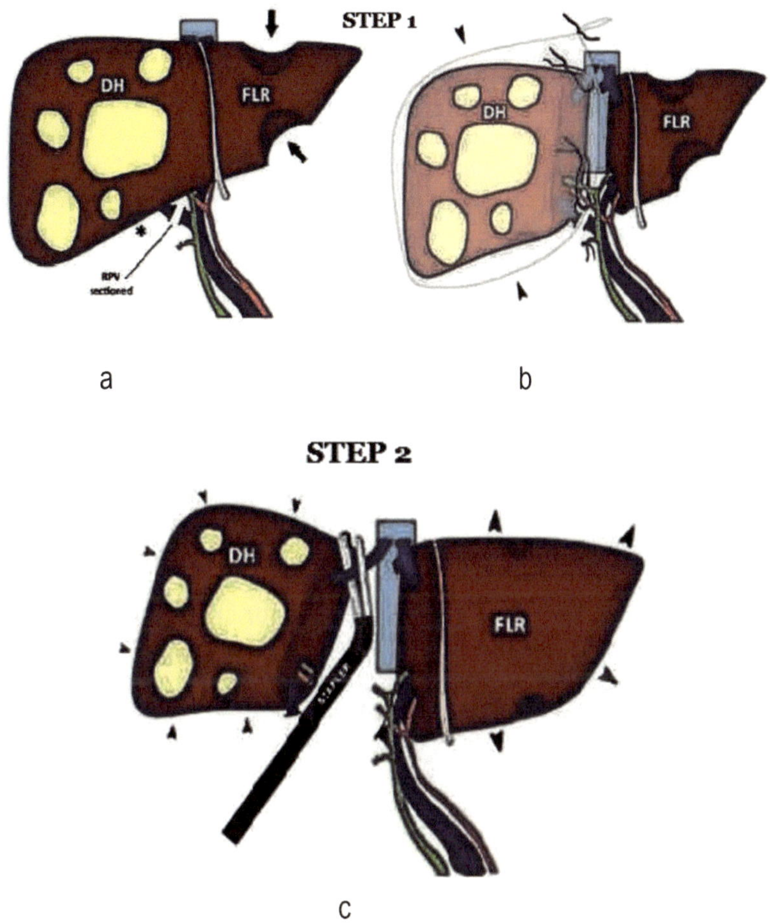

Figure 2.
ALPPS surgical technique ((a) Removal of the left liver metastases, (b) Parenchymal transection and right portal branch ligation, step 1; (c) Liver hypertrophy and parenchymal transection, step 2).

generated several controversies in the surgical community. In fact Schnitzbauer reported a mortality rate of 12% and a morbidity rate of close to 50%.

Over the following years, the technique has been refined trying to better clarify the indications and the various clinical scenarios, leading to steady improvements in safety.

During the 12th Biennial Congress of the European-African Hepato-Pancreato-Biliary Association, in the 10th ALPPS anniversary, some experts discussed indications, management, mechanisms of regeneration, and the pitfalls of the new technique [38].

First of all surgeons emphasized how an accurate knowledge of the vascular liver anatomy (especially that pertaining to the IV° segment [39]) was fundamental to avoid iatrogenic vascular damage resulting in failure of the procedure. It is necessary to assess liver function in addition to volume to avoid liver postoperative failure that occurred in 14 and 30% after stages 1 and 2, respectively [40]. The discrepancy between liver volume increases (up to 200%), and the high rate of liver failure may be attributed to a lack of maturity of the regenerating hepatocytes [41].

To obtain a proper functional study providing quantitative and visual information of the various regional hepatic districts, scintigraphy using ^{99m}Tc-labeled iminodiacetic acid derivatives should be performed. It provides a regional measure of the function of FLR. The use of scintigraphy for timing of stage 2 in ALPPS was compared with CT volumetry in 60 patients completing ALPPS in six centers. The results showed that often volumetry overestimated liver function [42].

Some technical aspects to improve ALPPS morbidity have been investigated in the last years. Interesting are the results of some studies on animal models that have evidenced as the reduction up to a minimum of 50% of the hepatic transection led to a rate of regeneration comparable to the complete transection of the parenchyma [43]. Partial transection offers comparable FLR hypertrophy but significantly lower morbidity, when compared with total transection (38.1 vs. 88.9%) and near-zero mortality [44].

Recent studies indicated that the presence of complications after phase 1 is to be considered predictive of mortality after phase 2 [40]. So during the interstage, the occurrence of complications is to be decisive for the outcome after ALPPS. In this respect some limitations in patient selection should be considered: in patients over 65 years of age or with biliary primary disease with associated cholestasis, the procedure should be contraindicated [43]. International ALPPS registry counts only 11 patients in whom the procedure has been performed for perihilar cholangiocarcinoma without obtaining encouraging results (90th mortality of 27%) [45]. Most recently, biliary tumors and elevated serum bilirubin (pre-stage 2) were identified as predictors of futile outcome after ALPPS [43].

With regard to the possible indication of ALPPS for hepatocellular carcinoma, although the liver's regenerative capacity is certainly less than a healthy liver [12], some group experience showed that ALPPS remains a possible approach to achieving an adequate FLR in patients with hepatitis-related hepatocellular carcinoma [46].

Colorectal liver metastases represent the main indications of ALPPS. Currently the mortality of the procedure in patients with colorectal liver metastases stands at 5% with a survival rate at 3 years around 50% [34, 47]. Although the recurrence rate compared to traditional surgery for colorectal liver metastases is high (only 13% of 3-year-old patients are disease-free), ALPPS is a surgical option for these patients otherwise unresectable.

As already mentioned the technique has undergone several modifications since its introduction focused on an attempt to reduce the complications and mortality of the "*classic*" ALPPS.

The proposed new technical variations have focused their attention on first-stage spitting of the liver parenchyma, on the use of ALPPS for salvage or rescue after TSH, as regard to prevent ischemia of segment IV°, on specific operative maneuvers (Pringle, hanging, anterior approach), on the use of laparoscopic approach at either stage, and on the methods to prevent and identify biliary complications and in the number and position of segments resected [48].

With the term "partial" ALPPS (**Figure 3a–d**), some authors [44, 49] described modification, which provided for the partial transection of the entire transection surface. The latter was carried out from 50–80% of the surface area. The authors reported no difference in liver hypertrophy between partial and full parenchymal splitting (60% vs. 61% median FLR hypertrophy), but a much greater morbidity after the first stage was reported when a full parenchymal split was used.

Associating liver tourniquet and portal ligation for staged hepatectomy (ALTPS). This technique reported in three studies [50–52] provided the positioning of a tourniquet around the future line of transection to ensure a parenchymal compression without having to perform the parenchyma splitting. The authors reported a median FLR growth of 61% over 7 days and a morbidity of 27 and 36% for stage 1 and stage 2, respectively. But a mortality rate of 9% in their series did not reflect a real improvement in terms of the patient's safety. An additional variation indicated with the name of "sequential" ALTPS was proposed by Robles Campos [50]. Unlike

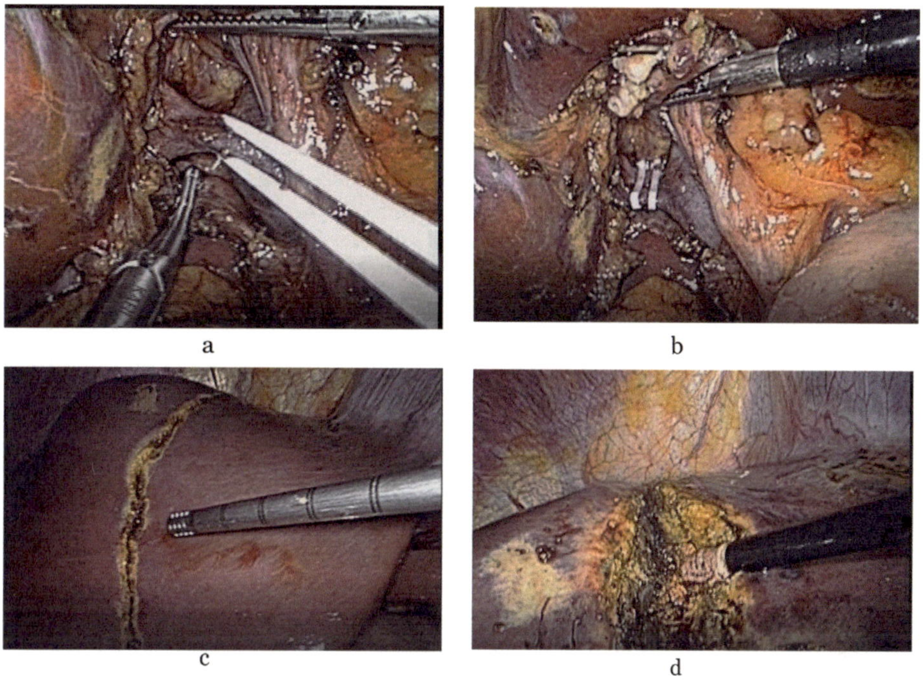

Figure 3.
Surgical steps of laparoscopic "partial ALLPS." (a) Isolation of the right portal branch. (b) Closing of the right portal branch with Hem-o-lock. (c) Demarcation of the section line. (d) Parenchymal transection.

the previous, they did not provide the portal ligature but the execution of portal embolization in the fourth postoperative days. The authors hypothesized that the delayed cessation of blood flow may be related to a decreased impact and severity of venous congestion in the FLR, possibly attenuating the risk of postoperative liver failure.

Conversion to ALPPS appears successful after both PVE and PVL with acceptable clinical outcomes. No differences in major complications showed by Truant [53] in patients who had no PVE before an in situ split.

There are also various technical measures proposed to avoid ischemia and the possible infectious risk at the level of IV° segment, recognized as one of the main causes of morbidity and mortality during the execution of ALPPS. Systematic use of antibiotic therapy has been proposed, partial transection was indicated with the role of generating less ischemic damage [54], and in addition, segment IV° has been resected [55]. Moreover some authors advise to minimize the surgical manipulation of the hepatic hilum to avoid hard surgical adhesions and to minimize the tumor progression during the second phase by means of an anterior approach or Pringle maneuver [46].

Laparoscopic ALPPS has been successfully performed both for two stages. At the expense of an increase in technical difficulty, fewer surgical adhesions were described during the second phase [56]. Although the number of patients treated is very limited, some series report 0% of mortality rate with no major complications and with postoperative hospital stay shorter than the open technique [57]. These results indicate that laparoscopic ALPPS is feasible and it is not inferior to the open approach.

"Hybrid" ALPPS. The technique consists of three main steps [58]: a surgical exploration with the parenchymal split in situ using the anterior approach, the execution of portal embolization using interventional radiology techniques, and right hepatectomy during the second surgical phase. Special care should be taken not to dissect the right hepatoduodenal ligament, and right liver mobilization should not be performed. The technique involves less manipulation to allow more accurate dissection and a greater oncological effectiveness during the second phase of the procedure. This approach was proposed for tumors involving biliary confluence, but although the technique is considered feasible, long-term survival data are still lacking.

Minimally invasive laparoscopic microwave ablation and portal vein ligation for staged hepatectomy (LAPS). On the basis that treatment with microwave thermal ablation/coagulation (MWA) represents a safe and effective treatment option for primary and metastatic liver malignancy, Gringeri [59] developed a novel ALPPS variation associating minimally invasive laparoscopic PVL and MWA on the future transection plane without in situ splitting. This allowed complete and satisfactory hypertrophy of the nonoccluded FLR (avoiding the development of porto-portal shunts) and an easier second step (liver resection) in a patient with hepatocellular carcinoma. With the use of intraoperative laparoscopic ultrasound guidance, the future transection plane was identified and marked with monopolar cautery. MWA antenna was then infixed into the parenchyma, positioning it at the right of the transection plane, applying a 5-minute ablation cycle. This maneuver was repeated step by step every 3 cm, proceeding from the inferior liver margin to the suprahepatic veins. This technique creates an avascular separation and a necrotic groove between the cancer and the FRL in the future transection plane.

Radiofrequency-assisted liver partition with portal vein ligation (RALPP). This technique first described by Gall [60] uses a radiofrequency ablation device to create a line of coagulative necrosis in the hepatic parenchyma instead of physical transection. In experimental study in animals, the procedure has also been performed percutaneously (*percutaneous radiofrequency-assisted liver partition with portal vein ligation* (PRALPPS)) [61].

Although there are still no data on the long-term outcome, as all surgical techniques developed in recent years, they appear to be feasible, inducing a sufficient hepatic hypertrophy with a lower rate of complications. Their execution, however, remains limited to highly specialized centers in liver surgery.

3. Conclusion

The improvement of surgical techniques made resectable, in selected cases, patients with disseminated liver disease, but the treatment of bilobar liver metastases still remains a surgical challenge. The achievement of an adequate residual liver volume to avoid postoperative liver failure was a key point of the procedures developed in recent decades. Since their birth TSH and ALLPS have undergone several changes in the attempt to reduce the rate of morbidity and mortality, and giant steps have been taken. The future of this surgery will be surely full of further innovations and encouraging for hepatobiliary surgeons, never forgetting that a justified nonoperative approach will always be less invasive than the least invasive surgical approach.

Conflict of interest

All authors declare no conflict of interest.

Author details

Fabio Uggeri[1,2]*, Enrico Pinotti[1,2], Mattia Garancini[2], Mauro Scotti[2], Marco Braga[1,2] and Fabrizio Romano[1,2]

1 School of Medicine and Surgery, University of Milan-Bicocca, Monza, Italy

2 Department of Surgery, San Gerardo Hospital, Monza, Italy

*Address all correspondence to: fabio.uggeri@unimib.it

IntechOpen

© 2019 The Author(s). Licensee IntechOpen. This chapter is distributed under the terms of the Creative Commons Attribution License (http://creativecommons.org/licenses/by/3.0), which permits unrestricted use, distribution, and reproduction in any medium, provided the original work is properly cited.

References

[1] Makuuchi M, Thai BL, Takayasu K, Takayama T, Kosuge T, Gunven P, et al. Preoperative portal embolization to increase safety of major hepatectomy for hilar bile duct carcinoma: A preliminary report. Surgery. 1990; **107**(5):521-527. PMID: 2333592

[2] de Baere T, Roche A, Elias D, Lasser P, Lagrange C, Bousson V. Preoperative portal vein embolization for extension of hepatectomy indications. Hepatology. 1996;**24**(6):13861391. DOI: 10.1053/jhep.1996.v24.pm0008938166

[3] Tanaka H, Hirohashi K, Kubo S, Shuto T, Higaki I, Kinoshita H. Preoperative portal vein embolization improves prognosis after right hepatectomy for hepatocellular carcinoma in patients with impaired hepatic function. The British Journal of Surgery. 2000;**87**(7):879-882. DOI: 10.1046/j1365-2168.2000.01439.x

[4] Wakabayashi H, Okada S, Maeba T, Maeta H. Effect of preoperative portal vein embolization on major hepatectomy for advanced-stage hepatocellular carcinomas in injured livers: A preliminary report. Surgery Today. 1997;**27**(5):403-410. DOI: 10.1007/BF02385702

[5] Adam R, Laurent A, Azoulay D, Castaing D, Bismuth H. Two-stage hepatectomy: A planned strategy to treat irresectable liver tumors. Annals of Surgery. 2000;**232**(6):777. PMID: 11088072

[6] Bismuth H, Adam R, Levi F, et al. Resection of nonresectable liver metastases from colorectal cancer after neoadjuvant chemotherapy. Annals of Surgery. 1996;**224**:509-522. PMID: 8857855

[7] Jaeck D, Oussoultzoglou E, Rosso E, Greget M, Weber JC, Bachellier P. A two-stage hepatectomy procedure combined with portal vein embolization to achieve curative resection for initially unresectable multiple and bilobar colorectal liver metastases. Annals of Surgery. 2004;**240**(6):1037. DOI: 10.1097/01.sla.0000145965.86383.89

[8] Shindoh J, Vauthey JN, Zimmitti G, Curley SA, Huang SY, Mahvash A, et al. Analysis of the efficacy of portal vein embolization for patients with extensive liver malignancy and very low future liver remnant volume, including a comparison with the associating liver partition with portal vein ligation for staged hepatectomy approach. Journal of the American College of Surgeons. 2013;**217**(1):126-133. DOI: 10.1012/j.jamcollsurg.2013.03.004

[9] Schnitzbauer AA, Lang SA, Goessmann H, Nadalin S, Baumgart J, Farkas SA, et al. Right portal vein ligation combined with in situ splitting induces rapid left lateral liver lobe hypertrophy enabling 2-staged extended right hepatic resection in small-for-size settings. Annals of Surgery. 2012; **255**(3):405-414. DOI: 10.1097/SLA.0b013e31824856f5

[10] de Santibanes E, Clavien PA. Playing play-Doh to prevent postoperative liver failure: The “ALPPS” approach. Annals of Surgery. 2012;**255**:415-417. DOI: 10.1097/SLA.0b013e318248577d

[11] Schlegel A, Lesurtel M, Melloul E, Limani P, Tschuor C, Graf R, et al. ALPPS: From human to mice highlighting accelerated and novel mechanisms of liver regeneration. Annals of Surgery. 2014;**260**:839-846. discussion 46–7. DOI: 10.1097/SLA.0000000000000949

[12] Schadde E, Ardiles V, Robles-Campos R, Malago M, Machado M, Hernandez-Alejandro R, et al. Early

survival and safety of ALPPS: First report of the international ALPPS registry. Annals of Surgery. 2014;**260**: 829-838. DOI: 0.1097/ SLA.0000000000000947

[13] Dahm F, Georgiev P, Clavien PA. Small for size syndrome after partial liver transplantation: Definition, mechanisms of disease and clinical implications. American Journal of Transplantation. 2005;**5**(11): 2605-2610. DOI: 10.1111/ j.1600-6143.2005.01081.x

[14] Balzan S, Belghiti J, Farges O, Ogata S, Sauvanet A, Delefosse D, et al. The "50-50 criteria" on postoperative day 5: An accurate predictor of liver failure and death after hepatectomy. Annals of Surgery. 2005;**242**(6):824. DOI: 10.1097/01.sla.0000189131.90876.9e

[15] Rahbari NN, Garden OJ, Padbury R, Brooke-Smith M, Crawford M, Adam R, et al. Posthepatectomy liver failure: A definition and grading by the international study Group of Liver Surgery (ISGLS). Surgery. 2011;**49**(5): 713-724. DOI: 10.1016/j.surg.2010. 10.001

[16] Golse N, Bucur PO, Adam R, Castaing D, Cunha AS, Vibert E. New paradigms in post-hepatectomy liver failure. Journal of Gastrointestinal Surgery. 2013;**17**(3):593-605. DOI: 10.1007/s11605-012-2048-6

[17] Mullen JT, Ribero D, Reddy SK, Donadon M, Zorzi D, Gautam S, et al. Hepatic insufficiency and mortality in 1,059 noncirrhotic patients undergoing major hepatectomy. Journal of the American College of Surgeons. 2007; **204**(5):854-862. DOI: 10.1016/j. jamcollsurg.2006.12.032

[18] Azoulay D, Castaing D, Smail A, Adam R, Cailliez V, Laurent A, et al. Resection of nonresectable liver metastases from colorectal cancer after percutaneous portal vein embolization. Annals of Surgery. 2000;**231**(4):480. DOI: 10.1097/00000658-200004000-00005

[19] Homayounfar K, Liersch T, Schuetze G, Niessner M, Goralczyk A, Meller J, et al. Two-stage hepatectomy (R0) with portal vein ligation-towards curing patients with extended bilobular colorectal liver metastases. International Journal of Colorectal Disease. 2009; **24**(4):409-418. DOI: 10.1007/ s00384-008-0620-z

[20] Viganò L, Procopio F, Cimino MM, Donadon M, Gatti A, Costa G, et al. Is tumor detachment from vascular structures equivalent to R0 resection in surgery for colorectal liver metastases? An observational cohort. Annals of Surgical Oncology. 2016;**23**(4): 1352-1360. DOI: 10.1245/s10434-015-5009-y

[21] Passot G, Chun YS, Kopetz SE, Zorzi D, Brudvik KW, Kim BJ, et al. Predictors of safety and efficacy of 2-stage hepatectomy for bilateral colorectal liver metastases. Journal of the American College of Surgeons. 2016; **223**(1):99-108. DOI: 10.1016/j. jamcollsurg.2015.12.057

[22] Naumov GN, Akslen LA, Folkman J. Role of angiogenesis in human tumor dormancy: Animal models of the angiogenic switch. Cell Cycle. 2006; **5**(16):1779-1787. DOI: 10.4161/ cc.516.3018

[23] Lam VW, Laurence JM, Johnston E, Hollands MJ, Pleass HC, Richardson AJ. A systematic review of two stage hepatectomy in patients with initially unresectable colorectal liver metastases. HPB: The Official Journal of the International Hepato Pancreato Biliary Association. 2013;**15**(7):483-491. DOI: 10.1111/j.1477-2574.2012.00607.x

[24] Rees M, Tekkis PP, Welsh FKS, O'Rourke T, John TG. Evaluation of long term survival after hepatic resection for

metastatic colorectal cancer: A multifactorial model of 929 patients. Annals of Surgery. 2008;**247**:125-135. DOI: 10.1097/SLA.0b013e31815aa2c2

[25] Minagawa M, Makuuchi M, Torzilli G, Takayama T, Kawasaki S, Kosuge T, et al. Extension of the frontiers of surgical indications in the treatment of liver metastases from colorectal cancer: Longterm results. Annals of Surgery. 2000;**231**:487-499. PMID: 10749608

[26] Abdalla EK, Vauthey JN, Ellis LM, Ellis V, Pollock R, Broglio KR, et al. Recurrence and outcomes following hepatic resection, radiofrequency ablation, and combined resection/ ablation for colorectal liver metastases. Annals of Surgery. 2004;**239**:818-825. DOI: 10.1097/01.sla.0000128305. 90650.71

[27] Narita M, Oussoultzoglou E, Jaeck D, Fuchschuber P, Rosso E, Pessaux P, et al. Two-stage hepatectomy for multiple bilobar colorectal liver metastases. The British Journal of Surgery. 2011;**98**(10):1463-1475. DOI: 10.1002/bjs.7580

[28] Wicherts DA, Miller R, de Haas RJ, Bitsakou G, Vibert E, Veilhan LA, et al. Long-term results of two-stage hepatectomy for irresectable colorectal cancer liver metastases. Annals of Surgery. 2008;**248**(6):994-1005. DOI: 10.1097/SLA.0b013e3181907fd9

[29] Yokoyama Y, Nagino M, Nimura Y. Mechanisms of hepatic regeneration following portal vein embolization and partial hepatectomy: A review. World Journal of Surgery. 2007;**31**(2):367-374. DOI: 10.1007/s00268-006-0526-2

[30] Adam R, Miller R, Pitombo M, Wicherts DA, de Haas RJ, Bitsakou G, et al. Two-stage hepatectomy approach for initially unresectable colorectal hepatic metastases. Surgical Oncology Clinics of North America. 2007;**16**(3): 525-536. DOI: 10.1016/j.soc.2007.04.016

[31] Blazer DG III, Kishi Y, Maru DM, Kopetz S, Chun YS, Overman MJ, et al. Pathologic response to preoperative chemotherapy: A new outcome end point after resection of hepatic colorectal metastases. Journal of Clinical Oncology. 2008;**26**(33):5344-5351. DOI: 10.1200/JCO.2008.17.5299

[32] Masi G, Loupakis F, Salvatore L, Fornaro L, Cremolini C, Cupini S, et al. Bevacizumab with FOLFOXIRI (irinotecan, oxaliplatin, fluorouracil, and folinate) as first-line treatment for metastatic colorectal cancer: A phase 2 trial. The Lancet Oncology. 2010;**11**(9): 845-852. DOI: 10.1016/S1470-2045(10) 70175-3

[33] Tsim N, Healey AJ, Frampton AE, Habib NA, Bansi DS, Wasan H, et al. Two-stage resection for bilobar colorectal liver metastases: R0 resection is the key. Annals of Surgical Oncology. 2011;**18**(7):1939-1946. DOI: 10.1245/ s10434-010-1533-y

[34] Baumgart J, Jungmann F, Bartsch F, Kloth M, Mittler J, Heinrich S, et al. Two-stage hepatectomy and ALPPS for advanced bilateral liver metastases: A tailored approach balancing risk and outcome. Journal of Gastrointestinal Surgery. 2019;**28**:1-10. DOI: 10.1007/ s11605-019-04145-9

[35] Simoneau E, Hassanain M, Shaheen M, Aljiffry M, Molla N, Chaudhury P, et al. Portal vein embolization and its effect on tumour progression for colorectal cancer liver metastases. The British Journal of Surgery. 2015;**102**(10): 1240-1249. DOI: 10.1002/bjs.9872

[36] Giuliante F, Ardito F, Ferrero A, Aldrighetti L, Ercolani G, Grande G, et al. Tumor progression during preoperative chemotherapy predicts failure to complete 2-stage hepatectomy for colorectal liver metastases: Results of

an Italian multicenter analysis of 130 patients. Journal of the American College of Surgeons. 2014;**219**(2): 285-294. DOI: 10.1016/j.jamcollsurg.2014.01.063

[37] Madoff DC, Hicks ME, Abdalla EK, Morris JS, Vauthey JN. Portal vein embolization with polyvinyl alcohol particles and coils in preparation for major liver resection for hepatobiliary malignancy: Safety and effectiveness—Study in 26 patients. Radiology. 2003; **227**:251-260. DOI: 10.1148/radiol.2271012010

[38] Lang H, de Santibañes E, Schlitt HJ, Malagó M, van Gulik T, Machado MA, et al. 10th anniversary of ALPPS—Lessons learned and quo Vadis. Annals of Surgery. 2019;**269**(1):114-119. DOI: 10.1097/SLA.0000000000002797

[39] Jin GY, Yu HC, Lim HS, Moon JI, Lee JH, Chung JW, et al. Anatomical variations of the origin of the segment 4 hepatic artery and their clinical implications. Liver Transplantation. 2008;**14**(8):1180-1184. DOI: 10.1002/lt.21494

[40] Schadde E, Raptis DA, Schnitzbauer AA, Ardiles V, Tschuor C, Lesurtel M, et al. Prediction of mortality after ALPPS Stage-1: An analysis of 340 patients from the international ALPPS registry. Annals of Surgery. 2015; **262**(5):780-786. DOI: 10.1097/SLA.0000000000001450

[41] Matsuo K, Murakami T, Kawaguchi D, Hiroshima Y, Koda K, Yamazaki K, et al. Histologic features after surgery associating liver partition and portal vein ligation for staged hepatectomy versus those after hepatectomy with portal vein embolization. Surgery. 2016; **159**(5):1289-1298. DOI: 10.1016/j.surg.2015.12.004

[42] Olthof PB, Tomassini F, Huespe PE, Truant S, Pruvot FR, Troisi RI, et al. Hepatobiliary scintigraphy to evaluate liver function in associating liver partition and portal vein ligation for staged hepatectomy: Liver volume overestimates liver function. Surgery. 2017;**162**:775-783. DOI: 10.1016/j.surg.2017.05.022

[43] Linecker M, Kambakamba P, Reiner CS, Nguyen-Kim TDL, Stavrou GA, Jenner RM, et al. How much liver needs to be transected in ALPPS? A translational study investigating the concept of less invasiveness. Surgery. 2017;**161**:453-464. DOI: 10.1016/j.surg.2016.08.004

[44] Petrowsky H, Gyori G, de Oliveira M, Lesurtel M, Clavien PA, et al. Is partial-ALPPS safer than ALPPS? A single-center experience. Annals of Surgery. 2015;**261**:e90-e92. DOI: 10.1097/SLA.0000000000001087

[45] Serenari M, Zanello M, Schadde E, Toschi E, Ratti F, Gringeri E, et al. Importance of primary indication and liver function between stages: Results of a multicenter Italian audit of ALPPS 2012–2014. HPB: The Official Journal of the International Hepato Pancreato Biliary Association. 2016;**18**:419-427. DOI: 10.1016/j.hpb.2016.02.003

[46] Chan AC, Poon RT, Chan C, Lo CM. Safety of ALPPS procedure by the anterior approach for hepatocellular carcinoma. Annals of Surgery. 2016;**263**: e14e16. DOI: 10.1097/SLA.0000000000001272

[47] Wanis KN, Ardiles V, Alvarez FA, Tun-Abraham ME, Linehan D, de Santibañes E, et al. Intermediate-term survival and quality of life outcomes in patients with advanced colorectal liver metastases undergoing associating liver partition and portal vein ligation for staged hepatectomy. Surgery. 2018;**163**:691-697. DOI: 10.1016/j.surg.2017.09.044

[48] Edmondson MJ, Sodergren MH, Pucher PH, Darzi A, Li J, Petrowsky H,

et al. Variations and adaptations of associated liver partition and portal vein ligation for staged hepatectomy (ALPPS): Many routes to the summit. Surgery. 2016;**159**(4):1058-1072. DOI: 10.1016/j.surg.2015.11.013

[49] Alvarez FA, Ardiles V, de Santibanes M, Pekolj J, de Santibanes E. Associating liver partition and portal vein ligation for staged hepatectomy offers high oncological feasibility with adequate patient safety: A prospective study at a single center. Annals of Surgery. 2015;**261**:723-732. DOI: 10.1097/SLA.0000000000001046

[50] Robles Campos R, Brusadin R, Lopez Conesa A, Parrilla Paricio P. Staged liver resection for perihilar liver tumors using a tourniquet in the umbilical fissure and sequential portal vein embolization on the fourth postoperative day (a modified ALTPS). Cirugía Española. 2014;**92**:682-686. DOI: 10.1016/j.ciresp.2014.07.006

[51] Robles R, Parrilla P, Lopez-Conesa A, Brusadin R, de la Pena J, Fuster M, et al. Tourniquet modification of the associating liver partition and portal ligation for staged hepatectomy procedure. The British Journal of Surgery. 2014;**101**:1129-1134. discussion 34. DOI: 10.1002/bjs.9547

[52] Cai X, Peng S, Duan L, Wang Y, Yu H, Li Z. Completely laparoscopic ALPPS using round-the-liver ligation to replace parenchymal transection for a patient with multiple right liver cancers complicated with liver cirrhosis. Journal of Laparoendoscopic & Advanced Surgical Techniques. Part A. 2014;**24**: 883-886. DOI: 10.1089/lap.2014.0455

[53] Truant S, Scatton O, Dokmak S, Regimbeau JM, Lucidi V, Laurent A, et al. Associating liver partition and portal vein ligation for staged hepatectomy (ALPPS): Impact of the inter-stages course on morbi-mortality and implications for management. European Journal of Surgical Oncology. 2015;**41**:674-682. DOI: 10.1016/j.ejso.2015.01.004

[54] Alvarez FA, Ardiles V, Sanchez Claria R, Pekolj J, de Santibanes E. Associating liver partition and portal vein ligation for staged hepatectomy (ALPPS): Tips and tricks. Journal of Gastrointestinal Surgery. 2013;**17**: 814-821. DOI: 10.1007/s11605-012-2092-2

[55] Andriani OC. Long-term results with associating liver partition and portal vein ligation for staged hepatectomy (ALPPS). Annals of Surgery. 2012;**256**:e5. author reply e16–9. DOI: 10.1097/SLA.0b013e318265fbbe

[56] Cillo U, Gringeri E, Feltracco P, Bassi D, D'Amico FE, Polacco M, et al. Totally laparoscopic microwave ablation and portal vein ligation for staged hepatectomy: A new minimally invasive two-stage hepatectomy. Annals of Surgical Oncology. 2015;**22**:2787-2788. DOI: 10.1245/s10434-014-4353-7

[57] Machado MA, Makdissi FF, Surjan RC, Basseres T, Schadde E. Transition from open to laparoscopic ALPPS for patients with very small FLR: The initial experience. HPB: The Official Journal of the International Hepato Pancreato Biliary Association. 2017;**19**:59-66. DOI: 10.1016/j.hpb.2016.10.004

[58] Li J, Kantas A, Ittrich H, Koops A, Achilles EG, Fischer L, et al. Avoid "all-touch" by hybrid ALPPS to achieve oncological efficacy. Annals of Surgery. 2016;**263**(1):e6-e7. DOI: 10.1097/SLA.0000000000000845

[59] Gringeri E, Boetto R, D'Amico FE, Bassi D, Cillo U. Laparoscopic microwave ablation and portal vein ligation for staged hepatectomy (LAPS): A minimally invasive first-step approach. Annals of Surgery. 2015;**261**: e42-e43. DOI: 10.1097/SLA.0000000000000606

[60] Gall TM, Sodergren MH, Frampton AE, Fan R, Spalding DR, Habib NA, et al. Radio-frequency-assisted liver partition with portal vein ligation (RALPP) for liver regeneration. Annals of Surgery. 2015;**261**:e45-e46. DOI: 10.1097/SLA.0000000000000607

[61] Gimenez ME, Houghton EJ, Davrieux CF, Serra E, Pessaux P, Palermo M, et al. Percutaneous radiofrequency assisted liver partition with portal vein embolization for staged hepatectomy (pralpps). ABCD: Arquivos Brasileiros de Cirurgia Digestiva (São Paulo). 2018;**31**(1):e1346. DOI: 10.1590/0102-672020180001e1346

Chapter 10

Management of Patients with Liver Transplantation in ICU

Areti Karapanagiotou, Achillefs Pitsoulis, Maria Vasileiou and Nikolaos Voloudakis

Abstract

Liver transplantation constitutes the most effective and indispensable treatment of end-stage liver disease (ESLD). Major advances in surgical techniques, anesthesiological management, postoperative care, immunosuppression, and diagnostic approach have led to increased overall survival of patients. Postoperative care poses a great challenge since detrimental occurrences that need prompt treatment may affect the graft or distant organ functionality. Adequate graft function is strongly associated with distant organ restoration and rapid patient recovery. In the ICU setting, the main focal points are hemodynamic stabilization, coagulation and electrolyte disturbances correction, respiratory support, early weaning from mechanical ventilation, and evaluation of graft functionality. It is of paramount importance to facilitate early graft recovery, recognize and promptly treat systematic complications and life-threatening sequelae, and individualize treatment protocols considering graft quality, donor's and recipient's health status, and potential co-morbidities. To achieve those goals, technological advancements in continuous patient monitoring, graft functionality, and its metabolic reserves must be assimilated and implemented in the ICU.

Keywords: liver transplantation, post-liver transplantation intensive care, immediate postoperative management, complications, infections prophylaxis, early postoperative complications

1. Introduction

In the past years, liver transplantation (LT) has made leaps and evolved from an endeavor in specialized centers to a worldwide definitive and gold standard treatment of the end-stage liver disease (ESLD), acute liver failure, and various cancer types [1, 2].

The advances in perioperative management, including the improvement of surgical techniques, preservation solutions, perioperative management, and monitoring, as well as advances in immunosuppression and postoperative care have led not only to an increased number of transplantations but also to better outcomes [2]. According to recent studies in the United Kingdom, the 1- and 5-year survival rate for liver transplant recipients has reached 92 and 80%, respectively [3]. However, there are still certain challenges in LT. Scarcity of allografts and disparity between supply and demand has led the transplantation community to expand the donor pool by utilizing split grafts, allografts from living donors after cardiac death and including marginal donors of older age and with extended steatosis [4].

IntechOpen

Additionally, recipients are sicker, given that priority of graft allocation is based on higher MELD scores, older and with co-morbidities such as metabolic syndrome, cardiac disease, and diabetes mellitus [5, 6]. Postoperative liver transplant patient care requires careful accounting of the recipient's pre-existing pathophysiology, intraoperative events, and donor's quality. Moreover, the implanted liver represents a unique biological entity that has undergone physiological changes and has to adapt to a new environment. This donor-recipient interaction is the key of a successful transplantation [7].

The intensivist's role is essential as a multifaceted approach is critical for optimal transplantation outcomes. The main hurdles to tackle are early recognition and immediate treatment of the hemodynamic and metabolic disorders, restoration of intravascular volume, avoidance of coagulation disorders, optimization of organs function affected by hepatic failure, prophylaxis and treatment of infections, early enteral nutrition, and evaluation of graft function. Technological advances offer the possibility of continuous cardiovascular and allograft function monitoring facilitating improved endpoint results.

2. General principles

The aim of immediate postoperative support is the adequate O_2 supply to tissues and graft by ensuring hemodynamic stabilization, fluid balance, restoration of diuresis, optimal ventilation, and supporting graft function. It should be noted that graft recovery depends primarily on the intrinsic hepatocyte recovery capacity and secondly on optimizing liver hemodynamics and preventing venous stasis.

3. Hemodynamic stabilization and monitoring

The primary goal of hemodynamic monitoring is to prevent inadequate cardiac filling and the subsequent tissue hypoperfusion, and also to avoid overloading leading to congestion of the lungs and sinusoids and hence allograft dysfunction [8]. The intravascular volume, cardiac output (CO), and systematic vascular resistance (SVR) are important parameters vital in determining the success of a LT. The treatment becomes even more complicated when renal and/or heart failure, portopulmonary hypertension, or hepatopulmonary syndromes are also present [9].

Successful management of patients with end-stage liver disease (ESLD) requires a complete understanding of their hemodynamic profile that is often characterized by high cardiac output (CO) with decreased systemic vascular resistance, depleted intravascular volume, and compensatory tachycardia with concomitant renal vasoconstriction and dilutional hyponatremia, due to excessive production of vasodilators during the development of hepatic failure [10]. Following LT, vasodilation and hyperdynamic circulation remain until the graft begins to function and excretes excess vasodilatory agents that are almost completely restored after 6 months [11].

Upon the arrival of a liver transplant recipient in the ICU, advanced monitoring, which estimates CO and volume status, additionally to standard hemodynamic monitoring, that is electrocardiogram, pulse-oximetry, and invasive blood pressure, are deemed essential [12].

Hemodynamic depression may be the result of hypovolemia, prolonged reperfusion syndrome, cardiac dysfunction, either caused by pre-existing or emerging ischemic cardiomyopathy, and metabolic disorders such as acidosis, hypocalcaemia, hypothermia, vasodilation due to sepsis, or graft dysfunction.

The assessment of the intravascular volume is of vital importance given that volume status can be affected by contradictory factors such hypovolemia or hypervolemia, both detrimental for graft and patient survival. Restoring volume status, a continually dynamic parameter, and achieving optimal CO are crucial in order to maintain the delicate balance between preload optimization and avoidance of pulmonary edema [13].

Hypovolemia, possibly due to continued bleeding, occult or overt, inadequate fluid replacement and/or loss in the third space, can lead to reduced preload and CO and hence hypoperfusion resulting in additional lesions in the newly transplanted liver [14]. The aim is to replace the intravascular fluid and maintain the circulating blood volume. There is still controversy over the type of fluids administered, with crystalloids gaining ground against the colloids (hydroxyl ethyl starches), which have been associated with renal injury and increased mortality in critically ill patients [15], a conclusion that is not supported by convincing evidence in LT. Nevertheless, the appropriate crystalloid should be carefully selected taking into account its special characteristics and based on its metabolism, electrolyte composition, pH and osmolarity, and considering patients' status [16]. Albumin (Alb) administration as a replacement fluid has been a matter of debate. In some centers, a large amount of Alb is exogenously administered following the LT to support circulatory stability. Moreover, a concentration of 25 g/L is considered necessary for the immunosuppressive drugs to be effective [17]. Beneficial properties were attributed to Alb in recent studies; whereas, postoperative hypoalbuminemia has been linked to the development of acute kidney injury (AKI) [18]. It has been found that during LT there is translocation of Alb, probably to the interstitial space, which persists until the third postoperative day and whose role has not been clearly clarified [19]. Certain centers choose to replace two-thirds of the required fluids with crystalloids and one-third of drain losses with albumin [14]. Although, blood and blood products transfusion strategies vary between institutions, it is considered that postoperative hematocrit (Hct) values, ranging between 25 and 30%, are safe for adequately transporting O_2 to the new graft [14]. The rational use of blood products depends on the monitoring of the coagulation mechanism. Whole-blood viscoelastic tests, such as thromboelastogram (TEG) and rotational thromboelastometry (ROTEM), that illustrate each step of thrombus formation and fibrinolysis are useful tools to guide transfusions and drug administration (anti-fibrinolytics, coagulation factors) [20, 21] by limiting the number of transfusions, as there has been an association between them and increased morbidity/mortality, prolonged stay in the hospital, postoperative sepsis, increased risk of acute rejection, and hepatic artery thrombosis [22–24].

Hypervolemia occurs either from intraoperative over-resuscitation or coexistence of renal dysfunction. It can result in capillary leak syndrome with loss of fluids in the third space, further congestion and graft edema due to vascular permeability disorder, caused by ischemia/reperfusion injury (I/R) that is more pronounced in grafts with higher preservation injury, greater steatosis, or in older donors [7, 25]. Studies also indicate that massive administration of fluids and blood is a risk factor for complications of the respiratory system postoperatively and is correlated with increased mortality [26]. On the contrary, conservative resuscitation strategy and negative fluid balance during the first three postoperative days, if hemodynamic stability has been achieved, act protectively. Codes et al. [27] concluded that a continuous positive balance in the first 4 days after surgery correlates with the development of AKI and the need for renal replacement therapy (RRT). Goal directed therapy (GDT) strategy, which has been successfully applied in major surgical interventions, is proposed. It aims at maintaining an adequate supply of O_2 to the end organs by a bundle of measures including fluid titration in conjunction with blood transfusions as well as administration of vasopressors and/or inotropic agents [28]. The hemodynamic targets are predefined and specific variables are used to control fluid adequacy, improvement of CO, and tissue perfusion. GDT has beneficial effects compared to liberal fluid administration, reducing postoperative ileus, mechanical ventilation time, and respiratory system complications, as it has been indicated in relevant, although limited, studies [29]. Jiang et al. [30] suggests the individualization of fluid administration in the perioperative period as an optimal recovery strategy. They estimated that transfusions >100 ml/kg and fluid balance ≤−14 ml/kg during the first postoperative days result in prolonged mechanical ventilation, extubation time, and ICU stay. Prudent use of vasopressor agents is proposed since they increase arterial tone and improve perfusion pressure avoiding overload. Noradrenaline (0.01–1 μg/kg/min) with mixed α-β-adrenergic effects is most commonly administered to maintain CO and organ perfusion. Vasopressin (0.5–0.6 U/h) and terlipressin (1.5 μg/kg/h) have also been used in recent years because of their modifying effect on visceral circulation, where approximately 37% of the total blood volume is located in cirrhotic patients, and of their ability to reduce pressure in the portal vein [31, 32].

Since there has been no consensus on hemodynamic monitoring in LT yet, there is a number of invasive and noninvasive CO monitors available in order to evaluate hemodynamic fluctuations (**Table 1**) [13, 36].

The pulmonary artery (PAC) catheter has traditionally been used for hemodynamic monitoring in LT. It provides the possibility of measuring the CO by the thermodilution method, which is considered the gold standard, but also the cardiac

Monitors	Principle	Advantages	Limitations
PAC	Thermodilution	Accurate continuous measures of CO Direct measures of PAP and RVEDVI Gold standard in POPH	Invasive CVP, PCWP static pressures measurement Unreliable indicators of volume status, SV and fluid responsiveness
PiCCO	Pulse contour analysis	Less invasive Continuous CO, SV measures ITBVI, EVLWI, PPV, SVV Reliable indicators of fluid responsiveness	Need for recalibration in marked changes of SVR Inaccurate CO measures in Child-Pugh Band C stages in cirrhosis Requires sinus rhythm and certain ventilator setting
LiDCO	Pulse contour analysis	Continuous CO, SV measures comparable to PAC measures PPV, SVV Indicative of volume status	Calibration with lithium Inaccurate CO measures in Child-Pugh Band C stages in cirrhosis
FlowTrac/Vigileo	Pulse contour analysis	No need for calibration Continuous CO, SV measures PPV, SVV, indicative of volume status	Not reliable in hyperdynamic circulation with very low SVR
TEE	Ultrasound, Doppler	Less invasive Direct visualization of cardiac function and volume status	Advanced training is required Risk of rupture in 3rd or 4th grade of esophageal varices

Table 1.
Hemodynamic monitoring in LT.

filling pressures, the CVP, and especially the PCWP for assessing the preload [33]. Numerous studies have shown that static preload measurements are indirect markers of the end diastolic volume and have a poor predictive value for fluid management, improvement of hepatic perfusion, and recovery guidance [34]. Although still under debate, current data favor the use of a modified pulmonary artery catheter, with an incorporated heating coil, that provide continuous measurement of CO (CCO) and right ventricular end diastolic volume (RVEDV) as the more reliable preload indicator. Patients with portopulmonary hypertension are highly benefited from PAC, as it is the method of choice for measuring and monitoring pulmonary artery pressures intraoperatively and directly postoperatively [13, 35].

In recent years, interest has shifted to the dynamic parameters and expanding data yielded from existing monitoring of blood pressure to assess the CO, the preload and the afterload. There is technology available to accurately analyze pressure waveforms and sufficient knowledge to generate algorithms that are interpreted by the complex pulse wave morphology [36, 37].

The PiCCO system (Pulsion Medical System, Munich, Germany) uses the method of transpulmonary thermodilution, single indicator technique, and arterial pulse contour analysis which by means of an algorithm can continuously calculate CO and preload markers: global end diastolic volume (GEDVI), extra vascular lung water index (EVLWI), and intrathoracic blood volume index (ITBVI) which is considered a reliable preload indicator in LT. In transplant patients, the CO measurements deriving from the PiCCO system are consistent with those of PAC [38, 39].

Furthermore, this system offers the capability of functional hemodynamic monitoring by detecting the changes in left ventricular pulse volume caused by changes in preload due to mechanical ventilation. Stroke volume variation (SVV) and pulse pressure variation (PPV) have been used successfully to assess the intravascular volume and fluid responsiveness in critically ill patients [12, 13, 40]. Certain LT studies have concluded that the SVV is a better indicator for RVEDVI than CVP, while a SVV greater than 9% is an indicator of low RVEDVI which means fluid responsiveness [41, 42]. However, there are always limitations deriving from the presence of arrhythmia and mechanical ventilation settings.

The LiDCO system (LiDCO Plus, Cambridge, United Kingdom) is similar to the PiCCO system, but in its case the lithium indicator dilution technique is applied in order to calibrate the arterial waveform analysis algorithm [40]·

The Flowtrac/Vigileo system (Edwards Lifesciences, Irvine, CA United States) is a special energy converter that links the arterial line with a CO monitor and uses arterial waveform analysis with an algorithm for real-time CO measurement in conjunction with patient demographics without the need for calibration. However, a poor correlation has been found between findings of waveform analysis CO when compared to PAC thermodilution, mainly in patients with cirrhosis B and C according to Child-Pugh classification [43, 44]. Biais et al. came to the same conclusion, using the recent third generation, FloTrac system, pointing out that there was great discrepancy in cases of significantly low SVR [45, 46].

In recent years, the use of transesophageal echocardiography (TEE) has been gaining ground not only because it is considered a noninvasive method, but also because it provides the ability to directly visualize the contractility of the left and right heart, preload status, and differential diagnosis of various pathological conditions such as pulmonary embolism, pleural, or pericardial effusion [47]. The CO can be estimated with measurements of flow across the cardiac valve, left ventricular outflow tract, or the flow in the main pulmonary artery. The ability to instantly display real-time preload is considered its biggest advantage. The functional application of TEE is limited by the risk of rupture of the third or fourth grade esophageal varices, but it is considered a reliable hemodynamic monitoring method when used by experienced intensivists [12, 13].

4. Liver allograft function

Assessment of graft function is necessary and is performed by combining clinical parameters, laboratory values, and imaging examinations. The first positive signs of adequate function of the new liver can be evident by the correction of metabolic acidosis, coagulation disturbances, hemodynamic stabilization, and temperature normalization in addition to diuresis restoration. Continuous monitoring in the postoperative period is required for the immediate recognition of early, subtle findings of graft dysfunction which necessitate aggressive treatment. Traditionally, the evaluation of liver function involves static and dynamic tests [48].

Static tests include hematology, coagulation, and biochemistry blood tests, in order to evaluate the main liver functions. The hepatic enzymes aspartate aminotransferase (AST) and alanine aminotransferase (ALT), which rather indicate hepatocyte necrosis, display a rise postoperatively reaching their peak during the first 2 days before they finally start decreasing. Their elevation is attributed to preservation injuries and/or prolonged cold ischemia time (CIT). A persisting elevated value raises concerns about liver function and requires further investigation. The canalicular enzymes γ-glutamyl transferase and alkaline phosphatase increase after day four and usually five-fold before their decline begins. The synthetic function of the liver is evaluated by the prothrombin time or international normalized ratio (INR), which estimate the production of coagulation factors by the liver. Bilirubin levels define the liver excretory function while its metabolic function is assessed by glucose and lactate levels. A resistant to the treatment hypoglycemia is an indicator of graft dysfunction. The levels of lactates should also be carefully considered, if increased, due to the fact that such result may derive from peripheral tissue hypoxia.

The dynamic tests express the ability of the liver to metabolize or excrete certain substances. The lidocaine conversion to monoethylglycinexylidide metabolite (MEGX test) assesses the metabolic capacity and the liver blood flow [48, 49].

The indocyanine green (ICG) clearance test is routinely used in several centers. The functional activity of the graft is assessed by ICG dye administration, which is almost exclusively eliminated from the liver into the bile without undergoing enterohepatic circulation. Its removal from the blood depends on the hepatic blood flow, parenchymal cell function, and biliary excretion. It is expressed as half-life time, blood clearance, or plasma disappearance rate (ICG-PDR) smaller than 15% associated with a higher rate of primary dysfunction [50]. The bedside ultrasound imaging methods with hepatic blood vessel Doppler examination are usually performed on the day of surgery or on the first postoperative one in order to evaluate the patency of the hepatic artery, the portal vein, and the hepatic vein. It is particularly useful in the presence of intraoperative technical difficulties or when there is graft dysfunction, with a view to identify vascular abnormalities that could be treated [51].

Recovery of the graft is a combination mainly of the severity of the recipient's condition, donor quality, intraoperative events, perioperative hemodynamic stability, and preservation injuries, while adequate blood flow to the organs and prevention of venous stasis in the new liver have to be ensured (**Table 2**) [49]. On the other hand, the risk of poor outcome is increased in case of ESLD-associated syndromes and co-morbidities coexistence, especially in sicker patients, as estimated by the MELD score [4, 7].

Donor quality has a major impact on the graft function since the use of marginal donors is now commonplace [4]. The prolonged time of cold ischemia for more than 12 h increases ischemia reperfusion injuries. Macrosteatosis greater than 30% reduces tolerances in such injuries, while the risk of rejection and PNF is increased. Grafts from donors older than 60 years of age are considered to be of higher risk for PNF or exhibit delayed recovery mainly owing to cholestasis, whereas grafts from donors older than 75 show reduced liver regeneration capacity [52–54].

Donor related	Recipient related	Intraoperative events	Allograft related
Donor age Macrovesicular steatosis >30% High dose of vasopressors Hypernatremia Prolonged ICU stay Prolonged CIT Donation after cardiac death	ESLD-associated syndromes Pretransplant HD/renal dysfunction Cardiovascular disease BMI < 18.5 kg/m^2	Massive transfusion Reperfusion syndrome High vasopressors dose	I/R Injury Graft inflow (Right HF, Hepatic vein stenosis/thrombosis) Graft outflow (Hepatic artery and portal vein patency) Small-for-size syndrome

Table 2.
Factors related to graft function.

Nevertheless, the results in the literature are contradictory; and in 2016, the donors older than 65 years old reached a percentage of 20.7%. In a recent study, Gilbo et al. concluded that older grafts can be safely used in older recipients without endangering their survival, if the remaining risk factors have been minimized [55]. The best practice for graft allocation is the use of scores that include donor and recipient data, such as the survival outcomes following liver transplantation (SOFT) and/or the BAR-score, which offer excellent prognostic ability for survival after transplantation and could lead to the final decision on using or rejecting the graft [56].

5. Ventilatory support and weaning from mechanical ventilation

The intraoperative use of short-acting anesthetics and neuromuscular blocking agents allows a prompt recovery of consciousness and facilitates the rapid release from mechanical support and early extubation (EE), which can occur in the operating theater or within the first three postoperative hours and is associated with shorter ICU and hospital stay. In a recent meta-analysis comparing early versus conventional extubation, the authors report a reduction in re-intubation rate, morbidity, respiratory complications, incidence of graft dysfunction, and ICU/hospital stay [57–59]. In a study published by Taner et al., it was exhibited that early extubation failed only in 1.90% of patients when performed on selected cases. According to these researchers, patients with HCC and low MELD score are appropriate candidates for EE [60].

Prolonged mechanical ventilation (MV) remains a critical risk factor for infections development, especially ventilator-associated pneumonia, tracheal trauma, prolongation of neuromuscular recovery, graft venous congestion due to positive intrathoracic pressures, and reduced venous return to the inferior vena cava and hepatic veins [61, 62]. It has also been correlated by Yuan et al. with the recipient's age, female gender, preoperative need for renal replacement therapy (RRT), ascites, higher MELD score, prolonged cold ischemia, and the number of transfusions [62].

Emphasis is placed on the fact that optimal selection criteria and timing of EE have not been clearly defined yet. Patients with encephalopathy, marked hypoxemia, obesity (BMI > 30), severe hemodynamic instability, pulmonary edema, cardiac or renal dysfunction, and multiple transfusions are not indicated for EE. The personalized and selective approach is likely to be the best strategy with a focus on avoiding delayed extubation, preserving hemodynamic stabilization, and ensuring graft functionality [63].

The criteria of weaning from MV applied to liver transplanted patients in ICU conform to those of the rest patient groups [64]. Distinct sequelae may often arise from ESLD-related disorders such as encephalopathy, massive transfusions, graft dysfunction, preoperative nutrition disorders, volume overload, and postoperative respiratory complications including pulmonary edema, pleural effusions, or pneumonia. During MV, lungs and liver allograft interaction should be taken into account with the aim of improving oxygenation without impairing the outflow of the liver graft. Implementation of daily withdrawal of sedation combined with spontaneous breathing trial facilitates weaning from MV [63].

Acute respiratory distress syndrome (ARDS), one of the prominent respiratory complications following LT, is usually attributed to reperfusion syndrome, substantial blood loss and transfusions, prolonged operation time, and early postoperative infections and sepsis. Lung-protective ventilator strategies with low tidal volumes (6 ml/kg IBW), higher respiratory rate, and positive end-expiratory pressure (PEEP) are recommended to limit lung injury from shear forces and atelectasis [64]. There is debate about optimum PEEP in LT since some consider that higher PEEP values impair venous return and visceral blood flow leading to hepatic edema. Evaluation of transpulmonary pressure has been proposed to optimize PEEP titration [65]. Saner et al. concluded that PEEP up to 15 cm H_2O affects neither blood flow to the liver, nor flow and velocity in the hepatic artery, right hepatic vein, and portal vein [66]. In refractory ARDS and persistent hypoxia, prone positioning, high frequency ventilation, and extracorporeal membrane oxygenation support have been utilized as rescue therapy [67–69].

There are certain syndromes related to ESLD characterized by severe hypoxemia which require special management in the ICU such as hepatopulmonary syndrome and portopulmonary hypertension.

Hepatopulmonary syndrome is caused by intrapulmonary capillary dilatation that leads to hypoxemia and shortness of breath. LT is considered the treatment of choice; however, in most cases, severe hypoxemia might persist for a 6–12 months period. In the ICU, fluids should be managed carefully and lung-protective strategies should be employed during MV. In persistent hypoxemia, high frequency ventilation and/or venovenous extracorporeal membrane oxygenation is recommended. Some authors suggest early extubation and the immediate application of noninvasive ventilation with high-inspired fraction of oxygen [70, 71].

Portopulmonary hypertension resulting from pulmonary vasoconstriction due to portal hypertension requires prevention of hypoxemia, maintaining oxygen saturation >90% and correcting factors involved such as acidemia, arrhythmia, and anemia. Administration of diuretics and/or renal replacement therapy is advised if volume overload cannot be avoided. MV can both compromise venous return from the allograft and increase pulmonary vascular resistance through alveolar overdistension; therefore, lung-protective ventilation is considered to be the most appropriate strategy. The use of pulmonary vasodilators, that can be both administered IV such as epoprostenol and orally, via nasogastric tube, such as phosphodiesterase V inhibitor or nonselective endothelin receptor antagonist, is recommended during ICU stay [71].

6. Immunosuppression

Advances in immunosuppression have greatly impacted the survival of patients following LT. The initial endpoint was to prevent rejection; but in recent years, the interest has also been shifted to avoiding long-term complications from immunosuppressant agents and relapsing of the disease. In spite of the latest developments in this field, most centers commence immunosuppression with calcineurin inhibitors (CNIs) and corticosteroids with or without an anti-proliferative agent depending on protocols [72, 73].

Calcineurin inhibitors: Tacrolimus and cyclosporine inhibit calcineurin by impairing interleukin-2 (IL-2) transduction. Used as first-line immunosuppressant, tacrolimus is considered 100 times more potent than cyclosporine, and is superior in graft and patient survival with fewer acute and steroid-resistant rejection episodes. The main side effect is nephrotoxicity, while hypertension, hyperkalemia, uremic hemolytic syndrome, and neurotoxicity have lesser incidence [72]. Corticosteroids are important both in the initial immunosuppressive therapy and in the treatment of acute rejection.

Mycophenolate mofetil has been widely used as an adjuvant and alternative immunosuppressive agent. It is a potential inhibitor of B- and T-cell proliferation. It is mainly utilized when a dose reduction or discontinuation of CNI is demanded due to certain adverse effects such as nephrotoxicity and neurotoxicity [72].

Mammalian target of rapamycin (mTor) inhibitors, sirolimus, and everolimus, prevent B- and T-cell proliferation prompting the cell to arrest at G1 to S phase of the cell cycle. Although accounted for wound healing delay incidents, they can be administered as primary and rescue immunosuppression therapy with the advantages of being renal sparing as well as reducing the need for high doses of steroids. The newer IL-2 receptor-blocking antibody preparations daclizumab (Zenapax) and basiliximab (Simulect) are often used to initiate immunosuppression and avoid CNIs, and can also play a part in steroid-resistant rejection [72].

7. Infection prophylaxis

Prevention of infections is a major problem as they are the leading cause of death following LT [74]. The most common ones in the immediate postoperative period are of bacterial or fungal origin and include bloodstream, catheter related, surgical site, pulmonary, urinary tract, *Clostridium difficile* infections, and intra-abdominal collections. The identification of risk factors and the stratification of patients according to them determine the prophylactic perioperative antimicrobial treatment [75, 76]. Antimicrobial chemoprophylaxis depends on the patient's immune status, intraoperative events, recent or recurrent hospitalization, and donor infections at the time of liver graft procurement while it has been tailored in accordance with the colonization of the patients, recently characterized by a prevalence of multidrug-resistant Gram-negative bacilli [76, 77]. Other recipient-related risk factors are malnutrition, re-operation, acute liver failure, biliary complications, and the existence of postoperative catheters, lines, and drains. Antibiotics right before surgery cover Gram-negative bacteria (*Pseudomonas* sp., *Enterobacter* sp., and *Klebsiella* sp.), Gram-positive organisms (*Staphylococcus aureus*), fungi, and viruses according to the center protocols and their epidemiology. Antifungal prophylaxis is administered to higher risk patients determined by factors such as renal dysfunction with a need for RRT, re-transplantation, multiple transfusions, prolonged ICU stay, colonization by *Candida*, and graft rejection incidents with administration of high doses of corticosteroids. In many centers, azoles or liposomal amphotericin are used [76–78]. Siddique et al. reported that the rate of post-transplant infections was 24.5% with no difference between deceased and living donors; however, mortality was higher in bacterial infections in deceased donor recipients [79].

Herpes family viral infections, due to immunosuppression mainly by administration of T-cell-specific agents, are adequately treated with acyclovir. Ganciclovir or valganciclovir is sufficient for CMV seronegative recipients with CMV-seropositive grafts, or after rejection treatment. In case of suspected infection during hospitalization, broad spectrum antimicrobial therapy is administered and reviewed according to cultures results [75].

8. Nutritional support in liver transplant recipients

Post-LT nutritional support in ICU is an essential adjunct to transplant recovery. Malnutrition, which characterizes many patients with ESLD being evident at rates of up to 80%, deteriorates with the progression of liver failure, and affects the patients' outcome [80]. On the other hand, it is associated with prolonged ICU and hospital stay, infections, respiratory complications, graft impairment, and mortality. Sarcopenia, defined as severe muscle wasting, is also a determining factor of the outcome, and it can be easily diagnosed with bioelectrical impedance. Patients with cirrhosis often present carbohydrate, fat, and protein disorders, characterized by elevated levels of aromatic amino acids and methionine while lowering plasma levels of branched-chain amino acids are detected [81, 82]. The immediate postoperative energy demands are increased, especially in patients with a high MELD score [82]. Factors such as operational stress, release of catabolic hormones, administration of immunosuppressants, mainly corticosteroids, as well as ICU factors including mechanical ventilation and hemodialysis, contribute to increased metabolic needs. For the above reasons, the aim is to ensure adequate intake of protein and calories in addition to protein breakdown protection [81]. An increase in nonprotein calories, estimated at 25–35% kcal/kg per day, is recommended when indirect calorimetry is not available. It should always be in accordance with the metabolic and inflammatory status, and it should be reviewed in hemodynamically unstable patients [83]. Due to elevated protein catabolism, it is necessary to obtain 1.5–2 g/kg of protein. Enteral nutrition (EN) has the edge over the parenteral one, assisting in maintaining intestinal integrity, by supporting the diversity of the microbiome, and helping the immune and metabolic response. The rapid onset of EN even 12 h after LT is recommended by some authors. It has been reported to reduce viral infections and contribute to a better N_2 balance. If postoperative encephalopathy remains, the amount of protein intake is not reduced but the type of nutrition is altered by the addition of branched-chain amino acid (BCCA) enriched formulae, while the administration of immunonutrition remains under discussion. Frequent screening of electrolytes is required to prevent and correct disorders, while re-feeding syndrome is also considered a risk factor for these disorders [83].

9. Renal dysfunction

Renal impairment is a very common complication after LT. Its presence ranges from 19 to 64%. Even with the application of the RIFLE and AKIN criteria, the percentage reaches from 39 to 54% [84, 85]. In cases of living donors, acute kidney injury (AKI) has been estimated at around 23% [86]. AKI occurrence is complex and multifactorial in origin, depending on the existence of the preoperative hepatorenal syndrome as well as various intraoperative and postoperative factors. High MELD score, perioperative transfusions, hemodynamic instability, vasoactive agents, graft dysfunction, infections, and nephrotoxic agents are mainly accountable for renal function deterioration [87]. Systematic evaluation of renal function is required with close monitoring of urine output, fluid balance, and hemodynamic parameters [18]. The treatment is mainly supportive and includes: restoring CO with sufficient preload for optimization of renal perfusion, administering loop diuretics, and efforts to avoid nephrotoxic agents. Renal replacement therapy is recommended in cases of volume overload, electrolyte disturbances, and acidemia in an attempt to avoid pulmonary edema and hepatic congestion. Immunosuppressants, antibiotics, and contrast agents are commonplace nephrotoxic agents. The dosage of CNIs should be minimized or they should be converted into mTOR inhibitors combined with anti-proliferative agents. In ICU, CVVDHF is the renal replacement therapy of choice and favors the outcome of patients [88].

10. Primary graft dysfunction

Primary graft dysfunction (PGD) is a major complication after LT and is associated with prolonged hospital and ICU stay jeopardizing graft viability, being responsible for its high rejection rates as well as higher mortality and morbidity. It describes different degrees of graft impairment which begins intraoperatively, divided into early or initial poor function (IPF) and primary nonfunction (PNF) [89–91]. IPF represents the clinical phenotype of severe ischemia-reperfusion injury due to various donor and/or recipient-related factors. Expanding the criteria to marginal donors has increased the use of allografts with a higher likelihood of initial malfunction. It affects the survival of both graft and patient, whether the transplant comes from living or deceased donors. Dysfunction may be transient and possibly reversible with appropriate supportive treatment. There are no clear definitions, nevertheless, there are suggested scores, such as MEAF and LGrAFT, that could help in early detection and classification of early hepatic impairment [92, 93]. On the contrary, PNF is a catastrophic injury characterized by hepatic necrosis, aminotransferase elevation, coagulation disorders, lactate elevation, hemodynamic instability, persistent hypoglycemia, and respiratory and renal failure with an incidence ranging from 0.9 to 7%. The treatment is immediate re-transplantation. There are certain risk factors related to donors, recipients, intraoperative events, and allograft preservation [91] (**Table 2**).

11. Rejection

Acute cellular rejection (ACR), usually mediated by T-cells, has decreased in recent years with the use of improved potent immunosuppressants, but still ranges from 15 to 25% and usually occurs 7–14 days after surgery [94]. Hyperacute liver rejection is controversial, but undoubtedly early accelerated rejection occurs in the first 7 days and is associated with preformed antibodies. Risk factors include adequacy, type, and level of immunosuppression, underlying immune disease, biliary complications, certain transplant-related features such as donor-negative recipient-positive CMV mismatch, sex mismatch with a female donor. ACR is not significantly associated with long-term graft failure unless it concerns HCV-positive patients in which case it may result in corticosteroid-resistant rejection and graft loss. Early ACR is associated with better graft outcomes [95]. It is even hypothesized that such activation of the immune system may be beneficial and may induce a degree of tolerance. Manifestations of ACR include elevated levels of aminotransferase, alkaline phosphatase, bilirubin, and fever in later stages. Hepatic artery or portal vein thrombosis, biliary leak, CMV infection, and delayed graft function should be excluded. Diagnosis is finally confirmed by percutaneous liver biopsy prior to initiation of treatment, which depends on patient severity and current immunosuppression [94]. Cyclosporine is converted to tacrolimus or the sub-therapeutic levels of tacrolimus are increased and/or mycophenolate mofetil is added. In moderate to severe ACR, high doses of corticosteroids, usually methylprednizolone, are administered as a first-line medicine in a dose ranging from 500 to 1000 mg for 1–3 days depending on the center protocol [94].

12. Cardiac complications after LT

Cirrhotic cardiomyopathy (CCM) is defined as cardiac dysfunction in patients with cirrhosis characterized by a blunted contractile responsiveness to stress and/or diastolic dysfunction and electrophysiological abnormalities in the absence of known cardiac disease [96]. Diagnostic features include a reduced ejection fraction (EF), an E/A ratio < 1, and electrocardiographic abnormalities such as a prolonged QTc interval. Diagnostic approaches involve transthoracic ultrasound, dobutamine stress echocardiography (DSE), as well as cardiac magnetic resonance (CMR). The concept of "ventriculo-arterial coupling" (VAC) has recently been suggested as a means of assessing cardiac function in ESLD. The VAC (ratio of ventricular elastance to arterial elastance) is measured conventionally by ultrasound and has been correlated with prognosis. Moreover, cardiac biomarkers such as troponin and brain natriuretic peptide (BNP) are deemed early markers [97].

It is difficult to define the exact impact of CCM due to the fact that its clinical course is usually silent, especially in early stages, due to the profound vasodilatation in cirrhosis and offloading of the left ventricle. It only becomes apparent in conditions of stress and increased afterload. LT is a cause of significant cardiovascular stress since there are marked variations in preload and afterload, cardiac workload increases and the existing underlying cardiac dysfunction may become overt heart failure during LT or several days postoperatively. Complete recovery has been recorded at 6 months [98].

Cardiac dysfunction and pulmonary edema are encountered in almost half of the patients within a week after LT. They have been identified as the third most important cause of mortality during the first year following the surgery. High MELD score and AKI have been considered as risk factors. Early diagnosis can prevent acute onset or deterioration of heart failure. An empirical and supportive therapeutic approach is applied which includes optimization of volume status and cardiac monitoring via echo and/or PAC [99, 100].

Prevalence of coronary artery disease (CAD) in cirrhosis reaches 5–26% and has been associated with poor prognosis. It has been correlated with a number of cardiac adverse events: myocardial infraction, arrhythmias, and cardiac death. LT can be postponed in cases with known CAD for medical optimization and/or revascularization [99, 100].

13. Neurological complications

Neurological complications (NC) are still common after LT with a 15–30% incidence rate. In recipients from living donors, this percentage does not exceed 20% [101, 102]. Major neurologic complications immediately postoperatively include alterations of consciousness, seizures, hepatic encephalopathy, CNI neurotoxicity, cerebrovascular complications, central nervous system infections, and central pontine myelinolysis (CPM) [103]. They can delay recovery and make immunosuppression and patient management difficult. Rapid patient recovery requires daily evaluation of mental status and neurological assessment in the ICU.

Immunosuppression-related neurotoxicity can range from headaches and convulsions to posterior reversible encephalopathy (PRES). Immunosuppressants have the potential to reduce the seizure threshold that is enhanced by electrolytic disorders mainly hypomagnesaemia and hypophosphatemia. CNIs are mainly implicated while incidents of PRES have been reported even in treatment with sirolimus. The treatment is conservative involving reduction of dosage and/or interchange with CNI-sparing regimens. Neurotoxicity of corticosteroids can be manifested either in the form of convulsions or myopathy and behavioral disorders [103].

Post-transplant encephalopathy is responsible for 12% of NC. It relates closely to metabolic disorders, CNS infections and/or septic encephalopathy, cerebrovascular events, history of severe encephalopathy, and graft dysfunction [78]. Seizures are one of the most common postoperative neurological consequences and may be the effect of various factors, mainly drug toxicity and metabolic disorders. Correction of underlying causes and administration of anti-convulsive medicines are the appropriate treatment.

Central pontine myelinolysis (CPM) represents a serious complication, with a low incidence of approximately 1–3.5% that may affect the postoperative course of patients. It has been associated with large fluid shift and rapid correction of prolonged hyponatremia. The indicated treatment is supportive and requires careful correction of severe hyponatremia (serum Na <125 mEq/L), which is encountered in approximately 17% of patients with ESLD, using sodium chloride and adjusting Na serum values to 8–10 mEq/L per day [104, 105].

14. Ischemia reperfusion injury

Ischemia-reperfusion injury is related with the degree of transaminitis and primary and/or delayed graft dysfunction. Mitochondria are more prone to I/R injuries with subsequent alterations that can lead to dysfunction or even to necrosis of hepatocytes following LT. Alternatively, machine reperfusion has been proposed to preserve the donor organ. It promises to restore energy balance, extend preservation time while offering the ability to "test" the organ performance [106, 107].

15. Postoperative surgical complications

15.1 Early surgical complications

In the early postoperative period, according to Parikh et al., 79.3% of patients are present with at least one complication with 62.8% of the recipients suffering severe

Complications	Diagnosis-treatment	Therapeutic approach
Abdominal bleeding	Anastomosis site Graft surface Diffusion bleeding	Re-operation
Biliary Complications	Biloma, Hemobilia Bile leaks Anastomosis necrosis Anastomotic stricture	ERCP, PTC, MRCP EUS-guided approach HIDA Digital Cholagiography or Surgical re-intervention

Table 3.
Immediate surgical complications after LT.

Vascular complications	Diagnosis	Treatment
Hepatic artery thrombosis (HAT) 2.9%	DUS, CT Angiography	Emergent revascularization (endovascular or surgical) or re-LT
Hepatic artery stenosis (HAS) 1–2%	DUS, CT Angiography	Endovascular intervention or surgical HA revision
Hepatic artery rupture (HAR) 0.64%	Angiography None in emergency	Emergent surgical hemostasis and surgical repair
Portal vein thrombosis (PVT) 5%	DUS, CT (portal phase) Venography	Surgical revision Endovascular intervention or re-LT
Portal vein stenosis (PVS) 2%	DUS, CT (portal phase) Venography	Endovascular intervention

Table 4.
Vascular complications after LT.

complications. The incidence of those related to surgical techniques range from 5 to 10% and can be categorized into abdominal bleedings, vascular complications, and biliary complications. Treatment can be determined by the severity of each case and its spectrum includes simple surgical interventions, or even re-transplantation. The main complications are illustrated in **Tables 3** and **4** along with diagnostic and therapeutic approaches [108, 109].

16. Conclusions

LT has been established as the gold standard treatment for patients with ESLD and following successful postoperative course, organs previously affected return to normal functionality in due time. Postoperative ICU stay is often imperative, especially in cases of adverse events during operation, delayed cardiovascular resuscitation, utilization of marginal donors, and distant organ dysfunction. Early recognition, evaluation, and treatment of hemodynamic instability, distant organ complications, impaired graft functionality, and use of optimal immunosuppressive agents are of paramount importance.

Prompt recognition and treatment of life-threatening sequelae following LT in addition with optimal management of immunosuppression are keys to successful postoperative care and have led to improved overall survival although recipients are in relatively worse condition and the use of marginal donors is more widespread.

Furthermore, overall survival of LT patients has improved dramatically in recent years due to the formation of LT specific centers and medical teams, which follow each patient from admission to the donor list up to the operation itself as well as during their postoperative course. Therefore, according to the authors, the creation of LT specific ICUs that provide a postoperative continuation of excellency in managing the intricacies of those patients is paramount. Those units will not only provide prompt treatment in cases of a complication but will also act as additional reinforcement against postoperative infections.

Author details

Areti Karapanagiotou[1,2*], Achillefs Pitsoulis[2], Maria Vasileiou[2] and Nikolaos Voloudakis[3]

1 Intensive Care Unit "Hippokratio" Hospital, Thessaloniki, Greece

2 Intensive Care Unit "G. GENNHMATAS" Hospital, Thessaloniki, Greece

3 Second Surgical Department AUTH, Thessaloniki, Greece

*Address all correspondence to: aretikarapan@gmail.com

IntechOpen

© 2019 The Author(s). Licensee IntechOpen. This chapter is distributed under the terms of the Creative Commons Attribution License (http://creativecommons.org/licenses/by/3.0), which permits unrestricted use, distribution, and reproduction in any medium, provided the original work is properly cited.

References

[1] Zanripar A, Busutil R. Liver transplantation: past, present and future. Nature Reviews. Gastroenterology & Hepatology. 2013;**10**(7):434-440. DOI: 10.1038/nrgastro.2013.88

[2] Adam R, Karam V, et al. 2018 annual report of the European liver transplant registry (ELTR) – 50-year evolution of liver transplantation. Transplant International. 2018;**31**(12):1293-1317

[3] Neuberger J. Liver transplantation in the United Kingdom. Liver Transplantation. 2016;**22**:1129-1135

[4] deLemos AS, Vageti PA. Expanding the donor Pool in liver transplantation: Extended criteria donors. Clinics in Liver Disease. 2013;**2**(4):156-159

[5] Karapanagiotou A, Kydona C, et al. Impact of the model for end-stage-liver-disease (MELD) score in Creece. Transplantation Proceedings. 2014;**46**(9):2312-2315

[6] Asrani S, Kamash P. Model for end-stage liver disease score and MELD exceptions 15 years later. Hepatology International. 2015Jul;**9**(3):346-354

[7] Markin N, Ringenberg K, et al. 2018 clnical update in liver transplantation. Journal of Cardiothoracic and Vascular Anesthesia. 10 Feb 2019. pii: S1053-0770(19)30106-5. DOI: 10.1053/j.jvca.2019.02.004

[8] Kramer D, Siegal E, et al. Perioperative management of the liver transplant recipient. Critical Care Clinics. 2019;**35**:95-105

[9] Utako P, Emyoo T, et al. Clinical outcomes after liver transplantation for hepatorenal syndrome: A systematic review and meta-Analysis. BioMed Research International. 24 May 2018;**2018**:5362810. DOI: 10.1155/2018/5362810. eCollection 2018

[10] Hori T, Ogura Y, et al. Systemic hemodynamics in advanced cirrhosis: Concerns during perioperative period of liver transplantation. World Journal of Hepatology. 2016;**8**(25):1047-1060

[11] Al-Hamoudi W, Alqahtani S, et al. Hemodynamics in the immediate post-transplantation period in alcoholic and viral cirrhosis. World Journal of Gastroenterology. 2010;**16**(5):608-612

[12] Singh S, Nasa V, et al. Perioperative monitoring in liver transplant patients. Journal of Clinical and Experimental Hepatology. 2012;**2**:271-278

[13] Rudnick MR, DeMarchi L, et al. Hemodynamic monitoring during liver transplantation: A state of the art review. World Journal of Hepatology. 2015;**7**(10):1302-1311

[14] Feltracco P, Barbieri S, et al. Intensive care management of liver transplanted patients. World Journal of Hepatology. 2011;**3**(3):61-71

[15] Zarychansky R, Abou-Setta AM, et al. Association of hydroxyethyl starch administration with mortality and acute kidney injury in critically ill patients requiring volume resuscitation. A systematic review and meta-analysis. JAMA. 2013;**309**(7):678-688

[16] Arshed S, Pinsky M, et al. Applied physiology of fluid resuscitation in critical illness. Critical Care Clinics. 2018;**34**:267-277

[17] Mukhtar A, Masry EL, et al. The impact of maintaining normal serum albumin level following living related liver transplantation: Does serum albumin level affect the course? A pilot study. Transplantation Proceedings. 2007;**39**:3214-3218

[18] Sang BH, Bang JY, et al. Hypoalbuminemia within two postoperative days is an independent risk factor for acute kidney injury following living donor liver transplantation: A propensity score analysis of 998 consecutive patients. Critical Care Medicine. 2015;**43**(12):2552-2561

[19] Amouzanden M, Nowak G, et al. Albumin mass balance and kinetics in liver transplantation. Critical Care. 2018;**22**:152-162

[20] Clevenger B, Mallett S, et al. Transfusion and coagulation management in liver transplantation. World Journal of Gastroenterology. 2014;**20**(20):6146-6158

[21] Zamper R, Amorim T, et al. Association between viscoelastic tests guided therapy with synthetic factor concentrates and allogenic blood transfusion in liver transplantation: A before-after study. BMC Anesthesiology. 2018;**18**:198

[22] Lisman T, Potre R. Rebalanced hemostasis in patients with liver disease: Evidence and clinical consequences. Blood. 2010;**116**(6):878-885

[23] Cywinski J, Alster J, et al. Prediction of intraoperative transfusion requirements during orthotopic liver transplantation and the influence on postoperative patient survival. Anesthesia and Analgesia. 2014;**118**:428-437

[24] Dunn LK, Thiete RH, et al. Duration of red blood cell storage and outcomes following Orthotopic liver transplantation. Liver Transplantation. 2012;**18**:475-481

[25] Keegan M, Cramer D, et al. Perioperative care of the liver transplant patient. Critical Care Clinics. 2016;**32**:453-473

[26] Carrier FM, Chasse M, et al. Effects of perioperative fluid management on postoperative outcomes in liver transplantation: A systematic review protocol. Critical Care. 2018;**7**:180-186

[27] Codes L, De Souza YG, et al. Cumulative positive fluid balance is a risk factor for acute kidney injury and requirement for renal replacement therapy after liver transplantation. World Journal of Transplantation. 2018;**8**(2):44-51

[28] Jin J, Lu D, et al. Clinical and economic impact of goal directed fluid therapy during elective gastrointestinal surgery. Perioperative Medicine. 2018;**7**:22-30

[29] Reydelle L, Blasco V, et al. Impact of goal-directed therapy protocol on postoperative fluid balance in patients undergoing liver transplantation; a retrospective study. Annales Françaises d'Anesthésie et de Réanimation. 2014;**33**:e47-e54

[30] Jiang GQ, Chen P, et al. Individualized peri-operative fluid therapy facilitating early phase recovery after liver transplantation. World Journal of Gastroenterology. 2012;**18**(16):1981-1986

[31] Wagener G, Gubitosa G, et al. Vasopressin decreases portal vein pressure and flow in the native liver during liver transplantation. Liver Transplantation. 2008;**14**:1664-1670

[32] Mukhtar A, Dabbous H, et al. Modulation of splanchnic circulation: Role in perioperative management of liver transplant patients. World Journal of Gastroenterology. 2016;**22**(4):1582-1592

[33] Hori T, Yamamoto C, Yagi S, et al. Assessment of cardiac output in liver transplantation recipients. Hepatobiliary & Pancreatic Diseases International. 2008;**7**:362-366

[34] Kumar A, Anel R, Bunnell E, et al. Pulmonary artery occlusion pressure

and central venous pressure fail to predict ventricular filling volume, cardiac performance, or the response to volume infusion in normal subjects. Critical Care Medicine. 2004;**32**:691-697

[35] Feltracco P, Biancofiore G, et al. Limits and pitfalls of haemodynamic monitoring systems in liver transplantation surgery. Minerva Anestesiologica. 2012;**78**:1372-1384

[36] Krenn CG, De Wolf AM. Current approach to intraoperative monitoring in liver transplantation. Current Opinion in Organ Transplantation. 2008;**13**:285-290

[37] Samgkum L, Liu G, et al. Minimally invasive or noninvasive cardiac output measurement: An update. Journal of Anesthesia. 2016;**30**(3):461-480. DOI: 10.1007/s00540-016-2154-9

[38] DellaRocca G, Costa MG, et al. Preload and haemodynamic assessment during liver transplantation: A comparison between the pulmonary artery catheter and transpulmonary indicator dilution techniques. European Journal of Anaesthesiology. 2002;**19**:868-887

[39] Monnnet X, Teboul JL. Transpulmonary thermodilution: Advantages and limits. Critical Care. 2017;**21**(1):147

[40] Teboul JL, Saugel B, et al. Less invasive hemodynamic monitoring in critically ill patients. Intensive Care Medicine. 2016;**42**:1350-1359

[41] Su BC, Tsai YF, et al. Stroke volume variation derived by arterial pulse contour analysis is a good indicator for preload estimation during liver transplantation. Transplantation Proceedings. 2012;**44**:429-432

[42] Kim SH, Hwang GS, et al. Is stroke volume variation a useful preload index in liver transplant recipients? A retrospective analysis. International Journal of Medical Sciences. 2013;**10**:751-757

[43] Biancofiore G, Critchley LA, et al. Evaluation of an uncalibrated arterial pulse contour cardiac output monitoring system in cirrhotic patients undergoing liver surgery. British Journal of Anaesthesia. 2009;**102**:47-54

[44] Krejci V, Vannucci A, et al. Comparison of calibrated and uncalibrated arterial pressure-based cardiac output monitors during orthotopic liver transplantation. Liver Transplantation. 2010;**16**:773-782

[45] Biais M, Nouette-Gaulain K, et al. Cardiac output measurement in patients undergoing liver transplantation: Pulmonary artery catheter versus uncalibrated arterial pressure waveform. Anesthesia & Analgesia. 2008;**106**:1480-1486

[46] Camporota L, Beale R. Pitfalls in haemodynamic monitoring based on the arterial pressure waveform. Critical Care. 2010;**14**:124

[47] Dalia A, Flores A, et al. A comprehensive review of transesophageal echocardiography during orthotopic liver transplantation. Journal of Cardiothoracic and Vascular Anesthesia. 2018;**32**:1815-1824

[48] Sakka SG. Assessing liver function. Current Opinion in Critical Care. 2007;**13**:207-214

[49] Fedovarious A, Charlton M. Abnormal liver tests after liver transplantation. Clinics in Liver Disease. 2016;**7**(4):73-79

[50] Sun Y, Yu L, et al. Predictive value of indocyanine green plasma disappearance rate on liver function and complications after liver transplantation. Medical Science Monitor. 2018;**24**:3661-3669

[51] Ren J, Zheng BW, et al. Application of contrast-enhanced ultrasound after liver transplantation: Current status and perspectives. World Journal of Gastroenterology. 2016;**22**(4):1607-1616

[52] Roullet S, Defaye M, et al. Liver transplantation with old grafts: A ten-year experience. Transplantation Proceedings. 2017;**49**:e2135-e2143

[53] Lué A, Solanas E, et al. How important is donor age in liver transplantation? World Journal of Gastroenterology. 2016;**22**(21):4966-4976

[54] Alamo JM, Olivares C, et al. Donor characteristics that are associated with survival in liver transplant recipients older than 70 years with grafts. Transplantation Proceedings. 2013;**45**(10):3633-3636

[55] Gilbo N, Jochmans I, et al. Age matching of elderly liver grafts with elderly recipients does not have a synergistic effect on long-term outcomes when both are carefully selected. Transplantation direct. 2019;**5**:e342

[56] Boecker J, Czigany Z, et al. Potential value and limitations of different clinical scoring systems in the assessment of short- and long-term outcome following orthotopic liver transplantation. PLoS One. 2019;**14**(3):e0214221

[57] Mandell MS, Stoner TJ, et al. A multicentre evaluation of safety of early extubation in liver transplant recipients. Liver Transplantation. 2007;**13**:1557-1563

[58] Rao JH, Zhang F, et al. Effects of multimodal fast-track surgery on liver transplantation outcomes. Hepatobiliary & Pancreatic Diseases International. 2017;**16**:364-369

[59] Li J, Wang C, et al. Immediate versus conventional postoperative tracheal extubation for enhanced recovery after liver transplantation IPTE versus CTE for enhanced recovery after liver transplantation. Medicine. 2018;**97**:45-55

[60] Taner CB, Willingham DL, et al. Is a mandatory intensive care unit stay needed after liver transplantation? Feasibility of fast-tracking to the surgical ward after liver transplantation. Liver Transplantation. 2012;**18**:361-369

[61] Razonable R, Findlay J, et al. Critical care issues in patients after liver transplantation. Liver Transplantation. 2012;**17**:511-527

[62] Yuan H, Tuutte-Newhall J, et al. Prognostic impact of mechanical ventilation after liver transplantation: A national database study. American Journal of Surgery. 2014;**208**(4):582-590

[63] Lui J, Spaho L, et al. Intensive care of pulmonary complications following liver transplantation. Journal of Intensive Care Medicine. Nov 2018;**33**(11):595-608

[64] Tobin MJ, Jubran A. Weaning from mechanical ventilation. In: Tobin MJ, editor. Principles and Practice of Mechanical Ventilation. 3rd ed. Chapter 58. The McGraw-Hill Companies, Inc.; 2013. pp. 1307-1351. ISBN: 978-0-07-173626-8

[65] Wu X, Zheng R, et al. Effect of transpulmonary pressure-guided positive end-expiratory pressure titration on lung injury in pigs with acute respiratory distress syndrome. Journal of Clinical Monitoring and Computing. 2019. DOI: 10.1007/s10877-019-00267-2

[66] Saner F, Steven O, et al. How far can we go with positive end-expiratory pressure (PEEP) in liver transplant patients? Journal of Clinical Anesthesia. 2010;**22**:104-109

[67] Jaber S, Lescot T, et al. Effect of noninvasive ventilation on tracheal

re-intubation among patients with hypoxemic respiratory failure following abdominal surgery: A randomized clinical trial. JAMA. 2016;**315**:1345-1353

[68] Lee KW, Cho CW, et al. Extracorporeal membrane oxygenation support for refractory septic shock in liver transplantation recipients. Annals of Surgical Treatment and Research. 2017;**93**(3):152-158

[69] Combes A, Pesenti A, et al. Is extracorporeal circulation the future of acute respiratory distress syndrome management? American Journal of Respiratory and Critical Care Medicine. 2017;**195**(9):1161-1170

[70] Cosarderelioglou C, Cosar AM, et al. Hepatopulmonary syndrome and liver transplantation: A recent review of the literature. Journal of Clinical and Translational Hepatology. 2016;**4**:47-53

[71] Aldenkortt F, Aldenkortt M, et al. Portopulmonary hypertension and hepatopulmonary syndrome. World Journal of Gastroenterology. 2014;**20**(25):8072-8081

[72] Jadiowiec C, Taner T. Liver transplantation: Current status and challenges. World Journal of Gastroenterology. 2016;**22**(18):4438-4445

[73] Pillai AA, Levitsky J. Overview of immunosuppression in liver transplantation. World Journal of Gastroenterology. 2009;**15**:4225-4231

[74] Baganate F, Beal E, et al. Early mortality after liver transplantation: Defining the course and the cause. Surgery. 2018;**116**:58-69

[75] Clark NM, Scott JC, et al. Infectious complications in liver transplantation UpToDate. Available from: http://www.uptodate.com/contents/infectious-complications in- liver-transplantation [Accessed: 01-October-2018]

[76] Karapanagiotou A, Cydona C, et al. Infections after orthotopic liver transplantation in the intensive care unit. Transplantation Proceedings. 2012;**44**:2748-2750

[77] Weiss E, Dahmani S. Early-onset pneumonia after liver transplantation: Microbiological findings and therapeutic consequences. Liver Transplantation. 2010;**16**:1178-1185

[78] Fernandez T, Gardiner P. Critical care of the liver transplant recipient. Current Anesthesiology Reports. 2015;**5**:419-428. DOI: 10.1007/s40140-015-0133-6

[79] Siddique O, Siddique A, et al. Effects of infection on post-transplant outcomes: Living versus deceased donor liver transplants. Journal of Clinical Experimental Hepatology. 2018;**4**(1):28-34

[80] Anastácio LR, Correia MI. Nutrition therapy: Integral part of liver transplant care. World Journal of Gastroenterology. 2016;**22**(4):1513-1522

[81] Arabi YM, Casaer MP, et al. The intensive care medicine research agenda in nutrition and metabolism. Intensive Care Medicine. 2017;**43**:1239-1256

[82] Fereira LG, Anastacio LR, et al. Assessment of nutritional status of patients waiting for liver transplantation. Clinical Transplantation. 2011;**25**:248-254

[83] Kaido T, Ogura Y. Effects of post-transplant enteral nutrition with an immunomodulating diet containing hydrolyzed whey peptide after liver transplantation. World Journal of Surgery. 2012;**36**:1666-1671

[84] Karapanagiotou A, Cydona C, et al. Acute kidney injury after orthotopic liver transplantation. Transplantation Proceedings. 2012;**44**:2727-2729

[85] Karapanagiotou A, Dimidriadis C, et al. Comparison of RIFLE and AKIN criteria in the evaluation of the frequency of acute kidney injury in post-liver transplantation patients. Transplantation Proceedings. 2014;**46**:3222-3227

[86] Hilmi I, Damian D, et al. Acute kidney injury after orthotopic liver transplantation using live donor versus cadaveric donor grafts: A propensity score-matched analysis. Liver Transplantation. 2015;**21**(9):1179-1185

[87] de Haan JE, Hoorn EJ, de Geus HRH. Acute kidney injury after liver transplantation: Recent insights and future perspectives. Best Practice & Research. Clinical Gastroenterology. 2017;**31**:161-169

[88] Papadopoulos S, Karapanagiotou A, et al. Causes and incidence of renal replacement therapy application in orthotopic liver transplantation patients: Our experience. Transplantation Proceedings. 2014;**46**:3228-3231

[89] Chen XB, Xu MQ. Primary graft dysfunction after liver transplantation. Hepatobiliary & Pancreatic Diseases International. 2014;**13**:125-137

[90] Neves DB, Rusi MB, et al. Primary graft dysfunction of the liver: Definitions, diagnostic criteria and risk factors. Einstein. 2016;**14**(4):567-572

[91] Xie Q, Zheng S. Risk factors for primary non-function after liver transplantation. HPB. 2018;**20**(2):S789-S790

[92] Pareja E, Cortes M, et al. A score model for the continuous grading of early allograft dysfunction severity. Liver Transplantation. 2015;**21**:38-46

[93] Agopian VG, Halander-Locke MP, et al. Evaluation of early allograft function using the liver graft assessment following transplantation risk score model. JAMA Surgery. 2018;**153**(5):436-444

[94] Dogan N, Husing-Kabar A, et al. Acute allograft rejection in liver transplant recipients: Incidence, risk factors, treatment success, and impact on graft failure. The Journal of International Medical Research. 2018;**46**(9):3979-3990

[95] Shindoh J, Akamatsu N, et al. Risk factors for acute liver allograft rejection and their influences on treatment outcomes of rescue therapy in living donor liver transplantation. Clinical Transplantation. 2016;**30**:880-896

[96] Liu H, Jayakumar S, et al. Cirrhotic cardiomyopathy: Implications for Liver Transplantation. Liver Transplantation. 2017;**23**:826-835 ASLD

[97] Shin WJ, Song JG, Jun IG, et al. Effect of ventriculo-arterial coupling on transplant outcomes in cirrhotics: Analysis of pressure-volume curve relations. Journal of Hepatology. 2017;**66**:328-337

[98] Carvalho MVH, Kroll PC, et al. Cirrhotic cardiomyopathy: The liver affects the heart Braz. Journal of Medical and Biological Research. 2019;**52**(2):e7809

[99] Kwon HM, Hwang GS, et al. Cardiovascular dysfunction and liver transplantation. Korean Journal of Anesthesiology. 2018;**71**:85-91

[100] Nicolau-Raducu R, Gitman M, et al. Adverse cardiac events after orthotopic liver transplantation: A cross-sectional study in 389 consecutive patients. Liver Transplantation. 2015;**21**:13-21

[101] Živković SA. Neurologic complications after liver transplantation. World Journal of Hepatology. 2013;**5**(8):409-416

[102] Saner FH, Gensicke J, et al. Neurologic complications in adult living donor liver transplant patients: An underestimated factor. Journal of Neurology. 2010;**257**:253-258

[103] Li C, Jin H, et al. Clinical analysis of neurological complications following liver transplantation. Biomedical Research. 2017;**28**(6):2471-2474

[104] Lening C, Agorian V, et al. Incidence, etiology, and outcomes of altered mental status in the perioperative setting of liver transplantation. The Neurohospitalist. 2018;**8**(3):124-128

[105] Karapanagiotou A, Kydona C, et al. The effect of hyponatremia on the outcome of patients after orthotopic liver transplantation. Transplantation Proceedings. 2012;**44**:2724-2726

[106] Cerera C, Narsalla D, et al. Normothermic machine preservation of the liver: State of the Art. Current Transplantation Reports. 2018;**5**:104-110

[107] Watson C, Jochmans I. From "gut feeling" to objectivity: Machine preservation of the liver as a tool to assess organ viability. Current Transplantation Reports. 2018;**5**:72-81

[108] Tan-Tam C, Segedi M, et al. Surgical complications of liver transplantation. AME Medical Journal. 2018;**3**:107-114

[109] Meek J, McDougal J, et al. Use of a mechanical thrombectomy device to treat early hepatic artery thrombosis after orthotopic liver transplant. Radiology Case Reports. 2018;**13**:522-526

Section 3

The Future of Hepatic Surgery

Chapter 11

Robotic Liver Surgery

Ricky Harminder Bhogal, Stephanos Pericleous and Aamir Z. Khan

Abstract

Robotic liver surgery is an evolving specialty within liver surgery. The robotic platform allows some of the limitations in both open and laparoscopic surgery to be overcome. Indeed as the technology develops there is scope for the number of robotic liver resections to increase as well as their complexity. In this chapter we discuss the current robotic platform, review the current role of robotics in liver surgery and review the available data in the literature on patient outcome.

Keywords: robotic surgery, liver surgery, liver metastasis, minimally invasive surgery, liver resection

1. Introduction

For many patients with liver tumours, whether benign or malignant, the optimal form of management is liver surgery. In the modern era with advancement anaesthetic techniques, improved understanding of liver pathophysiology and peri-operative patient management liver surgery has become a safe operation with excellent patient outcomes. Concomitant with this advancement in patient care has been a greater understanding of the nature of liver surgery and improving the precision of liver surgery. In particular surgery has followed the trend in other surgical disciplines and moved towards minimal access surgery. Building on the experiences of laparoscopic liver surgery hepatobiliary surgeons have begun to develop robotic liver surgical programs. Many institutes worldwide have performed complex liver procedures using robot-assisted surgery. This chapter summarises the nascent of field of robotic liver surgery and provides an overview of the current robot technology, surgical techniques and patient outcomes.

2. Liver anatomy

The liver is an accessory digestive gland located in the right upper quadrant of the abdomen. The liver's primary function is to produce bile that aids in the emulsification and digestion of dietary fat. The liver also serves many other critical functions including metabolism of drugs and toxins, removing degradation products of normal body metabolism and synthesis of many important proteins (e.g. clotting factors) and enzymes.

The liver is anatomically divided into two major lobes or into eight segments. Cantile line, which runs from the inferior vena cava (IVC) to the gallbladder fossa, marks the division between the left and right hemi-livers. Each hemi-liver can be divided further anatomically; the left liver can be divided into a left lateral section

IntechOpen

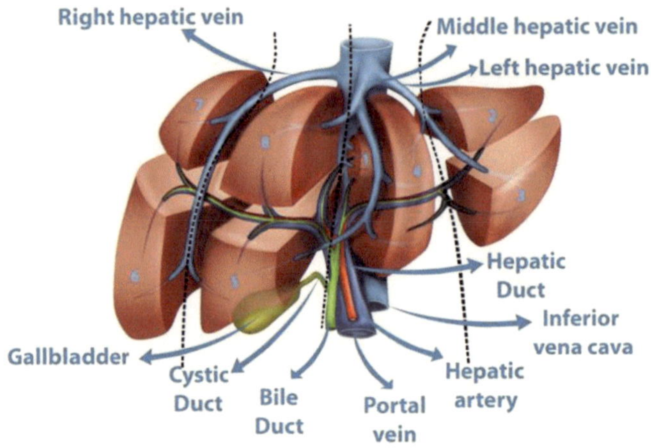

Figure 1.
The segmental anatomy of the liver. The liver derives its blood supply from the hepatic artery and portal vein. Both divide these structures divide into a left and right vessel to supply the respective side of the liver. The hepatic artery and portal veins divide into segmental branches to supply each of the segments within the liver. Correspondingly each segment has its own biliary duct and venous drainage. Importantly segment 1/caudate lobe is a specialised lobe of the liver and receives blood supply from both the left and right hepatic arteries with biliary drainage to both the left and right biliary ducts. Hence the left liver is made up of the segments 2, 3 and 4 and the right liver of segments 5, 6, 7 and 8.

(segments 2 and 3) and a left medial section or segment 4. The right hemi-liver can be divided into the right anterior section (segment 5 and 8) and right posterior section (segment 6 and 7). This segmental liver anatomy was originally described by Couinaud and is based upon the eight major divisions of the hepatic artery, portal vein and the biliary system (**Figure 1**). Segment 1 or caudate lobe is a unique liver lobe and is discussed below. Each Couinaud segment has its own arterial and portal blood supply, venous outflow and biliary drainage.

Blood enters the liver from two separate sources. Twenty percent of total liver blood flow is derived from the hepatic artery that is a branch of the coeliac artery. The remaining 80% is derived from the portal vein that is formed by the union of the Superior Mesenteric Vein and Splenic Vein behind the head of the pancreas. This venous blood brings nutrients and oxygen to liver parenchymal cells (e.g. hepatocytes, sinusoidal endothelial cells and cholangiocytes). Venous outflow of the liver is via the hepatic veins, which drain directly into the IVC and then the heart. This basic structure of the liver is integral to the planning of and performance of liver surgery.

3. Types of liver surgery and indications

3.1 Liver surgical procedures

There are important surgical principles and prerequisites that are mandatory when planning any liver operation. These are relevant for open, laparoscopic and robotic surgery. Most surgical procedures performed upon the liver involve the removal or resection of defined portion(s) of the liver. At the end of liver surgery there must be an adequate volume of liver of suitable quality left in-situ—termed future liver remnant (FLR)—that is generally considered to be 30% of original liver volume. In addition the FLR must have arterial and portal inflow, venous outflow and biliary drainage.

The different types of hepatectomies are illustrated in **Figure 2**. As discussed above as each segment of the liver has its own arterial and venous blood supply, biliary drainage and venous outflow, a single segment of the liver can be resected without significant risk to the patient (see below). Specifically resections that follow defined anatomical planes are referred to as anatomical resections (e.g. left hepatectomy or segment 7 resection) and those crossing anatomical planes are referred to as non-anatomical resections (NARs).

These liver procedures have traditionally been performed as open surgical operations but during the late 1990s there was a drive to perform these operations via minimally invasive techniques such a laparoscopic surgery and more recently via robotic-assisted surgery. These surgical approaches are discussed is more detail below.

3.2 Indications for liver surgery

Most liver operations are performed for the management of both benign and malignant hepatic tumours. **Table 1** demonstrates the frequency of these liver operations.

The vast majority of liver operations performed for metastatic liver disease are for colorectal liver metastasis, approximately 80% of all liver operations are performed for liver cancer. Other metastatic diseases considered for liver resection include neuroendocrine tumours and sarcoma. The most common primary malignant tumour of the liver is the hepatocellular carcinoma (HCC) and in patients with preserved liver function, hepatectomy can be considered. Importantly in patients were the liver is damaged or cirrhotic, liver surgery cannot be undertaken, as the liver will not regenerate. Cholangiocarcinoma is the other common primary liver tumour and in cases where there is no metastatic/extrahepatic disease hepatectomy as listed in **Figure 2** can be considered. Benign tumours include hepatocellular adenoma, hepatic haemangioma and focal nodular hyperplasia can be considered for liver resection in selected patients particularly if symptomatic. Hepatectomy may also be the procedure of choice to treat intrahepatic gallstones or parasitic

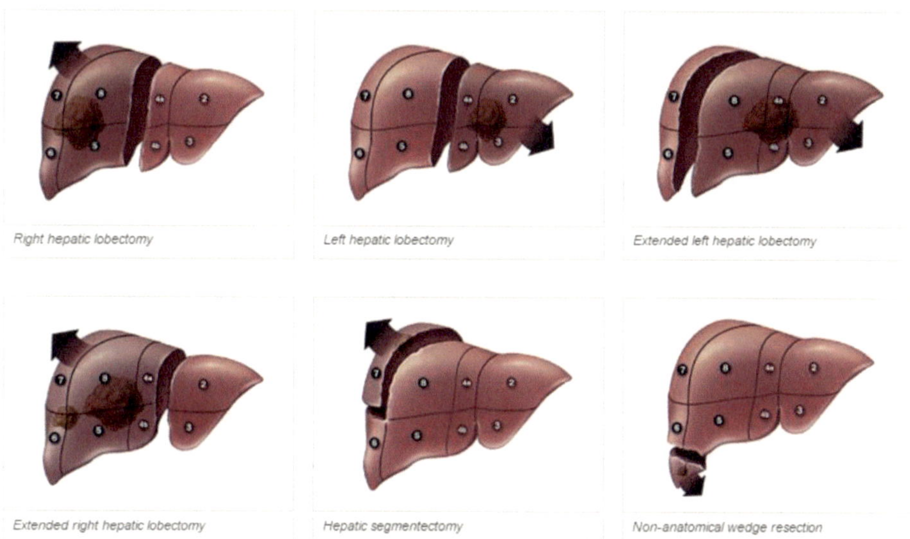

Figure 2.
The different types of hepatectomy. Liver resections are classified based upon the segments of the liver that are resected. A right hepatectomy/lobectomy is surgical resection of segments 5, 6, 7 and 8 whereas a left hepatectomy/lobectomy constitutes resection of segments 2, 3, 4. An extended left hepatectomy involves the further resection of segments 5 and 8. Combining a resection of segment 4 with a right hepatectomy is a classified as an extended right hepatectomy. Resection of a named segment is termed a segmentectomy and two contiguous segments a bi-segmentectomy. Resections crossing anatomical planes irrelevant of size are classified as non-anatomical resections.

Indication for liver surgery	Frequency (%)
Metastatic disease	51–55
Primary liver malignancy	14–16
Benign liver malignancy	8–11
Biliary tract malignancy	3–5
Benign liver disease	2–4
Benign biliary disease	1–4
Trauma	4–8
Other	3–6

Table 1.
Indications for liver resections.

cysts of the liver. Some of these pathologies such as HCC are also indications for liver transplantation but these indications and surgical techniques are outside the scope of this chapter. In the modern era liver surgery is safe when performed by experienced surgeons with appropriate technological and institutional support. As with most major surgical procedures, there is a tendency towards improved patient outcomes in high volume centres. Apart from liver surgery for trauma or HCC in cirrhotic patients where the mortality is high [1], the overall operative mortality for liver resections is now reported in the worldwide between 0 and 2% [2, 3]. This is a great advance in comparison to the mortality in liver surgery in early reports, which reached a mortality rate as high as 20% [4].

4. Evolution of robotic liver surgery

The German surgeon Carl Johann August Langenbuch was the first surgeon to perform a successful hepatic resection in 1888 [5]. The field of liver surgery did not advance significantly until the 1950s at which time liver surgery remained associated with high patient mortality with ill-defined surgical indications [6, 7] In 1952 Lortat Jacob published his surgical techniques of anatomical liver resection [8] whilst in 1956, Claude Couinaud [9, 10] published his seminal work on the segmental anatomy of the liver which forms the basis of modern liver surgery. The application of these findings was restricted due to the persisting high-risk nature of liver surgery and the inadequate nature of liver imaging. However the advent of intraoperative ultrasound (IOUS) in the early 1980s [11] allowed for the identification of smaller liver lesions that can be resected leading to the rapid expansion of open liver surgery [12]. The technique of IOUS allowed the surgeon to understand liver vasculature and biliary duct anatomy improving the precision and safety of surgery. Within the next decade the first reports of laparoscopic liver wedge resection were published [13] which was followed by laparoscopic major hepatectomy in the mid 1990s [14]. The Second International Consensus Conference in 2014 recommended that laparoscopic resection to be standard of practice for selected anterolateral minor liver resections [15]. This entailed that lesions in segments 2, 3, 4b, 5 and 6 should be considered for laparoscopic liver resection.

There is a common misconception that robotic liver surgery evolved from laparoscopic liver surgery but robotic surgery has developed in tandem with the former. Computer Motion Inc. and Intuitive Surgical Inc. independently developed robotic surgical systems in the 1990s. In 1999, Intuitive Surgical released the da Vinci robot in Europe. The da Vinci robot is made up of three components (**Figure 3**):

a surgeon console, a 4-armed patient cart that is docked against the operating table, and a vision cart. The robot as a high-definition 3-dimensional viewer, a footswitch that conveniently allows the surgeon to seamlessly move between the camera, retractors, and instrument control, and the Endowrist instruments. Importantly the Endowrist instruments are articulated in a manner that allows a greater degree of motion that the human wrist [16] (see below). In 2003, Intuitive Surgical and Computer Motion merged and during this time the first reports of robotic liver resections were published. Marescaux *et al*. reported the first transatlantic robot-assisted telesurgery in 2001, where a robotic cholecystectomy was performed by surgeons in New York, USA, and the patient in Strasbourg, France [17]. The second generation da Vinci S was released in 2006, and in 2014, the fourth generation da Vinci Xi robot was approved by the FDA, with a redesigned surgical arm cart, smaller, longer arms, and new camera system to allow more flexibility in cart position and port placement (**Figure 3**) [18].

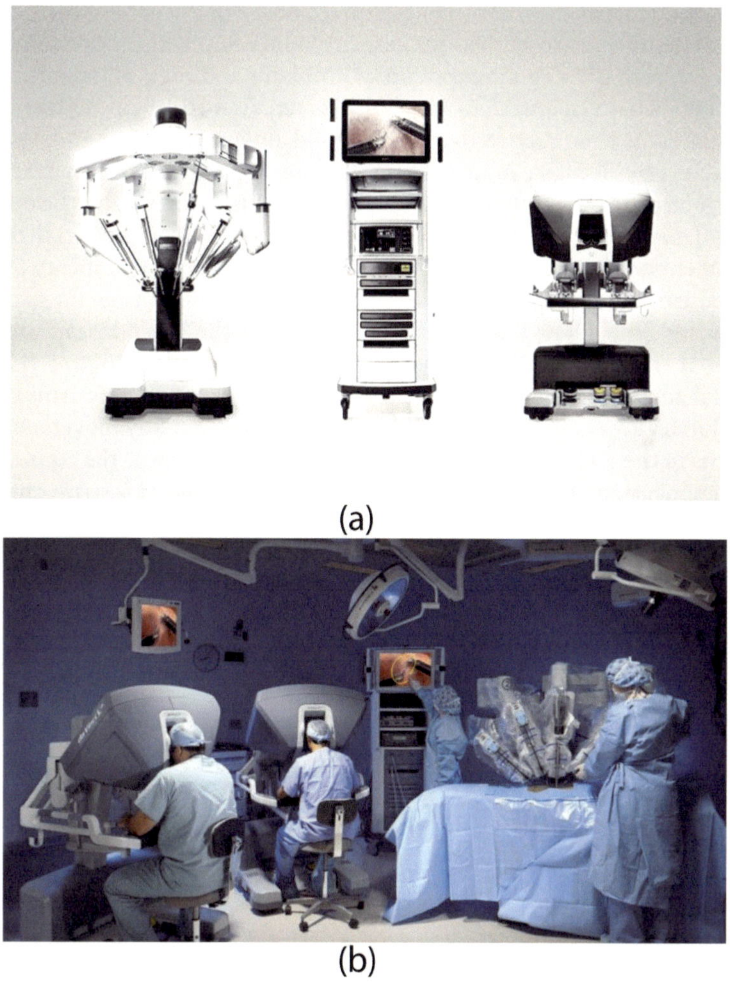

Figure 3.
The Da Vinci xi system. (a) Illustrates the current 4th generation da Vinci xi® robotic system. The system consists of three separate components; the patient cart, vision cart and surgeon cart (left to right). (b) Demonstrates the set-up of the robotic system in an operating theatre. Operating surgeons can sit unscrubbed at the surgeon console away from the operating table where the sterile patient cart is docked to the patient. The vision cart allows the other theatre staff to view the surgical field and allow the use of ancillary functions such as visual annotation and video recording.

5. The robotic assisted surgery components

As discussed above a surgical robot consists of three separate components all of which are integral to the safe execution of robotic liver surgery. A summary of each component is given below using the da Vinci Xi® system as an example.

5.1 Surgeon console

The surgeon console is the component of the robotic system where the operating surgeon sits and performs liver surgery. It is sometimes also termed the workstation. The surgeon console is located outside the immediate surgical field (**Figure 3**) and with the newer robotic systems there are dual surgeon consoles that also allow training robotic surgeons to be assisted and mentored during their learning curve. Before commencing surgery the operator is able to adjust the physical parameters of the console to ensure appropriate ergonomics. The operator is afforded a three dimensional view of the surgical field using the viewer (**Figure 4A**). The screen also provides details of the instruments that are in use in the patient cart, the type of energy systems that are applied to these instruments and also provide real-time alerts to the operator to pre-empt potential problems and suggest troubleshooting options. There is also an option to adjust the screen view to accommodate several images at the same time such as the surgical field alongside two other displays accommodated by auxiliary inputs. This setup ensures that the manoeuvres made by the surgeon are safer, more precise and steadier. Instruments and the endoscope are manipulated and manoeuvred using the finger controls that replicate tremor free movements within the abdomen (**Figure 4B**). The surgeon is able to control two robotic arms/instruments simultaneous. At base of the console the surgeon has various controls that allow the operator to manoeuvre the 3D endoscope with the camera pedal and the EndoWrist® instruments during surgery (**Figure 4C**). The toggle pedal allows the operator to switch between different robotic arms whilst the foot-clutch allows the finger controls to be reset without any movement of the instruments in the abdomen. There are also pedals at the base of the console that allow the application of electrocautery through desired robotic instruments. Using

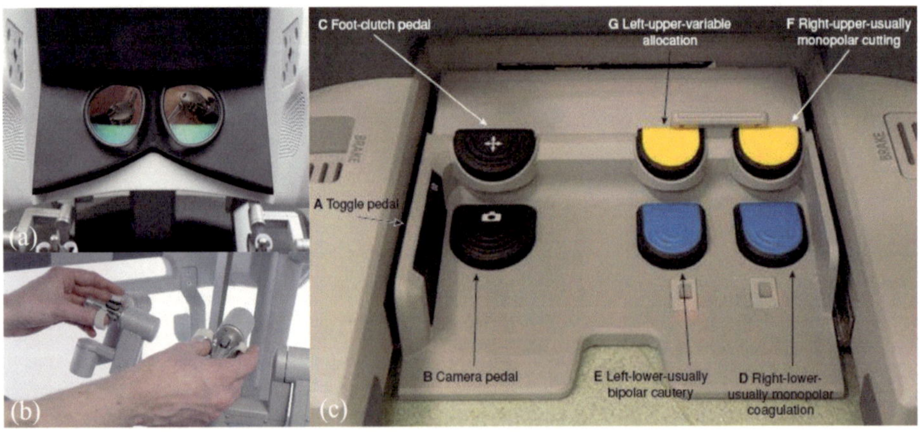

Figure 4.
The surgeon console. (a) The 3D viewer at the top of the surgeon console allow the operator to obtain an optimal view of the surgical field whilst being provided with contemporaneous information on instruments and energy devices. (b) Finger switches allow the operator to control the 3D endoscope, robotic instruments and allow advanced surgical manoeuvres such a suturing. (c) The base of the console allow the operator to control the endoscope in conjunction with the finger switches, switch between robotic instruments using the toggle pedal and allow electrocautery through the robotic instruments (both monopolar and bipolar).

the surgeon console the operator is able to simultaneously control the endoscope, instruments and energy application.

5.2 Patient cart

The patient cart is the component of the robotic system that is in direct contact with the patient and hence is required to be sterile draped prior to surgery. The patient cart consists of 4 robotic arms and makes up the surgical component of the robotic system. The patient cart has a display panel that allow for selection for the type of surgery to be undertaken (e.g. upper abdominal and pelvic) and needs to be selected prior to surgery. Once robotic ports have been inserted in an satisfactory manner (see below) the patient cart is manoeuvred into position using the handles (**Figure 5A**) and by utilising a spot laser in the helm of the cart the appropriate arm intended for the endoscope is positioned under the laser. This improves the position of the four robotic arms. A second assisting surgeon is stationed at the patient-side cart, in order to aid in the replacement of the robotic instruments and utilising assistant ports.

The 4 robot arms are latched deriving from a remote centre and fixed in space. This connection allows the surgical instruments and the endoscope to move freely reducing the force exerted on the patient's body to a minimum. Once the endoscope is engaged further instruments can be inserted in through other robotic ports after completion of docking (see below) and engaged in the remaining three robotic arms. Each robot arm has a port clutch at the base that allows docking of the robot port and for the instrument to swivel in a circular fashion and an instrument clutch at the base the allows the instrument to in and out of the abdomen to the desired length (**Figure 5B**). Pressing buttons on the instrument and replacing them with the desired instrument accomplish instrument changes—the robotic system allows the new instrument to be moved to within 3 mm of the position of the original instrument.

5.3 Vision cart

The visual cart is the final component of the robotic system (**Figure 3**). It contains an image-processing unit and a 24-inch touch screen monitor that allows live annotation of the screen and also allows other theatre staff to observe surgery.

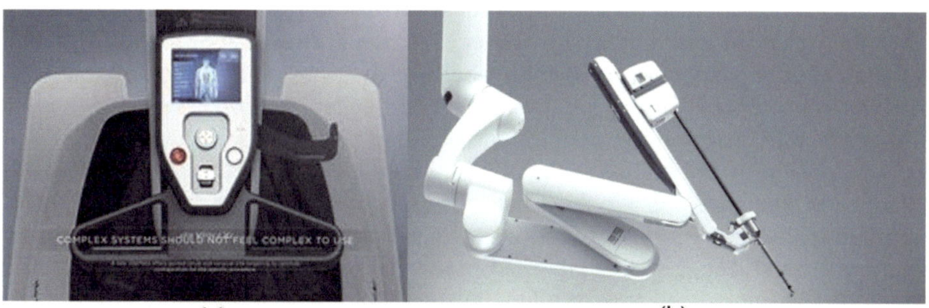

(a) (b)

Figure 5.
The patient cart. (a) The visual pad on the patient cart that allows operator to set the type of surgery to be performed and the handles that allows the patient cart to be moved around theatre. (b) A robotic arm with an instrument in place. The port and instrument clutches can be utilised to move the instrument into the correct position. Setting set-up it must be ensured that the robotic arms are in the correct alignment to avoid unnecessary collisions and clashes between arms.

The cart also contains an electrosurgical unit, the light source for the 3D endoscope and a series of racks for optional auxiliary surgical equipment such as recording facilities.

6. Robotic liver surgery

As experience with major laparoscopic operations such as splenectomy and colectomy has increased the interest in applying minimally invasive techniques to liver resection were developed in tandem. Technical developments such as more sophisticated energy devices and articulated laparoscopic staplers have enabled surgeons to tackle liver resection laparoscopically in line with international recommendations [15]. Specifically, as discussed above, lesions in the antero-medial segments of the liver are particularly favourable for this approach. Some of the major technical challenges in liver surgery include the access to the IVC and major hepatic veins, dissection of a difficult hepatic hilum coupled with the propensity for the liver to bleed during transection. These difficulties are magnified during laparoscopic surgery due to the limitations in depth perception, restricted movement with rigid instruments and fixed fulcrum at the ports, unnatural ergonomics that can compound suturing to the liver particularly in presence of haemorrhage. There is also a steep learning curve with laparoscopic liver surgery making its practice outside high-volume centres difficult although the same situation exists with robotic liver surgery. As a result, the uptake of minimally invasive hepatectomy has been understandably slow and cautious. However with increasing experience, surgeons have gradually increased the difficulty and complexity of liver surgery undertaken. This has developed from staging laparoscopy and de-roofing of simple liver cysts to resecting lesions in accessible parts of the liver such as the left lateral sector and wedge resections from the anteroinferior segments, to major hepatectomies. However, certain liver procedures are considered technically challenging. These include patient who have undergone previous surgery in particular upper abdominal surgery/liver surgery, resections involving the caudate lobe, lesions in the posterior portion of the liver and in patients requiring bile duct resection with reconstruction. In 2008 following a consensus conference experts recommended that laparoscopic resection should be considered in patients with solitary lesions, lesions 5 cm or less and/or those lesions located in segments 2–6 [19]. Furthermore the conference recommended that laparoscopic resection of liver segments 7, 8 and 1 was not standard practice. In part these recommendations were based upon the access to and visualisation of these areas of the liver and resection of these areas of the liver with rigid instruments. Moreover resection of liver lesions in the segments VII and VIII are particularly challenging because of issues with surgical access and the technical challenges in maintaining a curved transection lines throughout surgery thereby maintaining margins and obtaining R0 resection. Hence some evidence suggests that such lesions are more likely to be resected using right hepatectomy. Whilst oncologically this cannot be faulted it does necessitates the loss of a significant amount of normal functioning liver mass [20]. The most recent guidelines however still suggest that laparoscopic and by extension robotic liver surgery should not be considered for extended hepatectomies, when concomitant biliary reconstruction is needed or when lesions involve major vascular structures [15].

In theory, robotic surgery is an ideal platform for telesurgery. The indications for robotic hepatectomy are very similar to those for laparoscopic hepatectomy. Both benign and malignant tumours can be resected robotically. Robotic hepatectomy overcomes many of the problems inherent in laparoscopic surgery. In particular instruments allow curved transection lines and better visualisation of the liver [21].

Thus the greatest theoretical advantage of robotic hepatectomy may lie in sectoral, segmental, or subsegmental resections in difficult to access positions that mitigate against large incisions and extensive mobilisation required in an open approach. On the other hand, major hepatectomies for malignant conditions, such as hilar cholangiocarcinomas, where large incisions are required for specimen extraction may be better served by a traditional open approach although with improving robotic technology these may soon follow under the indications for robotic hepatectomy.

Image guided surgery is an evolving entity in liver surgery. The premise of this approach involves the use of pre-operative imaging being used to precision guide surgery. Some fields in surgery, such as orthopaedic surgery, have built up a significant amount of experience with this approach [22]. Essentially by using fixed bony landmarks on the body pre-operative images can be used as part of computer modelling systems to target organs and potentially lesion in real-time. Clearly the use of a mandatory console as part of robotic surgery means that such image-guided surgery can be made a routine part of surgery. For liver surgeons this would mean pre-emptive appreciation of vascular structures and the ability to carefully plan resection margins. However image-guidance surgery in hepatobiliary surgery remains a nascent field and further technological advances required before its use can be widely applied in robotic liver surgery.

7. Current advantages and disadvantages of robotic liver surgery

The utility of robotic liver surgery in part lies in the fact that it can overcome some of the inherent difficulties associated with laparoscopic liver surgery. For instances both these minimal access approaches to liver surgery entail long operative times and in the case of laparoscopic liver surgery this involves enduring unfavourable ergonomics during surgery primarily because of rigid laparoscopic instruments coupled with the primary operator having to remain scrubbed at the table side for extended periods of time. In the robotic liver surgery the primary operator being unscrubbed at the surgeon cart whilst operating and tailoring the console ergonomics to suit their individual preference overcomes these particular constraints. The benefits to the operating surgeon are clear namely operating in an ergonomically comfortable position with a 3-D view of the surgical field that aids depth perception. In addition the surgeon maintains control of the endoscope mitigating unnecessary camera movements and ensuring stable surgical views throughout the procedure. Robotic-assisted retractors are also controlled by the operating surgeon and maintain their position until further movement/retraction is required further avoiding inappropriate or ineffective retraction. Furthermore the use of articulated instruments that mimic the dexterity of the human hand allows for precise tissue manipulation and suturing in restricted surgical fields at angles not possible with rigid instruments. For instance Intuitive's multi-functional da Vinci instruments incorporate EndoWrist® technology (**Figure 6**).

The Endowrist® is incorporated into each Intuitive instrument (e.g. graspers, needle drivers and energy devices) and has a greater range of movement than the human hand. In addition robotic systems have in-built tremor reduction enhancing fingertip control. The Endowrist® technology also facilitates curved transection lines during liver surgery allowing for more complex liver resections to be performed. The technology also allows for the creation of biliary and enteric anastomoses in restricted surgical fields. During robotic surgery the surgeon's motions are scaled so that small, precise movements are effected at the patient's end which when fashioning a hepaticojejunostomy has significant advantages.

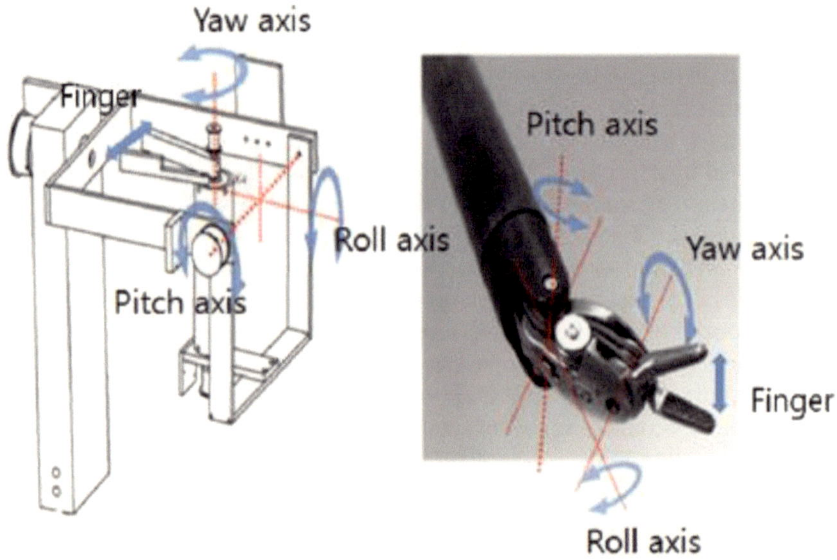

Figure 6.
Endowrist robotic instruments. Robotic instruments incorporate Endowrist technology that allows the operator to control various instruments via the fingers switches. The Endowrist allows more degrees of movement than the human hand.

Emerging reports suggests that the learning curve for robotic surgery may be shorter when compared with conventional laparoscopic surgery. However this may be due to the fact that many surgeons have previously obtained proficiency with laparoscopic surgery before engaging with robotic surgery. Currently complex laparoscopic liver resections are generally performed by surgeons who are experienced hepatobiliary/laparoscopic surgeons. Open surgical techniques are more readily translated to robotics and thus surgeons who are expert in open hepatobiliary surgery but not necessarily advanced laparoscopy may become proficient quicker with robotic hepatectomy. Robotic surgery lends itself well to computer based virtual reality training and as such trainee robotic surgeons may develop and attain significant competence with the robotic platform prior to operating on real patients. Such training systems have been developed and validated. Studies have found that structured training exercises improved simulator performance, although the translation to actual surgical performance has not been well studied [23]. Although the robotic dual console is also a teaching tool that could help accelerate proficiency. In addition port placement is more forgiving in robotic surgery as instruments are not completely restricted by a rigid fulcrum and also compensated for by the Endowrist®. The details of port placement are discussed further in Section 8 below.

Although the development of robotic surgery is developing quickly there are a number of disadvantages with the current operating systems. The current generation of robots require a large amount of space in theatre to accommodate each of the three components as well as the patient and anaesthetic equipment. In additions bulky arms can prove difficult to manoeuvre in the space between theatre operating lights. Spacious operating rooms are require and dexterity is limited by collision of robotic arms (**Figure 3**). Importantly a skilled assistant is needed for suction, change of instruments, application of argon plasma, and stapling. In addition if an assistant port is required this will need the assistant to operate an instrument through it and thus requires some element of laparoscopic skills. However newer robotic instruments such as robotic suction devices, sealers, and staplers has eliminated the routine need for accessory ports and necessity of a skilled bedside assistant. Although the robotic equivalent of CUSA is eagerly awaited which is likely to improve the division of the liver and the scope of liver surgery if and when available. Although there is improved depth perception with the robotic platform there is no tactile feedback and thus retraction force has to be judged and maintained by the operating surgeon. Although not strictly a problem limited to robotic surgery if the patient position requires adjustment this will often necessitates the robotic arms to be undocked, the robot to be moved and the robot arms to be redocked (see below). This will add time to the overall operating procedure and will also mean that an experienced theatre team is needed to carry this out smoothly with no loss of sterility. For similar reasons the ability to convert a robotic surgical procedure to an open procedure for emergencies such as bleeding requires a skilled team that can coordinate undocking of the robot, removal of the robotic instrumentation and conversion to laparotomy. The latest Intuitive Xi robot that allows a greater simplicity in manoeuvring the robotic components without having to move the operating table, patient cart or standard theatre equipment has overcome many of these logistical issues.

Robot and robotic malfunction is a known phenomenon and many of these problem require a replacement of robotic instruments [24]. One of the major disadvantages of robotic surgery is the high cost and this is multifaceted. Aside from the purchase of the platform and equipment there are costs incurred for consumables, surgeon and staff training as well as servicing costs for the robot. Although many of these may be offset by shorter length of ITU stay and shorter hospital stay. One of the limits of robotic HPB surgery is the need for specialised training, not only for the primary surgeon, but also for the assistant surgeon and OR nurses, although in some cases, the learning curve for specific robotic procedures has proven to be shorter than the laparoscopic equivalent [25]. A specific issue for liver surgeons is that at present only a limited number of instruments are available parenchymal transection such as harmonic shears. Although these remain an efficient tool as discussed above the development of a robotic CUSA would improve the mechanical steps of the operation.

8. Technique of robotic liver resection

8.1 General consideration for patients undergoing liver surgery

All patients considered for robotic liver surgery should have the same workup as for patients undergoing any form of liver surgery. Patients must have the physiological reserve to tolerate general anaesthesia and a prolonged pneumoperitoneum. In our institution all patients undergo cardiopulmonary exercise testing and routine haematology, coagulation and biochemistry as part of anaesthetic workup. General contraindications to laparoscopy such as uncorrected coagulopathy and cardio-respiratory compromise should be observed. Furthermore patients should be discussed in an appropriate multidisciplinary team meeting after cross-sectional imaging and staging. In our institution all patient undergo Computed Tomography (CT) of the thorax, abdomen and pelvis. We use MRI liver and CT-PET on a patient-dependent manner. Patients also give informed consent for robotic surgery and we quote a robot to open conversion rate of 10% in our unit based upon our unit prospectively collected data.

8.2 Patient positioning and robot docking

Following general anaesthesia the patient is placed in the supine position and strapped into position on the operating table. Depending upon the type of liver resection the patient may be kept in reverse-Trendelenburg position whilst supine or placed in this position with legs parted. With the patient in the desired position the optimal position for the ports is marked with a surgical pen. The general recommendation is the robotic ports should be placed 15–20 cm from the target liver segment/lobe. Importantly in laparoscopic surgery ports can be placed at various points within the abdomen however in robotic surgery the ports generally need to be placed in a horizontal line (**Figure 7**). Each port should be placed 7–10 cm apart depending upon the patient's abdominal girth. Additional assistant ports should be placed 7–10 cm caudal to this horizontal plane of robotic ports. Due to the limited degree of freedom of the Harmonic scalpel correct positioning of the instrument through the assistant port is critical in order to follow the transection line particularly for major liver resections. However with availability of the robotic Harmonic scalpel does make this less of an issue. The patient positioning and trocar placement vary depending upon the area of the liver to be resected. Trocars will be positioned very high subcostal and lateral for the posterior superior segments or closer to the transverse umbilical line for the anterior segments shifting towards the left or the right depending on the lesion location. The same basic principle that applies to laparoscopic surgery applies to robotic surgery that is to create adequate triangulation with enough space in between the ports to avoid instrument clashing and aid efficient movement of instruments. Sometimes this might require a switch of the instrument in between the left and right operative arm.

We recommend an open/Hassan technique to inserted the optical robotic port to establish pneumoperitoneum. Robotic ports are specialised metallatic ports. Once pneumoperitoneum is satisfactory a diagnostic laparoscopy is performed in order to

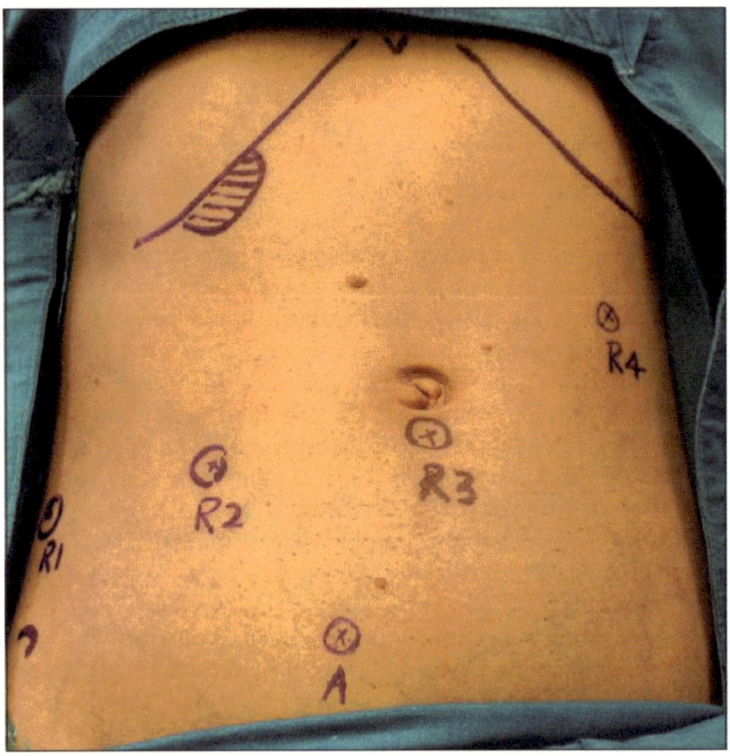

Figure 7.
The placement of robotic ports for liver resection. Demonstrates the robotic post placement for liver resection of segment 2, 3, 4, 5, 6 and cholecystectomy. R1–4 represent the robotic arms. Each of these robots ports can be used an optical port. Note the assistant port (A) is placed in the caudal position to provide optimal port placement.

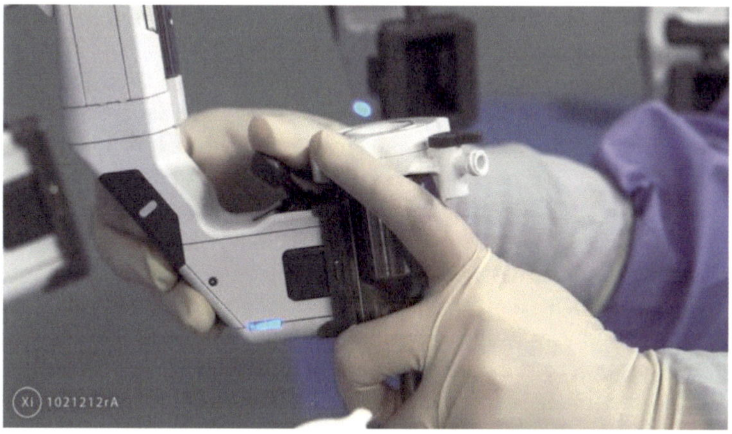

Figure 8.
Docking of the robotic ports. All robotic ports require to be docked to the robot arms on the patient cart prior to their use. The metallatic extension on the ports is engaged with the robot port using the port clutch in a process known as docking.

exclude the presence of metastases or occult disease. An IOUS is also performed in order to have a better understanding of the size, number and location of the lesions and their relationship to major vascular and biliary structures. Once confirmed that the resection is to proceed the patient cart is brought into the surgical field. A tracker laser is positioned over the optical robotic port to ensure that the robot is in the optimal position. Further robotic ports are then inserted under direct vision in the previously marked position. The metallatic extension on the robotic optical port (present on all robotic ports) is then engaged onto the robot arm using the port clutch—this procedure is known as 'docking' the robot (**Figure 8**). The endoscope is then placed through the robotic port and engaged onto the top of the robotic arm. By pressing the instrument clutch the endoscope is manovered into the peritoneal cavity and is then used to visualise the target anatomy (e.g. liver lesion). The targeting button is then pressed on to endoscope that then automatically places the remaining robotic arms into optimal positions. The remaining robot ports are then docked and the appropriate instruments inserted through the ports and engaged in the robotic arms.

8.3 Surgical procedure

The precise liver procedure to be performed will be dependent upon the type of liver resection to be performed. Below a description of anatomical and non-anatomical liver resections is discussed.

8.3.1 Anatomical/major robotic liver resection

Prior to any form of liver resection the central venous pressure is lowered to less than 5 mmHg in order to reduce blood loss that is used in conjunction with reverse Trendelenburg position for the same reason [26]. For anatomical or major robotic liver resection there are three surgical steps that have been recommended for safe resection outlined in **Table 2** and are similar to open liver surgery.

For major robotic liver resections the falciform ligament is usually divided with a vascular stapler or robotic stapler followed by a retrograde cholecystectomy using the same principles of laparoscopic cholecystectomy. In the case of left hepatectomy the left triangular ligaments can now be divided in order to mobilise the left lobe of the liver. A Nylon taped maybe passed at this point for future Pringle use although this is not necessary in all cases [27].

Next the relevant hepatic pedicle is then dissected using a combination of robotic monopolar hooks and/or bipolar forceps. For major hepatectomy the right or left hepatic artery is dissected first and clearly identified. IOUS may be utilised after selective clamping of the dissected artery to ensure satisfactory flow within the future liver remnant. Once satisfactory flow is confirmed the desired artery can be divided between prolene sutures, surgical clips or Hem-O-locks®. Next the relevant portal vein is completely dissected and selective stitches or ligatures are applied on the small branches if present. The portal vein is then divided between robotic clips/Hem-O-locks or sutured with either 4-0 or 5-0 prolene. Generally an extrahepatic dissection of the bile duct should be performed only when the anatomy is clear and confluence of the biliary ducts is low. In the latter ICG fluorescence can be easily used at any point and can help identify the biliary anatomy and used with the Firefly setting on the robotic system. For right hepectomy hepatocaval dissection the subsequent step following hilar dissection. Specifically the lateral reflection of the peritoneum is dissected using the hepatocaval plane as a guide. The third arm of the robot can then be used and a retractor deployed to lift the inferior surface of the right liver lobe to expose the IVC in analogous manoeuvre to open surgery. The retrohepatic veins can be divided using either sutures or surgical clips. Clips can also be placed for accessory hepatic veins of minor calibre or to further The liver is progressively dissected off the IVC until the inferior aspect of the right hepatic vein is visible and signals the end of this part of the dissection.

Transection of the liver is the last step of the operation. Parenchymal transection should follow the ischemic demarcation line and start at the anterior aspect of Cantile lines for a right hepatectomy. Many retraction measures can be employed to ensure effective retraction of the liver including stay sutures, rubber rings or surgical instruments. As discussed above many liver surgeons would consider robotic harmonic scalpel as the tool of choice for parenchymal transection. Liver transection is performed layer by layer proceeding in a superficial to deep manner in the same plane to maintain control of vessels and bleeding. Moreover superficial bleeding can be controlled with appropriate energy devices whilst larger vessels may require suturing and/or surgical clips. As the resection proceed deeper into the liver most surgeons would utilise surgical stapling devices to control venous structures such as segment 5 and 8 branches as well as the right/left hepatic vein. The liver is then completely mobilised by sectioning the remaining peritoneal attachments with assistance of the bedside surgeon. In the case of left lateral sectionectomy following left triangular division robotic resection can be completed by remaining lateral to the falciform ligament and completed parenchymal transection with robotic harmonic scalpel and vascular staplers. For segmentectomy the relevant portion of the liver is mobilised and IOUS used to identify selective pedicles prior to transection.

Following transection the raw surface of the remaining liver should then be examined for bleeding and bile leaks. At the end, haemostatic agents such as fibrin glue, Surgicel®, argon plasma can be applied to the remaining surface as a sealant.

Step 1	Division of the Falciform ligament ± cholecystectomy
Step 2	Portal pedicle dissection and liver mobilisation
Step 3	Liver transection

Table 2.
Suggested steps for major robotic liver resection.

Finally, the specimen is placed in an endoscopic bag and extracted through a small Pfannenstiel incision or through the site of a previous scar. Closed suction drains in the subhepatic and subdiaphragmatic area is used. The robotic cart is removed from the operative field, pneumoperitoneum is stopped and the trocars are extracted under direct laparoscopic vision.

8.3.2 Non-anatomical robotic liver resection

In our experience the Pringle manoeuvre has to be rarely used for NARs but when there is a need to secure more control on the liver inflow, the hepatic pedicle is prepared and a tourniquet is created using an umbilical tape. NARs are generally reserved for liver lesions that are superficial, subcapsular or easily visualised. As discussed above the main tool used for parenchymal transection is the robotic harmonic scalpel and it is ideally suited to perform NARs. Prior to commencing transection the resection line can be marked with diathermy which also allows the robotic harmonic scalpel to be positioned correctly and may mandate the switching of the robotic harmonic scalpel between different robotic arms. As described above transection is recommended to be performed in a layer-by-layer fashion. The fourth robotic arm can be used to aid retraction such that there is minimal traction on the lesion itself. Once the resection is completed haemostasis is achieved with a combination of the robotic energy instruments and topical haemostatic agents.

9. Current results of robotic liver surgery

Early experiences with using a robot in cholecystectomy demonstrated equivalent results to the laparoscopic approach. These early surgical reports served to show that robotic approaches were feasible for liver surgery [28, 29]. In most institutions robotic cholecystectomy is reserved for those surgeons completing approved training pathways/accreditation before commencing upon more complex procedures. Generally for cholecystectomy robotic surgery does not offer any significant advantage over the laparoscopic approach particularly when cost-benefit is considered. Below we discuss the current results for robotic liver resection. On reviewing the available literature it is evident that there are clear contraindications to the robotic liver surgery including invasion of major hepatic vessels and extension into the diaphragm necessitating diaphragmatic resection. There is no predetermined limit regarding the size of lesions that can be resected but very bulky tumours presented a technical challenge.

NAR/segmentectomy	87
Left lateral sectionectomy	51
Left hepatectomy	31
Bisegmentectomy	12
Right hemihepatectomy	51
Right trisectionectomy	3
Other	2
Total	237

Table 3.
Types and frequencies of robotic liver resections.

Authors	Year	n	Age	M:F	Resection type	Operative time (mins)	Blood loss (mins)	Conversion rate (%)	Transfusion rate (%)	Post-op stay (days)	Morbidity (%)	Mortality (%)	R0 (%)
Tsung et al. [31]	2014	57	58	42:58	37% major hepatectomy	253 (180–355)	200 (50–338)	7	4	4 (3–5.5)	20	0	95
Spampinato et al. [32]	2014	25	63	13:12	Major (16 RHH; 17LHH)	430 (240–725)	250 (100–19,000)	4	44	8 (4–22)	16	0	100
Tranchart et al. [27]	2014	28	66	13:15	All minor	210 (45–480)	200 (0–1800)	14	14	6 (1–15)	14	0	NR
Wu et al. [33]	2014	52	61	32:6	67% major hepatectomy	380	325	5	NR	8	8	0	NR
Boggi et al. [34]	2015	12	61	4:8	Superio-posterior segments	260	252	8	25	NR	33	0	100
Montalti R [35]	2016	36	62	21:15	Superio-posterior segments	306 (53–790)	415 (0–1500)	14	NR	6 (2–91)	19	3	89
Lee et al. [36]	2016	70	58	65:35	20% major hepatectomy	252 (97–620)	100 (2–2500)	6	5	5 (2—22)	12	0	98
Lai et al. [37]	2016	100	NR	NR	27% major hepatectomy	207	334	NR	NR	NR	14	0	96
Croner et al. [38]	2016	10	64	2:8	All malignant	321 (138–458)	306	NR	NR	7 (5–13)	10	0	100
Nota et al. [39]	2016	16	69	9:7	All minor (81% malignant	146 (60–265)	150 (5–600)	6	NR	4 (1–8)	43	0	NR

Authors	Year	n	Age	M:F	Resection type	Operative time (mins)	Blood loss (mins)	Conversion rate (%)	Transfusion rate (%)	Post-op stay (days)	Morbidity (%)	Mortality (%)	R0 (%)
Magistri et al. [40]	2017	22	61	18:4	10% major hepatectomy	318	400 (50–1500)	0	5	NR	59	0	96
Morel P [41]	2017	16	60	7:9	69% malignant (all minor)	352	NR	0	6	8	31	0	100
Wang et al. [42]	2018	63	NR	43:20	All HCC, 1 major hepatectomy	296	206	NR	NR	NR	11	NR	94
Ceccarelli et al. [43]	2018	70	NR	NR	26% malignant	NR	NR	10	NR	NR	NR	0	NR
Sucandy et al. [44]	2019	80	63	5:3	46% major hepatectomy	233	150	1	NR	3	14	1	NR

Table 4.
Recent results of robotic liver surgery.

9.1 Results from robot liver resection

Due to the less complex nature of surgery the most common robotic liver procedures performed globally are minor hepatectomy; segmentectomies (29%), left lateral sectionectomies (13%) and bisegmentectomies (9%). **Table 3** demonstrates the types and frequency of robotic hepatectomy.

This table illustrates the frequencies of the different types of robotic liver resections reported in the literature since 2013.

A recent meta-analysis published in 2013 has summarised the results of robotic liver resection up to 2013 [30]. The reader is directed here for the early results of robotic liver resection. In summary the number of major hepatectomies reported in the literature increased as experience with robotic surgery improved. The overall data suggested that robotic assisted liver surgery was comparable to both open and laparoscopic surgery in terms of peri-operative and postoperative outcomes, as well as oncologic efficacy. Complex procedures, such as extended liver resections were suggested to be technically easier due to the intrinsic advantages of the robotic system.

We discuss the results of robotic liver resection from 2013 to the current period. A number of selected studies reporting outcomes for robotic liver surgery since 2014 are shown in **Table 4**. This list is an exhaustive but highlights the progress that has been made worldwide in advancing robotic liver surgery. Achieving complete resection margins in liver surgery is critical for disease- and recurrence-free survival. It is currently still under investigation if minimal invasive techniques with reduced haptic feedback result in the same oncological results as open surgery. Unfortunately some studies still do not report complete resection rates (termed R0) in their data. However reviewing studies from 2014 onwards most report R0 resection rates of over 90% with many reporting 100%. The long-term outcome although is not well reported and many of these studies have not had the necessary follow-up time for this to be reported and this data is eagerly awaited. The limited studies that have been published appear to report equivalent disease-free and overall survival reported for HCC patients undergoing robotic-assisted versus laparoscopic liver surgery [37]. Although as discussed above robotic liver surgery carry increased costs the reported blood loss is in line with open and laparoscopic surgery and there is reassuringly low open conversion rate that is equivalent to laparoscopic surgery.

As the experience with robotic surgery has increased more recent studies have shown that the rate of major hepatectomy completed robotically has increased with low mortality. The morbidity however needs to be carefully interpreted as many studies report overall complications, that include minor complications, whereas as other has reported major complications only.

10. The future of robotic liver surgery

The robotic platform has distinct advantages over open and laparoscopic surgery and in some instances overcomes the limitations associated with these approaches. In particular the 3-D view, improved images and increased dexterity of operating improve the operators ability to carry out surgery without compromising patient safety. As demonstrated in this chapter the safety and feasibility of robotic liver surgery has been shown worldwide.

The future in robot liver surgery may lie in using this platform to perform more complex liver surgery such as extended liver resections or by incorporating digital technology into the operating system but most importantly the for the field to keep evolving there is a real need for randomised clinical trials. This will allow definition of benefits and demonstrate the real advantage of this approach for both patients and the surgical fraternity. The authors believe that will be the most effective route to the wider dissemination of this technology.

11. Conclusions

The current data suggest that both major and minor robotic hepatectomy is a safe and effective procedure with equivalent patient outcomes in terms of morbidity and mortality and oncological resection. There remain some important limitations to the wider dissemination of this technology principally around cost, some around training and so with the platform itself. It is hoped that collaborations between industry, academia and surgeons will overcome these problems allowing robotic liver surgery to be practiced widely and deliver patient benefit.

Conflict of interest

The authors have no conflict of interests to declare.

Author details

Ricky Harminder Bhogal*, Stephanos Pericleous and Aamir Z. Khan
The Royal Marsden Hospital, London, United Kingdom

*Address all correspondence to: ricky.bhogal@rmh.nhs.uk

IntechOpen

© 2019 The Author(s). Licensee IntechOpen. This chapter is distributed under the terms of the Creative Commons Attribution License (http://creativecommons.org/licenses/by/3.0), which permits unrestricted use, distribution, and reproduction in any medium, provided the original work is properly cited.

References

[1] Bismuth H, Eshkenazy R, Arish A. Milestones in the evolution of hepatic surgery. Rambam Maimonides Medical Journal. 2011;**2**(1):e0021

[2] Asiyanbola B, Chang D, Gleisner AL, et al. Operative mortality after hepatic resection: Are literature-based rates broadly applicable? Journal of Gastrointestinal Surgery. 2008;**12**:842-851

[3] Dimick JB, Cowan JA Jr, Knol JA, et al. Hepatic resection in the United States, indications, outcomes, and hospital procedural volumes from a nationally representative database. Archives of Surgery. 2003;**138**:185-191

[4] Almersjö O, Bengmark S, Hafström L. Liver resection for cancer. Acta Chirurgica Scandinavica. 1976;**142**:139-144

[5] Langenbuch C. Ein Fall von resecktion eines linksseitigen schnurlappens der leber. Berliner Klinische Wochenschrift. 1888;**25**:37

[6] Quattlebaum JK, Quattlebaum JK Jr. Technic of hepatic lobectomy. Annals of Surgery. 1959;**149**:648-651

[7] Fineberg C, Goldburgh WP, Templeton JY 3rd. Right hepatic lobectomy for primary carcinoma of the liver. Annals of Surgery. 1956;**144**:881-892

[8] Lortat-Jacob JL, Robert HG. Well defined technic for right hepatectomy. Presse Médicale. 1952;**60**:549-551

[9] Couinaud C. Lobes et segments hépatiques. Presse Médicale. 1954;**62**:709

[10] Couinaud C. Le foie. Paris: Masson; 1957

[11] Bismuth H, Castaing D. Peroperative echography in hepatobiliary surgery. Ann Gastroenterol Hepatol. 1984;**20**:221-223

[12] Bismuth H, Houssin D, Castaing D. Major and minor segmentectomies "réglées" in liver surgery. World Journal of Surgery. 1982;**6**:10-24

[13] Reich H, McGlynn F, DeCaprio J, et al. Laparoscopic excision of benign liver lesions. Obstetrics and Gynecology. 1991;**78**:956

[14] Hüscher CG, Lirici MM, Chiodini S, et al. Current position of advanced laparoscopic surgery of the liver. Journal of the Royal College of Surgeons of Edinburgh. 1997;**42**:219-225

[15] Wakabayashi G, Cherqui D, Geller DA, et al. Recommendations for laparoscopic liver resection: A report from the second international consensus conference held in Morioka. Annals of Surgery. 2015;**261**(4):619-629

[16] Lanfranco AR, Castellanos AE, Desai JP, et al. Robotic surgery: A current perspective. Annals of Surgery. 2004;**239**:14-21

[17] Satava RM. Surgical robotics: The early chronicles: A personal historical perspective. Surgical Laparoscopy, Endoscopy & Percutaneous Techniques. 2002;**12**:6-16

[18] Intuitive Surgical. Da Vinci Surgical Si System. Available from: http://www.intuitivesurgical.com/products/davinci_surgical_system/davinci_surgical_system_si/

[19] Buell JF, Cherqui D, Geller DA, et al. The international position on laparoscopic liver surgery: The louisville statement 2008. Annals of Surgery. 2009;**250**:825-830

[20] Cho JY, Han HS, Yoon YS, et al. Feasibility of laparoscopic liver

resection for tumors located in the posterosuperior segments of the liver, with a special reference to overcoming current limitations on tumor location. Surgery. 2008;**144**:32-38

[21] Casciola L, Patriti A, Ceccarelli G, et al. Robot-assisted parenchymal-sparing liver surgery including lesions located in the posterosuperior segments. Surgical Endoscopy. 2011;**25**:3815-3824

[22] Kingham TP, Scherer MA, Neese BW, et al. Image-guided liver surgery: Intraoperative projection of computed tomography images utilizing tracked ultrasound. HPB: The Official Journal of the International Hepato Pancreato Biliary Association. 2012;**14**:594-603

[23] Hung AJ, Patil MB, Zehnder P, et al. Concurrent and predictive validation of a novel robotic surgery simulator: A prospective, randomized study. The Journal of Urology. 2012;**187**:630-637

[24] Agcaoglu O, Aliyev S, Taskin HE, et al. Malfunction and failure of robotic systems during general surgical procedures. Surgical Endoscopy. 2012;**26**:3580-3583

[25] Ocuin LM, Tsung A. Robotic liver resection for malignancy: Current status, oncologic outcomes, comparison to laparoscopy, and future applications. Journal of Surgical Oncology. 2015;**112**:295-301

[26] Li Z, Sun YM, Wu FX, et al. Controlled low central venous pressure reduces blood loss and transfusion requirements in hepatectomy. World Journal of Gastroenterology. 2014;**20**:303-309

[27] Tranchart H, Ceribelli C, Ferretti S, et al. Traditional versus robot-assisted full laparoscopic liver resection: A matched-pair comparative study. World Journal of Surgery. 2014;**38**:2904-2909

[28] Gagner M, Begin E, Hurteau R, et al. Robotic interactive laparoscopic cholecystectomy. Lancet. 1994;**343**:596-597

[29] Himpens J, Leman G, Cadiere GB. Telesurgical laparoscopic cholecystectomy. Surgical Endoscopy. 1998;**12**:1091

[30] Ho CM, Wakabayashi G, Nitta H, et al. Systematic review of robotic liver resection. Surgical Endoscopy. 2013;**27**(3):732-739

[31] Tsung A, Geller DA, Sukato DC, et al. Robotic versus laparoscopic hepatectomy: A matched comparison. Annals of Surgery. 2014;**259**:549-555

[32] Spampinato MG, Coratti A, Bianco L, et al. Perioperative outcomes of laparoscopic and robot-assisted major hepatectomies: An Italian multi-institutional comparative study. Surgical Endoscopy. 2014;**28**:2973-2979

[33] Wu CY, Chen PD, Lee CY, et al. Robotic-assisted right posterior segmentectomies for liver lesions: Single-center experience of an evolutional method in left semi-lateral position. Journal of Robotic Surgery. 2019;**13**:231-237

[34] Boggi U, Caniglia F, Vistoli F, et al. Laparoscopic robot-assisted resection of tumors located in posterosuperior liver segments. Updates in Surgery. 2015;**67**:177-183

[35] Montalti R, Scuderi V, Patriti A, et al. Robotic versus laparoscopic resections of posterosuperior segments of the liver: A propensity score-matched comparison. Surgical Endoscopy. 2016;**30**:1004-1013

[36] Lee KF, Cheung YS, Chong CC, et al. Laparoscopic and robotic hepatectomy: Experience from a single centre. ANZ Journal of Surgery. 2016;**286**:122-126

[37] Lai EC, Tang CN. Long-term survival analysis of robotic

versus conventional laparoscopic hepatectomy for hepatocellular carcinoma: A comparative study. Surgical Laparoscopy, Endoscopy & Percutaneous Techniques. 2016;**26**:162-166

[38] Croner RS, Perrakis A, Hohenberger W, et al. Robotic liver surgery for minor hepatic resections: A comparison with laparoscopic and open standard procedures. Langenbeck's Archives of Surgery. 2016;**401**(5):707-714

[39] Nota CLMA, Molenaar IQ, van Hillegersberg R, et al. Robotic liver resection including the posterosuperior segments: Initial experience. The Journal of Surgical Research. 2016;**206**(1):133-138

[40] Magistri P, Tarantino G, Guidetti C, et al. Laparoscopic versus robotic surgery for hepatocellular carcinoma: The first 46 consecutive cases. The Journal of Surgical Research. 2017;**217**:92-99

[41] Morel P, Jung M, Cornateanu S, et al. Robotic versus open liver resections: A case-matched comparison. The International Journal of Medical Robotics. 2017;**13**. https://doi.org/10.1002/rcs.1800

[42] Wang WH, Kuo KK, Wang SN, et al. Oncological and surgical result of hepatoma after robot surgery. Surgical Endoscopy. 2018;**32**(9):3918-3924

[43] Ceccarelli G, Andolfi E, Fontani A, et al. Robot-assisted liver surgery in a general surgery unit with a "Referral Centre Hub & Spoke Learning Program". Early outcomes after our first 70 consecutive patients. Minerva Chirurgica. 2018;**73**(5):460-468

[44] Sucandy I, Schlosser S, Bourdeau T, et al. Robotic hepatectomy for benign and malignant liver tumors. Journal of Robotic Surgery. 2019. DOI: 10.1007/s11701-019-00935-0